The Measurement of Metabolic Bone Disease

MEASUREMENTS IN MEDICINE SERIES • VOLUME 1

SERIES EDITOR: M. Hobsley

The Measurement of Metabolic Bone Disease

Edited by

F. I. Tovey
Department of Surgery, University College
London, UK

T. C. B. Stamp
Royal National Orthopaedic Hospital
London, UK

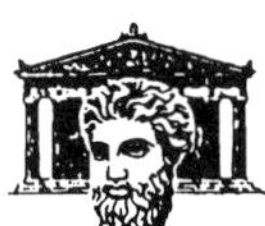

The Parthenon Publishing Group
International Publishers in Medicine, Science & Technology

NEW YORK LONDON

British Library Cataloguing in Publication Data
Metabolic Bone Disease. – (The Medical Measurements Series; Vol.1)
I. Tovey, F. I. II. Stamp, T. C. B.
III. Series
617.716

Library of Congress Cataloguing-in-Publication Data
The measurement of metabolic bone disease / edited by F.I. Tovey and
T.C.B. Stamp
p. cm. — (The medical measurements series ; v. 1)
Includes bibliographical references and index.
ISBN 1-85070-465-1 (hardback) : $58.00 (£30.00)
1. Bones—Metabolism—Disorders. 2. Bones—Metabolism— Measurement. 3. Bones—Pathophysiology. I. Tovey, F. I.
II. Stamp, T. C. B. III. Series.
[DNLM: 1. Bone Disease, Metabolic—diagnosis.
2. Bone Diseases, Metabolic—pathology.
3. Densitometry. WE 250 M484 1995]
RC931.M45M43 1995
616.7′107—dc20
DNLM/DLC
for Library of Congress 95-3667
CIP

ISBN 1-85070-465-1

Published in the UK and Europe by
The Parthenon Publishing Group Limited
Casterton Hall, Carnforth
Lancs. LA6 2LA

Published in North America by
The Parthenon Publishing Group Inc.
One Blue Hill Plaza
PO Box 1564, Pearl River
New York 10965, USA

First published 1995

Typesetting by AMA Graphics Ltd., Preston, England
Printed and bound by Butler and Tanner Ltd., Frome and London

Contents

List of contributors

J. E. Adams
Department of Diagnostic Radiology
Stopford Building
University of Manchester
Oxford Road
Manchester M13 9PT, UK

J. L. Berry
University of Manchester Bone Disease Research Centre
Department of Medicine
Manchester Royal Infirmary
Oxford Road
Manchester M13 9WL, UK

R. Eastell
Department of Human Metabolism and Clinical Biochemistry
Clinical Sciences Centre
Northern General Hospital
Herries Road
The University of Sheffield
Sheffield S5 7AU, UK

A. J. Freemont
University of Manchester Bone Disease Research Centre
Stopford Building
University of Manchester
Oxford Street
Manchester M13 9PT, UK

R. A. Hannon
Department of Human Metabolism and Clinical Biochemistry
Clinical Sciences Centre
Northern General Hospital
Herries Road
The University of Sheffield
Sheffield S5 7AU, UK

M. Hobsley
Department of Surgery
University College London
67–73 Riding House Street
London WIP 7LD, UK

E. B. Mawer
University of Manchester Bone Disease Research Centre
Department of Medicine
Manchester Royal Infirmary
Oxford Road
Manchester M13 9WL, UK

P. L. Selby
University of Manchester
Department of Medicine
Manchester Royal Infirmary
Oxford Road
Manchester M13 9WL, UK

T. C. B. Stamp
Royal National Orthopaedic Hospital
45–51, Bolsover Street
London WIP 8AD, UK

F. I. Tovey
Department of Surgery
University College London
67–73 Riding House Street
London WIP 7LD, UK

Foreword

Metabolic bone disease interests many and diverse groups of clinicians and medical scientists: specialists in internal medicine, rheumatology, orthopedic surgery, endocrinology, gynecology, pediatrics and geriatrics, researchers in anatomy, physiology, nutrition, biochemistry, pathology and imaging. The interest of all these workers is fanned by a combination of problems ranging from malnutrition in the emerging world through the aging populations of the developed world. Yet there is no field which has suffered more from nebulous concepts, difficult to pin down with watertight definitions, and from the difficulty of making the measurements one needs, even when one has been able to decide which those measurements are.

This particular field is therefore peculiarly apt for the first volume of a series entitled *The Medical Measurements Series*. The various contributions describe the anatomy and physiology of normal mature bone, the pathology of metabolic bone disease, the biochemistry of bone turnover and of overall calcium metabolism, and the methods available to quantify and categorise bone disease and its response to treatment.

Whether the reader approaches this book from the viewpoint of the clinician needing to understand how best he can treat his patients, the established researcher who wants an authoritative critique of present knowledge, or the newcomer to the field who needs a summary of the present position as an indication of possible areas for his own research endeavors, I believe he will find this book helpful.

M. Hobsley

Introduction

1

F. I. Tovey and T. C. B. Stamp

Several factors may influence the choice of a method for the measurement of metabolic bone disease. A major limiting factor will always be the equipment and methodology locally available, and also the availability of the required expertise and knowledge for the interpretation of the results. Another factor will depend on the type of information required. For instance, the most up-to-date measurements of bone density will detect osteopenia or loss of bone mass, but do not distinguish, for instance, between osteoporosis and osteomalacia. Measurements aimed at horizontal or cross-sectional studies of a community also may present considerably more problems than longitudinal studies involving individuals.

A cross-sectional study has the objectives of determining normal ranges of a population and of identifying abnormal groups outside those ranges, taking into account age, sex, menopausal status in women and ethnic origins. Other variables may need to be considered such as height, weight, body mass, total skeletal size, or individual variations in bone size. These factors may present considerable difficulties in the definition of normal ranges, which can be compounded further by variations in methods and equipment.

Longitudinal studies present fewer problems providing the same technique is used throughout in studying the progress of a patient or a group over a period of time and in assessing responses to treatment. The main difficulty is that of intra- or interobserver error, the amount depending on the method being used. The degree of error may be such that small changes in bone density over a short period of time are difficult to detect. This may mean that responses to treatment may only become detectable after sufficiently long periods have elapsed for any changes to be greater than the degree of error.

Problems may also arise when comparing results obtained from different studies, according to whether they relate to the appendicular or axial skeleton. Measurements obtained from cortical long bones cannot be compared without qualification with measurements obtained from cancellous trabecular bones of the axial skeleton. Changes may be more marked or may occur earlier in one than in the other.

For an understanding of the appropriate and relevant measurements of specific diseases a knowledge of the anatomical, pathological and biochemical changes that take place in different metabolic bone diseases is required. A prerequisite, however, is an initial understanding of the normal processes, bone resorption and accretion.

With this in mind, the next two chapters of this book describe the normal anatomy and physiology of bone and the different types of metabolic bone disease. These are followed by a description of the biochemical changes that characterize different metabolic bone diseases and their usefulness in the diagnosis and management of these diseases. A chapter on histomorphometry follows with details of the histological changes in the different disorders and their measurement.

The following chapters on radiogrammetry, nuclear methods, quantitative computer tomography and ultrasonic techniques deal largely with measurements of bone density. Radiogrammetric techniques giving measurements of cortical bone are of value primarily in the diagnosis and monitoring of cortical osteopenia with the exception of the Singh Index which is a measure of trabecular osteopenia. The other methods mostly give measurements of osteopenia involving cortical and trabecular bones, and do not differentiate between different causes of loss of bone density. Further biochemical or histomorphometric measurements are often required to distinguish between the various causes of osteopenia. In different sections relating to biochemistry mention is made either of plasma or of serum levels depending on the practice of the contributors' laboratories, but the results have similar interpretations.

In the concluding chapter the practical usefulness of the various methods in the diagnosis and management of metabolic bone diseases is evaluated. Particular attention is given to the methods of identifying people at risk, the prediction of bone loss and the selection of groups for treatment, particularly in the major social problem of osteoporosis.

Anatomy and physiology of normal bone turnover

2

P. L. Selby

INTRODUCTION

Since bone forms the major structural framework for the rest of the body there is a common perception that it is, like the girders in a building, a rather inert structure. Nothing could be further from the truth; bone is a dynamic biological tissue in which old tissue is constantly removed to be replaced by new. Indeed there is evidence to suggest that the structural integrity of the skeleton depends on this process since old bone is rather more brittle and liable to fracture than is new. Furthermore, these processes are vital to the second function of the skeleton which is to act as a buffer to ensure the correct mineral balance of the body. Any understanding of the way in which disease processes affect the skeleton must be based upon a knowledge of these processes. This chapter aims to give a brief introduction to the mechanisms of bone formation and resorption and the means by which they are controlled. In dealing with these processes only those that occur in the mature adult skeleton will be considered, the mechanisms of ossification and bone elongation which occur in the growing skeleton being beyond the scope of such a brief review.

THE STRUCTURE OF BONE

The majority of bones in the human body are formed by a process known as endochondral ossification in which the mineralized elements are laid down within a cartilaginous framework (for a review of this mechanism the reader is directed to standard textbooks such as ref. 1). This leads to a structure of bone which serves to maximize strength whilst minimizing weight in which there is a solid, usually tubular outer portion of compact or cortical bone with a core of spongy cancellous or trabecular bone. In the long bones this structure is confined to the ends of the bone and in the middle of the shaft there is no cancellous bone so that the bone at that site comprises only a dense cortical tube which is filled with fat known as yellow marrow.

It has been estimated that about 80% of the bone in the body is cortical. As stated above, the shafts of the long bones are almost entirely cortical and various postmortem studies have estimated the proportion of trabecular bone in a variety of different skeletal sites. Of those that are important for skeletal measurements it has been suggested that the distal forearm has 40–50% of its mineral within the trabecular compartment[2] and that less than 30% of a lumbar vertebra is trabecular bone[3]. However, this latter observation has been called into question by other workers who point out that the trabecular bone content of a lumbar vertebral body is of the order of 80%[4]. In order to try and reconcile these it must be remembered that in addition to the vertebral body, which does contain a considerable amount of trabecular bone, there is a lot of cortical bone in the neural arch, transverse and spinous processes as well as in association with the facet joints.

The two types of bone have different organization at the microscopic level; this reflects the different mechanisms by which bone turnover takes place. Cortical bone is remodeled by means of the concerted action of groups of cells which act together to resorb a cylinder of bone along the line of the capillaries, which, in turn, lie along the long axis of the bone. Almost immediately it has been resorbed the cavity is then refilled with new bone laid down and mineralized by osteoblasts. Thus, in longitudinal section there is the appearance of a cone of bone resorption traveling along the length of the bone which is filled in with osteoid which is then gradually mineralized. This process leads to the appearance of concentric rings at right angles to the long axis of the bone (Figure 1). These surround a canal which represents the original resorption cavity. The outer margin of these rings is marked by a so-called cement line which delineates a discrete package of bone known as an osteon. The canal is known as the Haversian canal and the osteon is frequently referred to as a Haversian system.

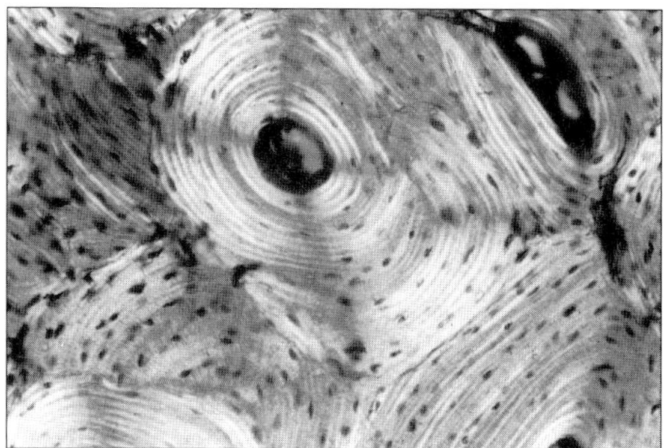

Figure 1 *Photomicrograph of cortical bone taken under polarized light to reveal the concentric lamellae of bone surrounding Haversian canals*

On the other hand, remodeling of trabecular bone mainly takes place on the surface of the trabecular bars and there are very few Haversian systems. There is still the same sequence of resorption closely followed by formation but this does not tunnel through the bone as in the cortex. Instead there is the production of a relatively shallow resorption cavity (also known as Howship's lacuna) which is then filled in from the base upwards by osteoid which is subsequently mineralized. In this case the appearance of the bone which is laid down is not that of the concentric circles of the Haversian system but of even lamellae running almost parallel with the surface of the trabecular bar (Figure 2).

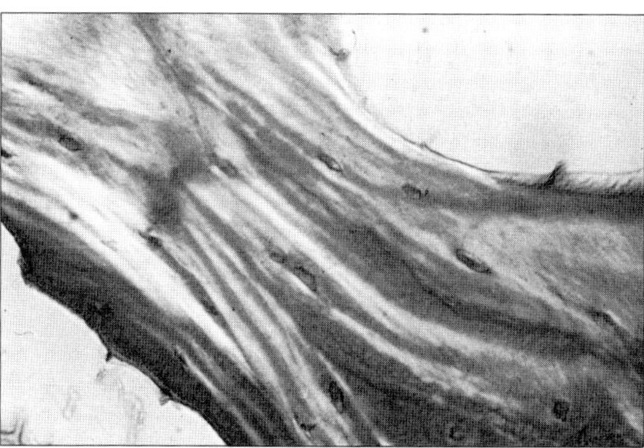

Figure 2 *Photomicrograph of trabecular bone taken under polarized light to reveal the lamellae running almost parallel to the bone surface*

It can be seen that these different means of bone remodelling have different implications for the replacement of bone that has been resorbed. Clearly, within the confines of a Haversian system there is no scope for putting back bone in excess of what was resorbed in the first place. On the other hand, given the mechanism of remodeling in trabecular bone it is at least possible for this to take place. However, this is rarely the case and in general, whatever the skeletal site, there is a slight deficit of formation over resorption in the remodeling cycle. These cumulate and together account for some of the gradual loss of bone which occurs with aging.

Since trabecular bone is laid down within a cartilagenous matrix which is no longer present in adult bone it is generally believed that it is not possible to replace the bars themselves once they have been lost as a result of aging or disease. This is clearly of some significance when it comes to consideration of the possibility of treatment to replace bone that has been lost as a result of disease, particularly osteoporosis, where not only is the thickness of the trabecular bars reduced but some of the trabeculae are lost. Even though it might be possible by means of some therapy to replace the amount of bone that has been lost it will not be possible to restore the trabecular architecture to its previous state. This will mean that one is left with fewer trabecular bars which are considerably thicker than previously. This is inherently a weaker structure than that produced by a greater number of thinner trabeculae. Thus, it can be seen that it is important to consider bone architecture as well as just the amount of mineral in bone when trying to consider the influence of any particular treatment on bone strength.

BONE MASS CHANGES DURING LIFE

At birth there is 25 g of calcium in the body, nearly all of which is in the skeleton. This rises to 1300 g at the time of skeletal maturity in early adult life. This not only represents the general growth of the skeleton along with the rest of the body but also the increased mineral content of the skeleton as it matures. The growth of the skeleton is not simply linear but parallels linear growth with particularly rapid skeletal growth in infancy and at the time of the pubertal growth spurt. In the past it was believed that following the attainment of full stature there was a period of perhaps as long as 15 years in which there was little net skeletal gain or loss; with the advent of more sensitive techniques for measuring the loss of bone it is now believed that bone loss, especially that affecting trabecular bone, begins within the third decade of life[5–7]. It is known that the production of an artificial menopause will lead to a marked acceleration of this rate of loss[8–11] and it is generally believed that the same is true following natural cessation of ovarian activity, although the evidence for this is less secure. However, cross-sectional studies would suggest that, like oophorectomy, menopausal ovarian failure causes an exponential increase in the rate of bone loss which subsequently declines to coincide with the steady loss in males over the next 10 years[12–14]. Overall, a woman might expect to lose 50% of her peak trabecular bone mass during adulthood whereas a man might only lose just under 40%.

In contrast, most investigators would now hold that cortical bone is well preserved until the fifth decade of life following which there is a virtually linear loss in both sexes such that over the rest of their life men will lose about one-quarter of their cortical bone whilst women will lose about one-third[15]. These changes appear to be the case when bone is measured at a predominantly cortical site such as the proximal forearm or using total body calcium measurement as a surrogate for the total amount of bone in the body, remembering that about 80% of this bone is cortical in the adult. Again there is some suggestion that this loss might be accentuated by the withdrawal of ovarian steroids at the time of the menopause.

In the long bones a further factor must be considered when looking at the changes with age, that is the change in shape of these bones with time. There is a gradual loss of bone from the endosteal (internal) surface of the bone but a concomitant deposition of bone on the subperiosteal (outer) surface. This results in the gradual thinning of the cortex of long bones with age but the widening of the bone itself.

There have been few studies that have examined the changes that occur in the skeleton in later life in any great detail; those that have, suggest that there may be an increase in bone mass with extreme old age although the clinical significance of this observation remains unclear[16].

THE MECHANISM OF BONE MASS CHANGES

It is likely that the precise mechanisms underlying bone loss differ according to both the skeletal site and also the type of bone involved (cortical or trabecular) although there is still a lot left to be discovered about these processes. Clearly, bone loss must be the final result of an imbalance between bone formation and resorption but how these processes are controlled in most circumstances remains unknown. The older techniques of radiocalcium kinetic studies suggested that there was a gradual decline in bone formation with age[17]. More recent studies using specific biochemical markers of bone turnover have borne this out. It is likely that the combination of these processes leads to the development of the age-related bone loss which occurs in both sexes. The more rapid loss of bone which occurs when ovarian function is lost is generally accepted as being the result of increased bone resorption[17]. The mechanisms whereby estrogen withdrawal might lead to increased bone breakdown will be discussed more fully later.

THE CELLULAR BASIS OF BONE TURNOVER

Bone turnover is largely determined by the action of cells within the bone. The most important of these are the bone-forming cells, osteoblasts, the bone-resorbing cells, osteoclasts, and the rather less well-characterized osteocytes which are buried deep in the substance of the bone.

Osteoblasts

Osteoblasts are the cells that both lay down the organic matrix of bone and control its mineralization. They are derived from progenitor cells of the marrow stromal lineage which are morphologically similar to fibroblasts. However, the active osteoblast has a very typical histological appearance. It is a cuboidal cell situated on the bone surface in close contact with other osteoblasts (Figure 3). The cell has an eccentric nucleus and bears the histological hallmarks of an active secretory mechanism in the form of prominent endoplasmic reticulum and Golgi apparatus.

The major secretory products are the structural proteins of bone. Of these, by far the most abundant is type I collagen. This forms the structural basis of the bone matrix and affords much of the strength of the skeleton through cross-links between adjacent strands. In addition to collagen, osteoblasts also produce a variety of other proteins which are important in the integrity of bone. Osteocalcin (bone Gla protein) is a vitamin K-dependent protein containing the unusual amino acid, γ-carboxyglutamic acid (Gla). These residues ensure that bone Gla protein has a tight affinity for the surface of calcium hydroxyapatite crystals in bone but the biological significance of this is uncertain. Although some bone Gla protein is tightly bound in this manner to bone the majority is free to enter the circulation where its concentration has recently been developed as a marker of osteoblast activity.

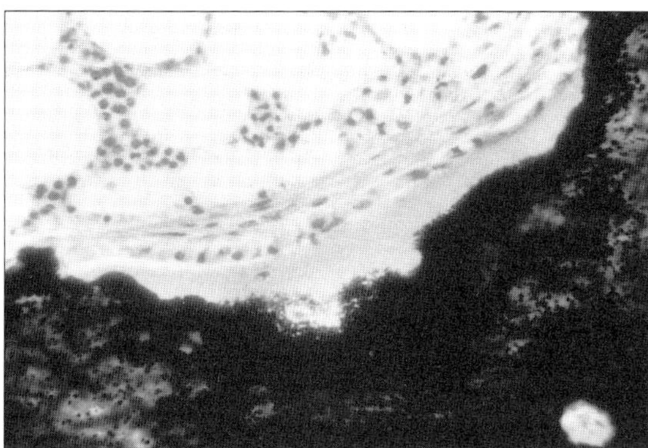

Figure 3 *Osteoblasts in an area of bone formation. The mineralized bone is the dark area at the bottom of the picture. In the middle lies a crescentic grey area which is the unmineralized osteoid and this is covered with a single layer of cuboidal osteoblasts*

Other non-collagenous proteins secreted by osteoblasts include osteonectin, osteopontin and a variety of phosphoproteins and proteoglycans. The function of these compounds remains obscure.

In addition to secreting the matrix on which mineralization takes place, osteoblasts also appear to have a major role in controlling the mineralization process. There is still considerable doubt about the precise mechanisms by which this is brought about. Whilst on the one hand it is clear that the physicochemical properties of the collagen fibrils in bone are conducive to the deposition of calcium hydroxyapatite in association with the 'hole' zones which occur periodically along the molecule; it is equally clear that some mineral deposition is actively controlled by the osteoblasts. This occurs in the form of calcium-rich structures known as 'matrix vesicles' which bud off from the membrane of osteoblasts in areas of bone mineralization. Calcium phosphate is also found in the mitochondria of osteoblasts in actively mineralizing bone.

The matrix vesicles are rich in alkaline phosphatase which is an enzyme which has for long been associated with osteoblastic activity. This is a glycoprotein enzyme which splits organic phosphate bonds. It is clearly of importance during the mineralization of bone although its precise role remains uncertain. Activity of the enzyme in plasma was, for many years, one of the few available biochemical measures of osteoblast activity. However, alkaline phosphatase is not unique to osteoblasts, it is also found in the liver, kidney, placenta and small intestine. The enzymes from these various sites have the same amino-acid structure to that in bone but differ in their glycosylation allowing the determination of the source of origin of alkaline phosphatase activity from analysis of isoenzyme types.

When the bone is not actively undergoing turnover the osteoblasts lose their plump shape and form a layer of closely opposed flattened lining cells upon the bone surface. These cells form a barrier between the surface of the bone and the surrounding environment and restrict the access of any potentially bone-resorbing cell or substance. In order to initiate bone resorption the lining cells must either separate or be removed and so it is likely that, in addition to the effect of osteoblasts on bone formation they might also have a major effect, as lining cells, on the induction of bone resorption.

Osteoclasts

Osteoclasts are the main agents of bone resorption. They are derived from hemopoietic stem cells and although they bear some similarity to giant cells derived from macrophages it is now generally accepted that they do not share identical origins although they clearly share a common ancestor in the form of a primitive hemopoietic stem cell.

Morphologically, osteoclasts are very characteristic in that they generally form multinucleate giant cells in resorption pits or lacunae on the bone surface (Figure 4). This is not essential for bone resorption and given the correct circumstances mononuclear osteoclasts are able to resorb bone. It is believed that the multinuclear cells arise from the fusion of cells rather than from the division of the cell nuclei.

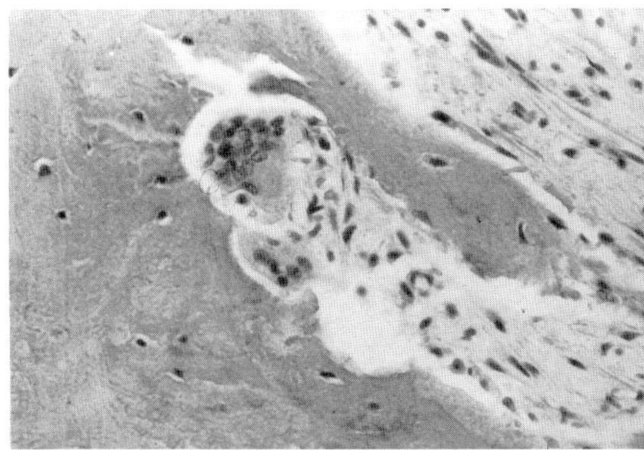

Figure 4 *Osteoclastic bone resorption; two multinucleate osteoclasts are seen in the middle of the picture*

In addition to being multinucleate, osteoclasts have other characteristic histological features. The central part of the cell membrane is in close contact with the bone surface and forms a structure descriptively known as the ruffled border on account of the many folds in the plasma membrane. This is a highly metabolically active region rich in mitochondria and lysozymes. Surrounding this area is an area of much lower metabolic activity virtually devoid of organelles known as the clear zone. It is believed that this fixes the osteoclast firmly to the bone surface rather like a suction cup and keeps the products of the ruffled border in close contact with the bone surface. Osteoclasts produce a variety of lysozymal enzymes to resorb bone but, perhaps surprisingly, they do not produce collagenase. The most abundant of these enzymes is tartrate-resistant acid phosphatase. The resorptive enzymes produced by osteoclasts operate at acid pH levels and the osteoclast has a mechanism for producing an acid environment within the region of the ruffled border in the form of carbonic anhydrase to generate protons and an ATP-linked proton pump to develop the proton gradient necessary to maintain this acidic state.

These mechanisms give osteoclasts the probably unique property of being able to form resorption pits in bone. Other cells, notably macrophages, are able to release calcium from bone in tissue culture but it is only osteoclasts that lead to the development of these well-defined areas of resorption. In addition, osteoclasts have a variety of surface immunological markers which mark them out as being separate from giant cells.

Osteocytes

These cells are situated in lacunae buried deep within the substance of the bone. Their most remarkable feature is the presence of an interconnecting network of dendritic processes. It is believed that osteocytes are formed from osteoblasts which become buried in the bone during the process of formation. This view is supported by the observation that the osteocytes' processes interact with osteoblasts and lining cells on the surface of the bone. It is generally held that through the network of dendritic processes osteocytes are able to transmit information about the internal milieu of bone to the bone-forming cells on the surface. Perhaps the most important part of such information is that relating to the mechanical stresses to which the bone is subject.

In the past it was thought that osteocytes had a role in the resorption of bone. Apart from some rather tenuous evidence that under certain circumstances of increased resorption osteocyte lacunae might increase in size there is no real support for this notion.

Interaction between bone cells

Under normal physiological circumstances there is a roughly constant amount of bone in the body. Since about 6 mmol of calcium is removed from the skeleton each day by resorption it is necessary that a similar amount is returned by formation unless the body is to lose bone. To avoid this there is a process, known as coupling, whereby the activities of osteoclasts are able to influence the amount of bone laid down by osteoblasts. The basis of this mechanism is not clear but it is likely to be the result of some chemical mediator. Various compounds have been suggested as possible coupling factors but none has received universal acceptance. Clearly it cannot be 100% effective since some bone is lost progressively throughout life.

It is, however, clear that there is co-operation between bone cells at the microscopic level. This is best seen in the process of remodeling be it in the Haversian systems of cortical bone or the Howship's lacunae of trabecular bone. In the early seventies, as a result of careful histomorphometric studies, Frost put forward the hypothesis that bone remodeling took place as the result of the concerted action of both bone-forming and resorbing cells which he termed the 'basic multicellular unit'[18]. He suggested that there was an initial activation of a basic multicellular unit which resulted in the recruitment of osteoclasts which resorbed a given amount of bone either in the form of a Haversian canal or Howship's lacuna depending on where they were situated. This phase lasted for about 14 days following which there was a so-called reversal phase in which a layer of mucopolysaccharide, the cement line, was laid down over the surface of the resorbed bone over about 14 days. After this there was a recruitment of osteoblasts which replaced the resorbed bone with osteoid which they subsequently mineralized. This phase of the cycle takes around 3–6 months.

Similarly, it is clear that there is a marked influence of osteoblasts on the activity of osteoclasts. This takes place in two ways. In the first place it is clear that the initiation of bone resorption is dependent on the bone-lining cells, which are inactive osteoblasts, allowing osteoclasts access to the bone surface. Indeed there is some evidence to suggest that osteoclasts are unable to remove the thin layer of unmineralized bone that covers the bone surface and that this must be removed by neutral proteases produced by osteoblastic cells before osteoclastic resorption can occur. The second mechanism will be explored in more detail later but can be summarized by stating that it appears that many of the actions of hormones which appear to act on osteoclasts are, in fact, mediated through the paracrine involvement of osteoblasts.

HORMONAL INFLUENCES ON THE SKELETON

At least three different types of hormone are known to act upon the skeleton:

(1) The classical calcium-regulating hormones, parathyroid hormone, calcitriol and calcitonin;

(2) Other classical hormones such as the gonadal steroids, corticosteroids and thyroxine; and

(3) Locally acting cytokines and other factors.

Although this latter group is very important in the regulation of bone turnover it is an area in which there is still much controversy regarding the precise roles of virtually every compound which has been described and so detailed discussion of it is outside the scope of this chapter.

Calcium-regulating hormones

Parathyroid hormone

This is an 84-amino-acid peptide hormone produced by the four parathyroid glands which are situated behind the thyroid in the neck. Its primary function is to maintain plasma calcium concentration within the physiological range. This is achieved by both stimulating net calcium release from bone and, more importantly, by promoting calcium reabsorption in the renal tubule. Parathyroid hormone probably has no direct effect on the gut.

Although the net effect of parathyroid hormone on bone is to increase bone resorption its effects on the skeleton are complex and involve all three bone cell types described above.

Parathyroid hormone stimulates osteoclastic bone resorption both by increasing the activity of osteoclasts that are already present and also by increasing the production of osteoclasts from their precursors. These actions do not appear to result from a direct effect of parathyroid hormone upon the osteoclast itself. In cell culture isolated osteoclasts will not respond to parathyroid hormone and no specific parathyroid hormone receptors have been isolated upon osteoclasts. Instead it would appear that a further cell is necessary to translate the parathyroid hormone signal into a paracrine stimulus to osteoclast activity; the most likely candidate for this cell is the osteoblast[19,20].

In addition to this, parathyroid hormone also has an effect on the osteoblast itself. There appears to be some contradiction between what is observed in isolated cells where parathyroid hormone appears to inhibit collagen production by osteoblasts, and in patients with hyperparathyroidism in which there is an increase in bone turnover, including bone formation. There is no definite explanation for this discrepancy, perhaps the most likely explanation is that bone formation is increased in hyperparathyroidism as a result of the release of coupling factors secondary to increased bone resorption. This would not explain the observations of some groups that bone mass can be increased in patients with osteoporosis by the administration of parathyroid hormone injections[21].

Parathyroid hormone has a further effect on the quiescent osteoblasts which comprise the bone-lining cells. In this particular population it leads to retraction of the cells and hence allows bone-resorbing cells access to the bone surface.

Calcitriol

It has been known for many years that vitamin D is essential for skeletal health. More recently it has become recognized that it is not the native vitamin D derived either from diet or the effect of sunlight on the skin which exerts this effect but rather more active hydroxylated derivatives. The activation of vitamin D takes place in two stages: an initial hydroxylation at position 25 in the liver is followed by a further hydroxylation, this time at position 1, in the kidney. The hepatically derived 25-hydroxyvitamin D (25-OHD; calcitriol) is the major circulating form of vitamin D but is still only weakly biologically active. It is the second hydroxylation to 1,25-dihydroxyvitamin D (1, 25-(OH) 2D; calcitriol) which imparts the major biological activity. Since this final step is under feedback control, mainly by the trophic action of parathyroid hormone on the renal hydroxylase, it is correct to think of calcitriol as a hormone rather than a vitamin.

25-hydroxyvitamin D can also be hydroxylated in the kidney at position 24 to yield 24,25-dihydroxyvitamin D. This probably has no biological activity but there is still some dispute as to its role, if any.

The major effect of calcitriol is to stimulate the absorption of calcium from the gastrointestinal tract. In itself this is important for the skeleton for an adequate supply of mineral is essential for normal bone formation. Indeed, it is likely that the failure of mineralization (osteomalacia) which is seen in vitamin D deficiency relates more to a lack of adequate mineral supply to the bone than to a direct effect of vitamin D on bone formation. Calcitriol does, however, exert direct effect on bone cells when it stimulates bone turnover.

On the one hand calcitriol is a potential stimulator of osteoclastic bone resorption, both increasing the activity of osteoclasts and also increasing their formation from precursors. Once again it would appear that this is not the result of a direct action on the osteoclast itself but is mediated through the paracrine influence of another cell, probably the osteoblast. On the other hand, osteoblast activity is itself directly stimulated by calcitriol in addition to any effect it may have on bone formation through increased fluxes of mineral.

In addition to these activities it is now well-recognized that calcitriol has a host of activities outside the calcium and bone homeostatic pathway. These are mainly in the field of cell division and differentiation but they are outside the scope of this chapter. They have recently been reviewed extensively by Walters[22] and Bikle[23].

Calcitonin

The third major calcium-regulating hormone is calcitonin. This is a 32 amino-acid peptide hormone derived from the parafollicular cells (C cells) of the thyroid. It has a direct effect *in vitro* to inhibit osteoclast activity and has been shown to inhibit both normal and abnormal bone resorption when given in pharmacological doses. These effects are usually short lived and there is little evidence to suggest that calcitonin has any major role to play in the regulation of normal bone turnover.

Other classical hormones

With the exception of the gonadal steroids it is unlikely that any of the other classical hormones play a major role in normal skeletal physiology. Thyroid hormones, corticosteroids and growth hormone are all capable of exerting a profound effect on the skeleton in disease states but there is little evidence that, other than their general effect on the health of many cell types, these hormones have bone-specific actions.

Gonadal steroids

These are important both as determinants of bone growth and maturation at the time of puberty and also in the maintenance of skeletal integrity throughout adult life. Estrogen withdrawal at the time of the menopause is associated with a marked increase in the rate of bone resorption and subsequent rapid loss of bone. These changes can be prevented or, to some extent, reversed by the administration of estrogen replacement in postmenopausal women. The mechanisms by which estrogen brings about these changes is not clear. Whilst estrogen receptors have been detected in bone cells these have only convincingly been demonstrated in osteoblasts and then at rather low concentrations. This raises the question as to whether, like calcitriol and parathyroid hormone, the action of estrogen on bone resorption is indirectly mediated via the paracrine influence of osteoblasts[24]. Recently there has also been some evidence coming to light to suggest that, independent of its effects on bone formation, estrogen might stimulate osteoblastic differentiation and collagen synthesis suggesting that in addition to being anticatabolic estrogens might be positively anabolic for bone.

Less is known about the precise actions of androgens upon the skeleton. From studies of bone turnover in hypogonadal males treated with testosterone it would appear that their major effect in the mature skeleton is anabolic[25].

ACKNOWLEDGEMENT

I am grateful to Dr A. J. Freemont, Professor of Osteoarticular Pathology in the University of Manchester, for the provision of the illustrations for this chapter.

References

1. Aaron JE. Histology and micro-anatomy of bone. In: Nordin BEC, ed. Calcium, Phosphate and Magnesium Metabolism. Edinburgh: Churchill Livingstone, 1976; 298–356.
2. Schlenker, RA, Von Seggen WW. The distribution of cortical and trabecular bone mass along the lengths of the radius and ulna and implications for *in vivo* bone mass measurements. Calcif Tiss Res 1976; 20: 41–52.
3. Nottestad SY, Baumel JJ, Kimmel DB, Recker RR, Heaney RP. The proportion of trabecular bone in human vertebrae. J Bone Min Res 1987; 2: 221–9
4. Eastell R, Mosekilde L, Hodgson SF, Riggs BL. Proportion of human vertebral body bone that is cancellous. J Bone Min Res 1990; 5: 1237–41.
5. Stevenson JC, Banks LM, Spinks TJ, Freemantle C, MacIntyre I, Hesp R, Lane G, Endacott JA, Padwick M, Whitehead MI. Regional and total skeletal measurements in the early post-menopause. J Clin Invest 1987; 80: 258–62.
6. Buchanan JR, Myers C, Lloyd T, Greer RB. Early vertebral trabecular bone loss in normal pre-menopausal women. J Bone Min Res 1988; 3: 583–7.
7. Mazess RB, Barden HS, Etinger M, Johnston C, Dawson-Hughes B, Baran D, Powell M, Notelovitz M. Spine and femur density using dual-photon absorptiometry in US white women. J Bone Min Res 1987; 2: 211–19.
8. Aitken JM, Armstrong E, Anderson JB. Osteoporosis after oophorectomy for non-malignant disease in premenopausal women. Br Med J 1973; 2: 325–8.
9. Aitken JM, Hart DM, Lindsay R. Oestrogen replacement therapy for the prevention of osteoporosis after oophorectomy. Br Med J 1973; 3: 515–18.
10. Horsman A, Simpson M, Kirby PA, Nordin BEC. Non-linear bone loss in oophorectomised women. Br J Radiol 1977; 50: 504–7.
11. Genant HK, Cann CE, Etinger B, Gordan GS. Quantitative computed tomography of vertebral spongiosa: a sensitive method for detecting early bone loss after oophorectomy. Ann Intern Med 1982; 97: 699–705.
12. Johnston CC, Hui SL, Witt RM, Appledorn R, Baker RS, Longcope C. Early menopausal changes in bone mass and sex steroids. J Clin Endocrinol Metab 1985; 61: 905–11.
13. Nilas L, Christiansen C. Bone mass and its relationship to age and the menopause. J Clin Endocrinol Metab 1987; 65: 697–702.
14. Slemenda C, Hui SL, Longcope C, Johnston CC. Sex steroids and bone mass. A study of changes about the time of the menopause. J Clin Invest 1987; 80: 1261–9.
15. Riggs BL, Wahner HW, Melton LJ, Richelson LS, Judd HL, Offord KP. Rates of bone loss in the appendicular and axial skeleton of women. J Clin Invest 1986; 77: 1487–91.
16. Hui SL, Wiske PS, Norton JA, Johnston CC. A prospective study of change in bone mass in post-menopausal women. J Chronic Dis 1982; 35: 715–25.
17. Heaney RP, Recker RR, Saville PD. Menopausal changes in bone remodelling. J Lab Clin Med 1978; 92: 964–70.
18. Frost HM. Bone Remodelling and its Relationship to Metabolic Bone Disease. Springfield, Illinois: Charles C. Thomas, 1973.
19. Rodan GA, Martin TJ. Role of osteoblasts in hormonal control of bone resorption – a hypothesis. Calcif Tiss Int 1981; 33: 349–51.
20. Braidman IP, Anderson DC, Jones CJP, Weiss JB. Separation of two bone cell populations from fetal rat calvaria and a study of their responses to parathyroid hormone and calcitonin. J Endocrinol 1983; 99: 387–99.
21. Reeve J, Meunier PJ, Parsons JA, Bernat M, Bijvoet OLM, Courpron P. Anabolic effect of human parathyroid fragment on trabecular bone in involutional osteoporosis: a multicentre trial. Br Med J 1980; 280: 1340–4.
22. Walters MR. Newly identified actions of the vitamin D endocrine system. Endocr Rev 1992; 13: 719–64.
23. Bikle DD. Vitamin D: new actions, new analogs, new therapeutic potential. Endocr Rev 1992; 13: 765–84.
24. Selby PL. Studies into the action of sex steroids on bone in the postmenopausal woman [MD Thesis]. University of Cambridge. 1990.
25. Francis RM, Peacock M, Aaron JE, Selby PL, Taylor GA, Thompson J, Marshall DH, Horsman A. Osteoporosis in hypogonadal men: role of decreased plasma 1,25 dihydroxy-vitamin D, calcium malabsorption and low bone formation. Bone 1986; 7: 261–8.

Metabolic bone diseases

3

F. I. Tovey and T. C. B. Stamp

The term 'metabolic bone disease' was introduced by Albright and Reinfenstein[1] in 1948 to describe diseases of the whole skeleton resulting from disturbances of factors which were mostly, but not all, metabolic. These may result from a defect in mineralization and/or an imbalance between resorption and bone formation. As a result bone architecture becomes disturbed.

In these conditions there may be a change of bone density. Loss of bone density (osteopenia) occurs in most forms of osteomalacia and all forms of osteoporosis. In the former there is usually a reduction of mineral content but the volume is normal, whereas in the latter there is reduced bony tissue per unit volume (Figure 1).

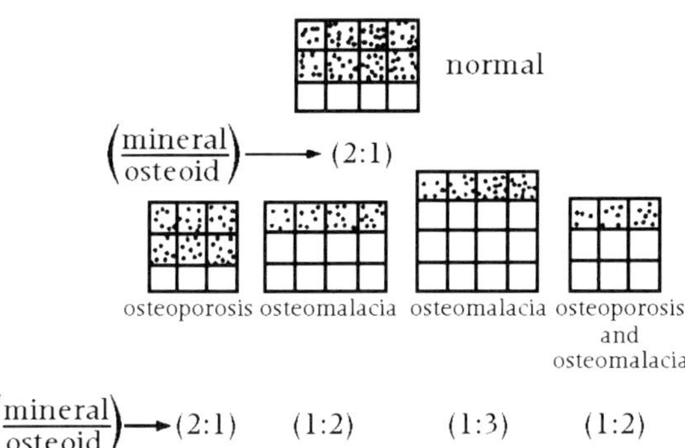

Figure 1 *Schematic representation of bone mass and mineral–osteoid relationships in osteoporosis and osteomalacia. Each block represents a hypothetical bone segment. The stippled areas denote mineralized osteoid; the clear areas poorly mineralized or non-mineralized osteoid. The total number of small blocks in each hypothetical segment represents individual bone units. Note that the bone mass is always decreased in osteoporosis, although the mineral–osteoid ratio is normal. Although bone mass may be normal, increased, or (when associated with osteoporosis) decreased in osteomalacia, the mineral–osteoid ratio is always decreased. Adapted from reference 21*

These two conditions constitute the main problems in clinical practice. A less frequent problem are Paget's disease, in which there is usually an increase in bone density, and conditions associated with parathyroid dysfunction.

This book is concerned with methods of measurement affecting the diagnosis, the progress and the response to treatment of metabolic bone diseases. Such measurements involve not only those of bone density, but also of histological and biochemical changes. The subsequent discussions of the various metabolic bone diseases lay emphasis on those parameters which are measurable and assist in the diagnosis and management of the conditions. The discussion concentrates on the more common clinical problems and less frequent and more obscure problems are omitted.

OSTEOPOROSIS

The term osteoporosis[2,3] refers to too little qualitatively normal bone per unit volume. Primarily this bone loss may be physiological in the sense that it describes normal bone loss due to aging and bone loss in excess of the above in postmenopausal osteoporosis in women.

The normal rate of bone loss in males over 40 years and females between the age of 40 and menopause is 0.3–0.4% a year, but in postmenopausal women it may rise to at least double this level.

In osteoporosis, resorption exceeds bone formation. The increased resorption affects trabecular bone, where the rate of bone turnover is greater, and to a lesser extent compact cortical bone. When pathological fractures occur they are seen most frequently in the vertebral bodies, proximal femur and distal radius. The trabeculae become thinner and more widely spaced. Resorption of cortical bone occurs particularly on its endosteal surface and the cortex becomes thinner. The endosteal surface is less well defined. There is reduction in the width of osteoid seams and there is reduced osteoblastic activity and mineralization as shown by double tetracycline labeling. Calcium and phosphate levels are usually within the normal range. The 24-h urinary calcium output and urinary total hydroxyproline are usually in the normal range (except in very acute disease), but are significantly higher in the group as a whole than in normal subjects.

In addition to primary or idiopathic osteoporosis related to aging or menopausal estrogen loss as described above, there are various secondary causes of osteoporosis (Table 1).

OSTEOMALACIA OR RICKETS

Osteomalacia or rickets[4,5] is primarily a defect involving the parathyroid–vitamin D axis resulting in deficient mineralization of bone. Most frequently it is due to inadequate activity of vitamin D resulting in secondary hyperparathyroidism. This may be the result of several causes and is more often privational in Third World countries and Asian immigrants in Britain.

Table 1 *Secondary causes of osteoporosis*

Endocrine	e.g. hyperthyroidism
Nutritional	low calcium intake protein malnutrition alcoholism
Gastrointestinal	gastrectomy malabsorption
Liver disease	
Renal disease	chronic renal failure hemodialysis
Drugs	corticosteroids anticonvulsants methotrexate heparin
Immobilization	
Rheumatoid arthritis	

In children, during the growing phase, it causes rickets. The rapid growth areas are most affected with defective mineralization of the growth plates.

Defective provisional calcification in the growing bone is associated with a lengthened zone of hypertrophy. There is distortion of the longitudinal cell columns in the zones of hypertrophy and maturation. There is lack of normal vascularization and excessive osteoclastic resorption in the primary spongiosa. This results in expanded widened growth plates.

Trabecular bone shows increased osteoid and/or osteoid seams. There is defective mineralization, and a reduced calcification front, as demonstrated by double tetracycline labeling.

Clinically, the classical appearance is a child with swollen epiphyses, beading of the costochondral junctions (ricketty rosary), a Harrison's sulcus due to pull of the diaphragm on the thorax, softening of the bones resulting in bowing of the tibia and fibula in younger children or genu valgum at an older age. There may be bone pain and tenderness. Proximal myopathy with weakening, particularly of the thigh muscles, may occur as a result of a defect in calcium ion transport needed for muscle contraction.

The radiological appearances of cupped expanded radial epiphyses and costo-chondral junctions are characteristic. There may be subperiosteal erosions of the phalanges or the spine may show codfish vertebrae with symmetrical biconcavity of the vertebrae and ballooning of the discs.

In adults, the clinical picture is more insidious, the patient may complain of non-specific bone pains and tenderness or of muscle weakness due to proximal myopathy. The weakness of the thigh muscles may show itself in difficulty in getting up from the sitting position. X-rays, apart from loss of bone density, may be nonspecific or may show Looser zones – transparent lines at right angles to the cortex with possibly a slight periosteal reaction. These are thought to be pseudofractures. Actual pathological fractures may occur, often involving the metatarsals. Spinal X-rays may show increased density of the vertebral end plates (Rugger jersey spine).

X-rays of the hands may show subperiosteal erosions of the phalanges, particularly the radial border of the index middle phalanx. The endosteal surfaces of the metacarpals may appear woolly.

Histologically, increase in trabecular bone surface covered by osteoid or in osteoid volume is seen, with defective mineralization and reduced calcification fronts, as shown by toluidine blue staining or single or double tetracycline labeling.

Biochemically, raised plasma alkaline phosphatase due to increased osteoblastic activity is found in the majority of cases. Although calcium absorption is impaired, plasma calcium levels, although low in growing children, are usually in the lower range of normal in adults as a result of the secondary hyperparathyroidism. Phosphate levels tend to be low (normal) but rise rapidly in response to vitamin D treatment.

The cardinal distinctive features of osteoporosis and adult osteomalacia due to vitamin D deficiency are shown in Table 2.

As mentioned, the majority of cases of osteomalacia or rickets are due to vitamin D deficiency as a result of privation, poor dietary intake, lack of sunlight, or malabsorption as a result of gastrectomy, intestinal bypass, short bowel syndrome, or steatorrhoea due to pancreatic deficiency. Other less frequent causes are listed in Table 3. Some of these are more suitable for a larger exposition on metabolic bone disease, and the subsequent discussion will be restricted to those conditions where methods of measurement may influence the diagnosis, management, or monitoring of progress.

Defective 25-hydroxyvitamin D synthesis due to drugs

The anticonvulsants primidone, phenytoin and carbamazepine[6] may induce liver enzymes which hydroxylate vitamin D to inactive metabolites.

Table 2 *Comparison of osteoporosis and osteomalacia (privational and malabsorption) measurable parameters*

Parameter	*Osteoporosis*	*Osteomalacia*
Bone density	↓	↓ or occasionally ↑
Radiological	low cortical indices Singh Index	none specifically measurable except subperiosteal resorption due to secondary hyperparathyroidism, and/or radioisotope scans showing areas of increased uptake, or Looser zones if present
Histomorphometry	trabecular thinning and reduction	increased osteoid reduced calcification front
Calcium ions	normal	normal or low
Phosphate	normal	low normal rise in response to vitamin D
Plasma alkaline phosphatase	normal	↑ fall in response to vitamin D
Urinary total hydroxyproline	high normal	↑ or normal
24-h urinary calcium	high normal	↓
Plasma 25-hydroxyvitamin D	normal	normal or ↓
Parathyroid hormone	normal	↑

Table 3 *Other causes of rickets and osteomalacia (excluding privation and malabsorption of vitamin D)*

Defective 25-OHD synthesis (hepatic)	
acquired	drug-induced hepatic damage (rare)
Defective 1,25(OH)$_2$D (calcitriol) synthesis	(Renal)
acquired	chronic renal damage primarily affecting tubules obstructive uropathy Fanconi syndrome
hereditary	vitamin D-dependent rickets type 1
Target organ resistance to 1,25(OH)$_2$D (calcitriol)	celiac disease vitamin D-dependent rickets type 2
Hypophosphatemia	
acquired	tumor-induced adult sporadic Fanconi syndrome
hereditary	X-linked (autosomal) Fanconi syndrome
Acidosis	
acquired	renal tubular disease
hereditary	renal tubular acidosis
Hypophosphatasia	
hereditary	autosomal recessive autosomal dominant
Intoxication (inhibiting mineralization)	
diphosphonate	
fluoride	
aluminium	
gallium nitrate	

25-OHD, 25-hydroxyvitamin D; 1,25(OH)$_2$D, 1,25-dihydroxyvitamin D (calcitriol)

Defective 1,25-dihydroxyvitamin D synthesis (calcitriol)

This occurs with certain forms of proximal tubular damage in the kidney. This may be the result of obstructive uropathy in which surgical interventions such as ileal conduit or ureterosigmoidostomy may feature. The Fanconi syndromes will be discussed later in the context of hypophosphatemia.

Vitamin D-dependent rickets

This may present as type 1 or type 2.

Type 1[7–9]

This involves an enzyme defect of renal 25-hydroxyvitamin D 1α-hydroxylase and appears in infancy. It results in gross calcitriol deficiency and severe secondary hyperparathyroidism.

Type 2

End organ resistance to 1,25-dihydroxyvitamin D (calcitriol) occurs as a result of various hereditary abnormalities of intracellular receptor protein causing severe hypocalcemia and secondary hyperparathyroidism.

Hypophosphatemia

This is characterized by a renal tubular phosphate leak with low plasma phosphate, but normal calcium and normal or low 1,25-dihydroxyvitamin D levels. It may be part of a Fanconi syndrome, but apart from this there are two types, one occurring in infancy and one in adults.

The first type is due to an abnormal dominant X-linked gene. Females may not develop rickets, but in males there is progressive bowing of the legs and decreased growth rate. Unexpectedly, myopathy is absent. There is increased bone density, with progressive thickening of the cortices progressing into adult life. A variable progressive calcification occurs in the paraspinal ligaments and tendon insertions (enthesopathy). Dental root hypoplasia is not uncommon and apical abscesses may occur.

The adult type[10–12] is either idiopathic or associated with a mesenchymal tumor. The patient develops osteomalacia with severe demineralization. Severe bone pains and myopathy are a feature. The patient may have pathological fractures or show Looser zones on X-ray. Resection of a mesenchymal tumor often produces a remission but long-term follow-up is required.

Both types respond to calcitriol with calcium supplements. Phosphate supplements may be required in children subject to response to calcitriol, but are mandatory in adults.

Fanconi syndromes

These syndromes involve multiple proximal tubular resorptive defects. These chiefly involve phosphate, glucose, amino acids and bicarbonate but may extend to calcium, potassium, urate, or water in the proximal or other parts of the tubule. There may be impairment of synthesis of calcitriol. As a result the subject may develop rickets or osteomalacia with variable combinations of hypophosphatemia, acidosis and defective calcitriol production.

The treatment involves vitamin D and adequate supplements of sodium bicarbonate, potassium and phosphates as indicated.

Renal tubular acidosis

Two types of renal tubular acidosis are seen[13]. In type 1 there is defective hydrogen ion secretion in the distal tubules, and in type 2 there is partial failure to reabsorb bicarbonate in the proximal tubule. Both lead to acidosis with a urine pH of over 5.6. It may present as rickets or osteomalacia, as urolithiasis, or as a hypokalemic paralysis.

The treatment in type 1 is to give a supplement of sodium bicarbonate.

Hypophosphatasia

In hypophosphatasia[14,15] there is a hereditary defect of alkaline phosphatase. This enzyme regulates the local concentration of phosphate and pyrophosphate required for mineralization. In infancy this may cause severe rickets, hypercalciuria, nephrocalcinosis and uremia with a high mortality. In older children and adults it may be less severe with osteoporosis, osteomalacia and fractures. At the moment there is no satisfactory treatment.

Drugs which inhibit mineralization

Certain drugs or poisons inhibit mineralization and histological appearances of osteomalacia are encountered at times with chronic fluoride ingestion, with chronic etidronate overdosage, aluminium and gallium nitrate toxicity.

OTHER CONDITIONS ASSOCIATED WITH CHANGES IN BONE ARCHITECTURE

Paget's disease

Characteristically there are areas of greatly increased bone turnover. Increased resorption occurs as a result of increased activity of osteoclasts. This is accompanied by increased osteoblastic activity. Lamellar bone becomes replaced by woven bone and there is a loss of Haversian systems. The bone architecture becomes disorganized with increase in osteoid showing normal calcification fronts. There may be areas of gross osteolysis.

The picture is one of new bone formation, sclerosis, bony expansion, coarse trabeculation and cortical thickening. Plasma alkaline phosphatase may be grossly raised and 24-h urinary hydroxyproline output is increased. Plasma calcium and phosphate levels are normal. Radiologically the changes are focal and may be monostotic or polyostotic. The appearance is that of expanded bone with irregular thickened cortices and a coarse distorted trabecular pattern. There may be cortical fractures. The bones may bend. The patient may complain of bone pain and may develop secondary osteoarthritis. Nerve compression syndromes may occur affecting cranial nerves, the brain stem, spinal cord, or roots. There may be cardiac failure due to osseous hyperemia. Occasionally malignant change to a chondro-, osteo- or fibro-sarcoma may be seen.

Some benefit may be obtained from calcitonin which inhibits resorption.

Conditions associated with parathyroid dysfunction

Primary hyperparathyroidism (osteitis fibrosa)[16]

In 85–90% of cases this is due to a solitary adenoma and in 10–15% there is hyperplasia of all four glands, leaving only 1% due to carcinoma. In some cases a solitary adenoma is associated with a multiple endocrine adenoma syndrome (Type I). The plasma calcium is raised with a low phosphate level. A minority of patients (5–10%) may complain of pain, especially in the knees and ankles. There may be pathological fractures. Urolithiasis may develop. The bone shows increased resorption, noticeable as subperiosteal erosions. Peritrabecular fibrosis occurs and there is increased synthesis of immature woven bone. Occasionally degenerative joint lesions may develop.

Hypoparathyroidism[17,18]

Three types occur: idiopathic; post-thyroidectomy; and pseudohypoparathyroidism.

The idiopathic form may occur from infancy to early adult life. The hypocalcemia manifests itself as epilepsy, tetany, carpopedal spasm, laryngeal stridor, cataract and may be associated with mental retardation. Bone density tends to increase.

Post-thyroidectomy hypoparathyroidism due to damage or inadvertent removal of the parathyroid glands usually manifests on the 4th or 5th day (earlier in thyrotoxic patients) as hypocalcemia with paraesthesiae, tetany and carpopedal spasm. Following the earlier days of ^{131}I treatment for thyrotoxicosis the onset of more insidious latent hypocalcemia was reported[9,20].

Pseudohypoparathyroidism is associated with a target organ resistance of the bones and kidneys to parathyroid hormone. The clinical features include short stature, rounded facies and variable brachydactyly (particularly shortening of the fourth metacarpal). There may be ectopic subcutaneous calcification. The condition is twice as common in females as males.

CONCLUSION

This review is selective and of necessity brief. An attempt has been made to describe those features which can be subjected to measurement. Selected references are given which would be helpful if more information is required.

References

1. Albright F, Reifenstein EC. The Parathyroid Glands and Metabolic Bone Disease. Baltimore: Williams and Wilkins, 1948.
2. Dixon, A StJ, Russell RGB, Stamp TCB, eds. Osteoporosis: A Multidisciplinary Problem. Roy Soc Med Int Congress and Symposium Series 1983: No 5. London: Academic Press.
3. Garn SM. The Earlier Gain and Later Loss of Cortical Bone. Springfield Illinois: Charles C, Thomas, 1970.

4. Peacock M. Osteomalacia and rickets. In: Nordin BEC, ed. Metabolic Bone and Stone Disease. London: Churchill-Livingstone, 1987: 71–111.
5. Stamp TCB. Metabolic bone disease. In: Scott JD, ed. Coperman's Textbook of the Rheumatic Diseases. 6th edn. London: Churchill-Livingstone, 1986: 992–1023.
6. Stamp TCB, Flanagan RJ, Richens A, Round JM, Thomas M, Dupre P, Jackson M. Anticonvulsant osteomalacia. In: Copp DH, Talmage RV, eds. Endocrinology of Calcium Metabolism. Amsterdam: Excerpta Medica, 1978: 16–22.
7. Rasmussen H, Anast C. Familial hypophosphataemia (vitamin D-resistant rickets). In: Stanbury JB, Wyngarden JB, Frederickson DS, eds. The Metabolic Basis of Inherited Disease. New York: McGraw-Hill, 1978: 1537–62.
8. Thakker RW, O Riordan JLH. Inherited Forms of Rickets and Osteomalacia. Baillières. Clin Endocrinol Metab 1988; 2: 157–91.
9. Fraser D, Kooh SW, Kind HP, Holick MF, Tanaka Y, De Luca HF. Pathogenesis of hereditary vitamin D dependent rickets; an inborn error involving defective conversion of 25OHD to $1{,}25(OH)_2D$. N Engl J Med 1973; 289: 817–24.
10. Dent CE, Stamp TCB. Hypophosphataemic osteomalacia presenting in adults. Quart J Med 1971; 40: 303–24.
11. Reid IR, Hardy DC, Murphy WA, Teitelbaum SL, Bergfeld MA, Whyte MP. X-linked hypophosphataemia; a clinical, biochemical and histopathologic assessment of morbidity in adults. Medicine (Baltimore) 1989; 68: 336–52.
12. Weidner N, Santa-Cruz D. Phosphaturic mesenchymal tumours. A polymorphous group causing osteomalacia or rickets. Cancer 1987; 59: 1442–54.
13. Morris JC Jr. Renal tubular acidosis. N Engl J Med 1982; 304: 418–20.
14. Rasmussen H, Bartter FC. Hypophosphatasia. In: Stanbury JB, Wyngarden JB, Frederickson DS, eds. The Metabolic Basis of Inherited Disease. New York: McGraw-Hill, 1978; 1340–9.
15. Whyte P, Murphy WA, Fallon MD. Acute hypophosphatasia with chondrocalcinosis and arthropathy. Variable penetrance of hypophosphatasemia in a large Oklahoma kindred. Am J Med 1982; 72: 631–41.
16. Davies DR, Dent CE, Watson L. Idiopathic calciuria and hyperparathyroidism. Br Med J 1971; i: 108.
17. Nusnyowitz ML, Frami B, Kolb FO. The spectrum of the hypoparathyroid states. Medicine (Baltimore) 1976; 55: 105–18.
18. Nagant de Deuxchaisnes, Krane SM, eds. Metabolic Bone Disease. Vol II. New York: Academic Press, 1978: 217–445.
19. Adams PH, Chalmers TM. Parathyroid function after I^{131} therapy for hyperthyroidism. Clin Sci 1965; 29: 391–5.
20. Eipe J, Johnson SA. Hypoparathyroidism following I^{131} therapy for hyperthyroidism. Arch Intern Med 1968; 121: 270–2.
21. Avioli LV, Lindsay R. In : Avioli LV, Krane SM, eds. Metabolic Bone Disease. Philadelphia: WB Saunders Co, 1990; 398, Figure 12.1.

Biochemical markers of bone turnover

4

R. A. Hannon and R. Eastell

INTRODUCTION

Bone is constantly being remodeled at discrete locations in the skeleton. This is achieved by the 'coupled' processes of bone resorption, carried out by the osteoclasts, followed by bone formation, which is carried out by the osteoblasts. Bone mass remains constant when both processes are balanced; however, if the 'coupling' between balance and formation is altered there can be a net change in bone mass. During growth, aging and in metabolic bone disease, the relationship between bone formation and resorption may differ from that found in the healthy young adult.

Direct measurements of resorption and formation can be made by bone histomorphometry. However, this technique is invasive, time-consuming and not suitable for repeated measurements on individual subjects or for use in studies of large populations. Furthermore, it only measures formation and resorption in a small area of trabecular bone rather than in the entire skeleton. Another direct technique is the use of calcium kinetics: again this is a complex technique to carry out, results depend on the model used, and it is not suitable for repeated measurements. These limitations to the established techniques for measurement of bone remodeling have led to the increased use of biochemical markers of bone turnover.

An ideal marker of bone turnover would be bone-specific, reflect either resorption or formation but not both, and correlate well with the appropriate direct measurements of bone turnover. Biochemical markers of bone turnover fall into two categories: formation markers and resorption markers which reflect osteoblast and osteoclast activity, respectively. As bone turnover is a 'coupled' phenomenon, markers of formation and resorption will correlate to a greater or lesser degree with each other. Since the main function of the osteoblast in bone formation is the synthesis of type 1 collagen, and a major function of the osteoclast in bone resorption is the degradation of collagen, products or by-products of these processes should be good markers of bone turnover.

Type 1 collagen is the major type of collagen found in bone, representing 90% of the organic matrix[1], where it is synthesized by osteoblasts. Type 1 collagen is a trimeric protein comprising two α_1(I) and one α_2(I) polypeptide chains. It is synthesized in a precursor form, procollagen, which is then modified extracellularly to produce collagen (Figures 1 and 2). As the three polypeptides which make up the procollagen molecule are synthesized they enter the cisternae of the rough endoplasmic reticulum where they undergo a series of post-translational modifications. Firstly, 'signal' sequences are removed from the N-terminal end. The next event is the hydroxylation of the proline and lysine residues of the nascent procollagen chains by specific enzymes. This is followed by the glycosylation of hydroxylysine. Galactose is added to some of the hydroxylysine residues yielding galactosylhydroxylysine residues, some of which are further glycosylated to glucosylgalactosylhydroxylysine (Figure 1a). Once translation is complete, the propeptide chains come together and are stabilized by the formation of disulphide bridges (Figure 1b). At the N-terminus these are intrachain bridges whereas at the C-terminus

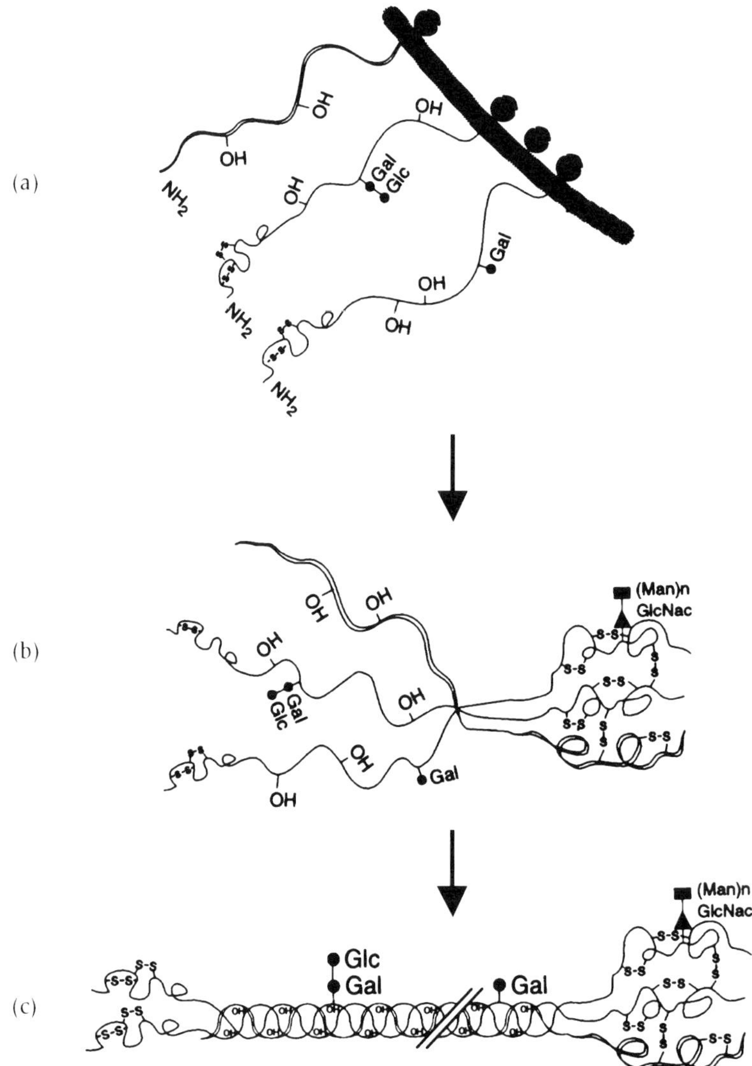

Figure 1 *Intracellular post-translational modifications of procollagen propeptides illustrating the origin of some collagen markers of bone turnover. (a) Hydroxylation and glycosylation of lysine residues; (b) disulfide bridge formation in the C-terminal region in preparation for the folding of a helix; (c) complete procollagen molecule which is secreted into the extracellular space; modified with permission from Prockop and colleagues*[2]

there are both inter- and intrachain bridges. The C-terminal interchain bridges, which are formed first, facilitate the rapid formation of the triple helix (Figure 1c). The procollagen molecule is then secreted into the extracellular space where the N-terminal propeptide and then the C-terminal propeptide are cleaved by specific peptidases[2–4] (Figure 2a). The resulting collagen molecules assemble in a quarter-stagger array which is stabilized by intramolecular and intermolecular cross-links (Figure 2b). Cross-link formation occurs between lysyl and hydroxylysyl residues of the telopeptide regions and the ε-amino group of lysyl, hydroxylysyl, or glycosylated hydroxylysyl residues of other polypeptide chains. The resulting Schiff base-type cross-links

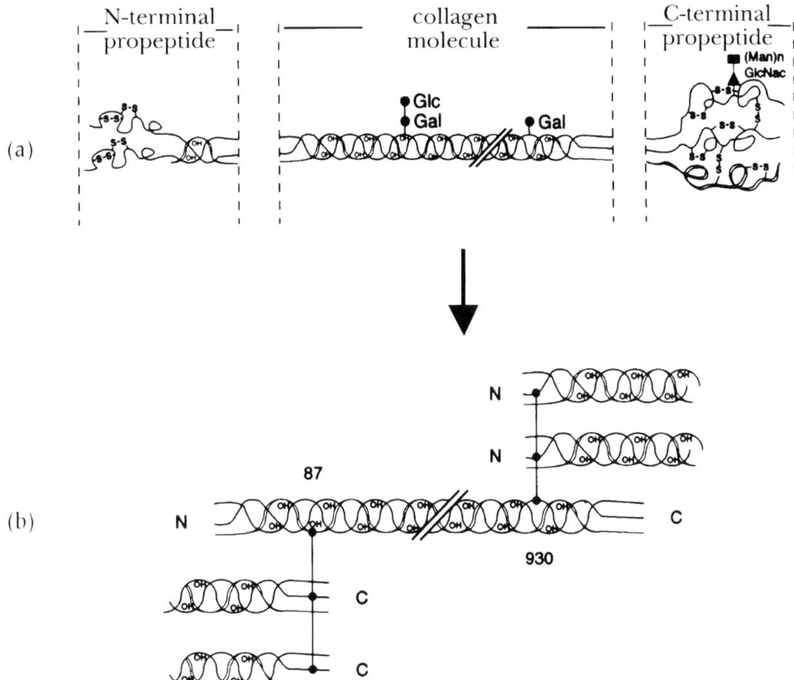

Figure 2 *Extracellular modification of procollagen and collagen illustrating the origin of some collagen-based markers of bone turnover: (a) cleavage of the N- and C-terminal propeptides; (b) formation of pyridinium cross-links between aligned collagen molecules during fibril formation; modified with permission from Prockop and colleagues[2] and Hanson and colleagues[5]*

are further stabilized by a reduction step, during collagen maturation[6].

The C-propeptide produced by the cleavage of the procollagen molecule is released in an amount equimolar to the amount of collagen formed and is not incorporated into the bone matrix. It therefore is a potential marker of bone formation. The N-terminal propeptide is not stabilized by interchain disulfide bridges and therefore once released is probably circulating as three separate chains[7] a proportion of which are known to be incorporated into the bone matrix.

Collagen is broken down by the action of lysosomal enzymes including cathepsins. The cross-links are released intact into the circulation and are not further degraded before excretion in the urine, 50% being free and the other 50% being bound to collagen fragments[8]. The hydroxylysylglycosides are also released intact and excreted as such[9]. Hydroxyproline is also released, but 90% is metabolized by the liver and only 10% is excreted in urine. These degradation products largely fulfil the criteria of markers of bone resorption.

Table 1 *Major biochemical markers of bone turnover*

Formation markers
Serum osteocalcin (bone Gla-protein)
Serum alkaline phosphatase
Serum bone-specific alkaline phosphatase (BAP)
Serum procollagen type I carboxyterminal propeptide (PICP)
Resorption markers
Serum tartrate-resistant acid phosphatase (TRAP)
Urinary hydroxyproline
Urinary pyridinium cross-links
Urinary hydroxylysine glycosides

These products and by-products of collagen biosynthesis, together with other osteoblast and osteoclast enzymes and other proteins (Table 1), provide a range of markers of bone turnover which can be used, with greater or lesser effect, to investigate bone metabolism.

MARKERS OF BONE FORMATION

Alkaline phosphatase

Alkaline phosphatase is an orthophosphoric-mono-ester phospho-2-hydrolase which shows optimum activity at alkaline pH. Robinson showed in 1923 that alkaline phosphatase activity was associated with osteoblast activity[10]. Since that time serum alkaline phosphatase has been accepted as a marker of bone formation.

Several authors[11,12] have demonstrated that serum total alkaline phosphatase correlated well with mineralization rate as measured by ^{47}Ca kinetic methods. The precise role of alkaline phosphatase in mineralization relationship is unclear although two mechanisms have been suggested. Firstly, alkaline phosphatase releases inorganic phosphate which is required for the formation of calcium–phosphate complexes which are deposited in the matrix during mineralization. Secondly, alkaline phosphatase may hydrolyse inorganic pyrophosphate which is a potent inhibitor of hydroxyapatite crystal formation and dissolution[13].

Assay

Serum total alkaline phosphatase is routinely measured by an automated colorimetric method using *p*-nitrophenyl phosphate as substrate[6].

Bone alkaline phosphatase

Circulating alkaline phosphatase is not derived solely from bone. Several isoforms of alkaline phosphatase exist. Four alkaline phosphatase genes have been located: the genes for germ cell, placental and intestinal isoforms are on chromosome 2 and the gene for the tissue non-specific isoform is on chromosome 1[14]. The tissue non-specific gene codes for liver, kidney and bone alkaline phosphatase. The difference between these isoforms is the post-translational glycosylation[15]. The most abundant isoforms found in serum from normal adults are bone and liver in approximately equal amounts[16]. The liver and bone forms have different electrophoretic mobilities, although the difference in mobility is very small[17]. They also differ in their resistance to inactivation by heat and urea, bone being the more sensitive isoform[18]. Total alkaline phosphatase relates well to other measurements of bone formation and has been used extensively as a marker of bone formation in metabolic bone diseases. However, measurement of bone-specific alkaline phosphatase can be superior to measurement of total alkaline phosphatase. Changes in bone-specific alkaline phosphatase may be observed even if changes in total alkaline phosphatase are absent. In situations where liver isoform is increased both isoforms must be measured specifically.

Brixen and colleagues[19] have shown, in patients with different metabolic bone diseases, that bone alkaline phosphatase is a better predictor of bone mineralization, as measured by ^{47}Ca kinetics, than total alkaline phosphatase. However, serum osteocalcin correlates better with mineralization than either total or bone alkaline phosphatase. In normal women there is a significant correlation between bone formation rate, measured by histomorphometry, and serum concentration of bone alkaline phosphatase[20].

Assay

Measurement of bone alkaline phosphatase in serum relies on quantifying differences between the liver and bone isoenzymes. Moss and Whitby[21] developed a heat inactivation method based on the determination of half-inactivation time of liver alkaline phosphatase at 56°C and hence derived the bone alkaline phosphatase activity indirectly.

Several quantitative electrophoretic methods have been described, using a variety of supporting media, including agarose[22], polyacrylamide[23–25] and cellulose acetate[26]. In some of these methods, the electrophoretic separation of the bone and liver isoforms is enhanced by incorporation of wheat germ lectin into the supporting medium or by a short pretreatment of the sample with neuraminidase. Wheat germ lectin is a carbohydrate-binding protein which binds preferentially to the N-acetylglucosamine residues of the bone isoform. Neuraminidase preferentially digests the sialic acid residues of the bone isoform, thereby altering the relative electrophoretic mobilities of two isoforms[23]. Van Hoof and co-workers[22] compared a lectin-affinity electrophoresis method on cellulose acetate with electrophoresis on agarose, with and without neuraminidase pretreatment. Bone alkaline phosphatase activity as measured by electrophoresis on agarose without neuraminidase pretreatment correlated well with the activity measured with neuraminidase pretreatment ($r = 0.86$). The correlation between agarose electrophoresis and cellulose acetate lectin affinity electrophoresis was not as good ($r = 0.6$). The bone activity was systematically higher when measured by the cellulose acetate affinity method. This may be due to the lack of specificity of the lectin binding.

Rosalki and Foo[26] developed a method of estimating bone alkaline phosphatase depending on the selective precipitation of the bone isoenzyme by wheat germ lectin. Wheat germ lectin is a carbohydrate-binding protein which preferentially binds to the *N*-acetylglucosamine residues on the bone isoform of alkaline phosphatase. Serum samples are incubated with wheat germ lectin, and the alkaline phosphatase activity measured in the precipitate (bone) and supernatant (liver). In subsequent modifications of this method[27,28], total alkaline phosphatase activity and the alkaline phosphatase activity in the supernatant (liver) are measured and the bone alkaline phosphatase activity calculated, indirectly. Different batches of wheat germ lectin, even from the same supplier, differ in their affinity for bone alkaline phosphatase and therefore each batch must be standardized to precipitate 50% alkaline phosphatase activity from a standard pool of adult serum[28]. In liver disease, biliary alkaline phosphatase may co-precipitate with bone alkaline phosphatase. This interference is removed by pretreatment with Triton-X[26]. However, the treatment itself may increase total alkaline phosphatase activity[29] which gives negative interference for the bone estimation of bone alkaline phosphatase.

Day and colleagues[29] have compared the wheat germ precipitation method with two electrophoretic methods. They suggest that although it is a good method for determining the main source of alkaline phosphatase, the wheat germ lectin precipitation method lacks the accurate quantification of the electrophoretic methods. Behr and Barnert[27] found, as we do in our laboratory, that the wheat germ lectin precipitation method is a rapid and technically simple method.

Recently, several groups have turned their attention to measuring bone alkaline phosphatase using monoclonal antibodies. Lawson and colleagues[30] isolated two monoclonal antibodies, one (B4-50) of which has a five times greater affinity for liver alkaline phosphatase than for the bone isoform, whereas the other monoclonal antibody (B4-78) has equal affinity for both forms. Using these antibodies, a solid-phase immunoassay was developed to measure proportions of liver and bone alkaline phosphatase in mixtures of the two. Seabrook and associates[31] developed a plate capture assay using a monoclonal antibody BAP 1/9 which preferentially bound bone alkaline phosphatase vs. liver alkaline phosphatase. In 1989 Hill and Wolfert[32] reported the preparation of monoclonal antibodies which preferentially reacted with bone alkaline phosphatase rather than liver alkaline phosphatase. Two of these antibodies were used to develop an immunoradiometric bead assay. Garnero and Delmas have demonstrated that this assay is a reliable and sensitive method for the measurement of bone alkaline phosphate in normal subjects and in patients with metabolic bone diseases[33]. The cross-reactivity with the liver isoform is in the order of 15%.

Bone alkaline phosphatase in normal subjects

At birth, and in the 1st year of life, the predominant isoform of alkaline phosphatase found in serum is the bone form[16]. In childhood, bone alkaline phosphatase levels may be ten times those in normal adults. These levels peak three times during childhood, between the ages of 1 and 2 years, 6 and 7 years and during puberty, after which levels fall to those of the adult[34]. The same is true for total alkaline phosphatase which reaches adult levels at age 20 years for males and 18 years for females[35]. Several groups have shown that bone alkaline phosphatase, measured by wheat germ lectin precipitation, is higher in men than in women[26,28]. However, Behr and Barnert[27] found no significant difference in levels between men and women. Others[34,36] have found that levels of bone alkaline phosphatase are lower in women than in men under the age of 50 years but higher in women than in men over the age of 50 years. Duda and co-workers[37] reported that bone alkaline phosphatase increases in both sexes after the sixth decade (Figure 3).

Bone alkaline phosphatase exhibits variation through the menstrual cycle, being higher during the luteal phase than the follicular phase by 14% ($p < 0.05$)[38].

Nielsen and colleagues[39] have shown that there is a circadian rhythm in serum alkaline phosphatase concentration. Bone alkaline phosphatase peaks at 14.30 and 23.30 with a nadir level at 06.30, the difference between peaks and nadir being 30% ($p < 0.05$). Total alkaline phosphatase shows similar circadian variation with a nadir at 06.30 but the difference between peak and nadir levels was only 23%. Total alkaline phosphatase also shows a seasonal variation, low levels being found in the summer and high levels in the winter[40]. This is probably due to changes in the bone isoform of alkaline phosphatase as no changes in liver function were found. The variation correlates negatively with serum levels of 25-hydroxyvitamin D.

Bone alkaline phosphatase in metabolic bone disease (Figures 4 and 5)

Osteoporosis In postmenopausal osteoporosis total alkaline phosphatase levels and bone alkaline phosphatase levels are elevated[37,41]. The mean Z-score for total alkaline phosphatase was + 0.96 in a group of 62 women with osteoporosis[42]. The mean Z-score for bone alkaline phosphatase was + 1.90, in a similar group of women[37]. Sorensen[28] showed that after 1 year of cyclic hormone treatment in normal healthy postmenopausal women total and bone alkaline phosphatase levels fell significantly whereas liver alkaline phosphatase remained constant. Bone alkaline phosphatase increased in a parallel untreated group.

Hyperparathyroidism Several groups have shown a significant increase in total alkaline phosphatase in patients with primary hyperparathyroidism[43,44]. Minisola and colleagues[43] reported a mean Z-score of + 3.88 for total alkaline phosphatase in patients with primary hyperparathyroidism. Duda and colleagues[37] showed similar results for bone alkaline phosphatase. The mean Z-score for patients with primary hyperparathyroidism is + 3.6. However, Gonchoroff and associates[45] used a high-performance affinity chromatography method for measuring the bone isoenzyme and found that only two out of seven patients had Z-scores greater than + 2.

Hyperthyroidism Broulik and associates[46] showed that in 20 out of 28 patients with hyperthyroidism the total alkaline phosphatase was significantly increased above the normal range whereas 24 of these patients had bone alkaline phosphatase levels above the normal range. This discrepancy between the two measurements serves to illustrate the point that an elevated bone alkaline phosphatase level may be masked when only the total alkaline phosphatase con-

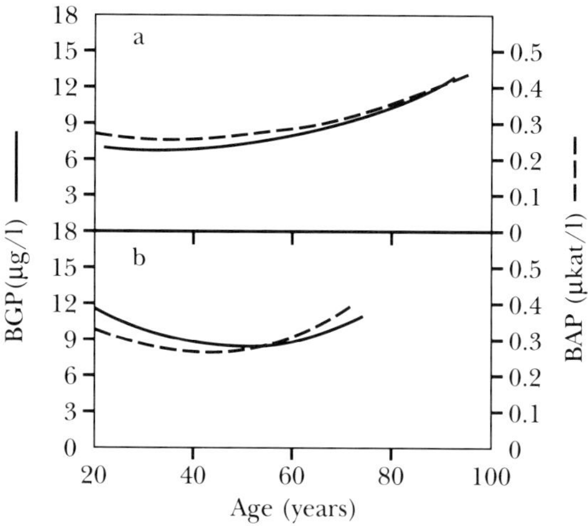

Figure 3 *Regression of values for serum osteocalcin (bone Gla protein, BGP) and serum bone alkaline phosphatase (BAP) on age: (a) for normal women; (b) for normal men; modified with permission from Duda and colleagues*[37]

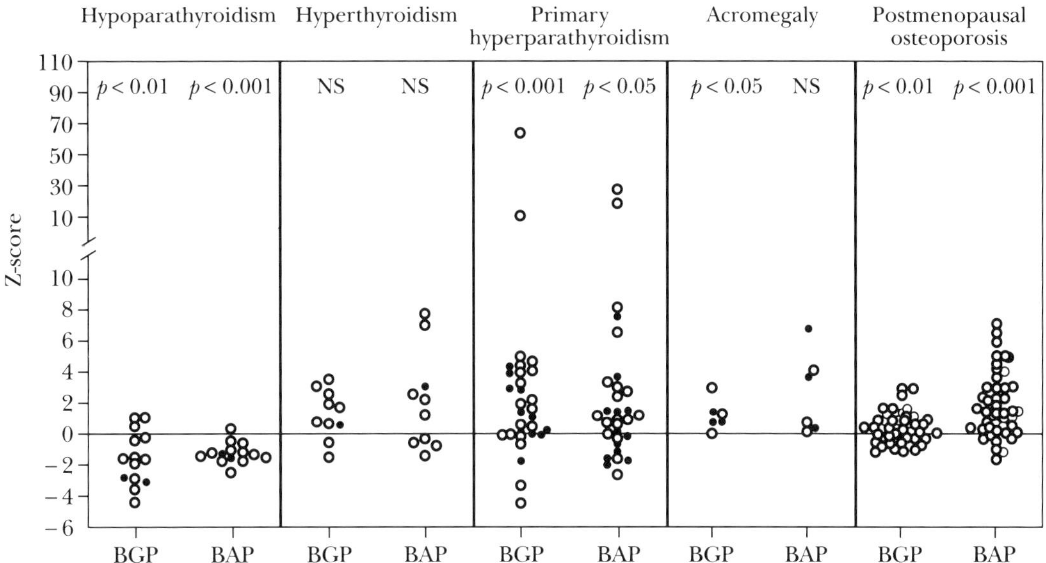

Figure 4 *Individual serum osteocalcin (bone Gla protein, BGP) and bone alkaline phosphatase (BAP) values gave concordant results in patients with hypoparathyroidism, hyperthyroidism, primary hyperparathyroidism, acromegaly and postmenopausal osteoporosis. The Z-score is SD from the predicted mean for normal subjects obtained from sex-specific regression equations that predicted serum concentration as a function of age (see Figure 3): open circles, women; closed circles, men; modified with permission from Duda and colleagues*[37]

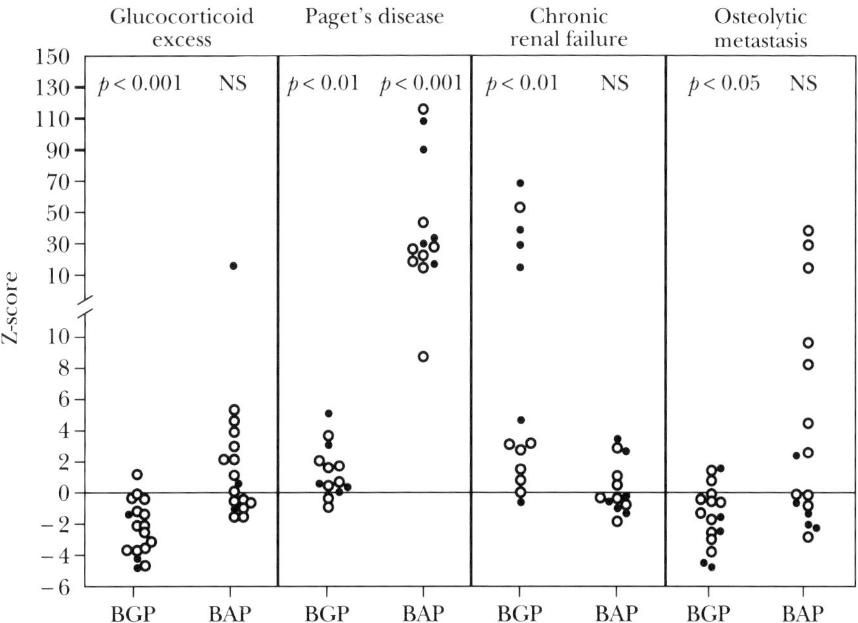

Figure 5 *Individual serum osteocalcin (bone Gla protein, BGP) and bone alkaline phosphatase (BAP) values gave discordant results in patients with glucocorticoid excess, Paget's disease, chronic renal failure and osteolytic metastasis. The Z-score is SD from the predicted mean for normal subjects obtained from sex-specific regression equations that predicted serum concentration as a function of age (see Figure 3): open circles, women; closed circles, men; modified with permission from Duda and colleagues*[37]

centration is measured. Tibi and colleagues[47] reported a significant increase in liver alkaline phosphatase in hyperthyroidism patients in addition to the increase in bone alkaline phosphatase. Both decreased after treatment. Duda and colleagues[37] reported that there was only a small increase in bone alkaline phosphatase levels in hyperthyrodism. This increase was not significant, possibly due to the fact that only ten patients were studied (Figure 4).

Osteomalacia Serum levels of total and bone alkaline phosphatase are increased in patients with vitamin D deficiency osteomalacia[48,49]. Since alkaline phosphatase is thought to have a role in mineralization this increase is difficult to explain. Demiaux and associates[49] have shown that serum alkaline phosphatase correlates positively with matrix formation, measured by histomorphonetry, but negatively with mineral apposition rate ($r = -0.77$, $p < 0.05$). Although mineralization is decreased in osteomalacia, matrix formation is increased as indicated by increased serum levels of osteocalcin. The increase in alkaline phosphatase may reflect increased osteoblast activity. Treatment with vitamin D results in an initial increase and then a decrease in alkaline phosphatase over a period of several months[50].

Paget's disease Bone alkaline phosphatase increases dramatically in Paget's disease with Z-scores of + 20 to + 41[36,37,44,45,50]. Osteocalcin (the other established marker of bone formation) does not increase to the same extent[51].

Metastatic bone disease Torres and colleagues[44] reported significantly increased levels of total alkaline phosphatase, but decreased levels of osteocalcin, in patients with hypercalcemia of malignancy. This is in agreement with Duda and associates[37] who reported a small increase in bone alkaline phosphatase and significant decrease in osteocalcin in 16 patients with osteolytic metastasis to bone of whom four were hypercalcemic (Figure 5).

Osteocalcin

Osteocalcin or bone Gla protein is the most abundant non-collagenous protein found in bone and is also found in dentin[52]. It is a small protein of 49 residues with a molecular weight of 5.8 kDa. An important feature of the primary structure is the presence of three γ-carboxyglutamic acid residues at positions 17, 21 and 24. These residues are derived from the post-translational carboxylation of glutamic acid residues. They have two important roles: first, as potent binders of calcium ions which are required to stabilize the α-helical region of the molecule, and second in the binding of the molecule to the hydroxyapatite of the mineralized bone[53]. Osteocalcin biosynthesis, which occurs in the osteoblast, is vitamin K-dependent and is stimulated by 1,25-dihydroxyvitamin D_3[54]. Price and colleagues[55] calculated that 60–90% of the osteocalcin synthesized is incorporated into the bone, the rest is released into the circulation and is rapidly degraded by metalloenzymes in the liver and kidneys[56]. Intact osteocalcin is not released into the circulation as a result of bone resorption. Taylor and co-workers[57] have shown that circulating osteocalcin comprises intact molecules together with smaller fragments. These fragments are produced during bone resorption or result from the catabolism of the circulating protein. The elevated levels of serum osteocalcin in patients with severe renal failure[58] are due, at least partially, to decreased renal filtration since some fragments found in uremic serum are the same as those found in normal urine[59].

Although the precise function of osteocalcin remains unclear several roles for this protein have been proposed. It may have a role in the maturation stage of bone mineral formation[59]. It may also act as a messenger for 1,25-dihydroxyvitamin D3 in the process of osteoclast activation and as such could act as a 'coupling' factor between osteoblast activity and osteoclast activity[54,60].

The use of serum osteocalcin as a marker of bone formation has been validated by bone histomorphometry and calcium kinetics. In women with postmenopausal osteoporosis, serum osteocalcin levels correlate significantly with bone formation rate ($r = 0.66$, $p < 0.001$) but not with bone resorption[61]. In this study osteocalcin was superior to serum alkaline phosphatase as a marker of bone formation as there was no significant correlation between serum alkaline phosphatase concentration and bone formation rate. Eastell and colleagues[20] confirmed these findings in normal women and also demonstrated a significant correlation between serum osteocalcin levels and kinetically determined calcium accretion rate. No significant correlation was found between serum bone alkaline phosphatase and calcium accretion rate. Similar results have been reported for several endocrine diseases[12,19,62].

Assay

Many immunoassays have been developed to measure serum osteocalcin[63–66] (for full review *see* Power and Fottrell[67]). The antisera used in many of these assays are directed against bovine osteocalcin, in particular the C-terminal region of the molecule[68]. Ideally, human osteocalcin should be used as a source of reagents for the assay, but it tends to be unstable. Bovine osteocalcin has been used because of the great degree of homology between bovine and human osteocalcin; bovine osteocalcin differs by only five residues, at the N-terminus, from human osteocalcin[67]. Price and Nishimoto[63] demonstrated 100% cross-reactivity with human osteocalcin using an antiserum against bovine osteocalcin. Similarly, ovine osteocalcin differs from human by only five residues, however there is a longer region of identity with human osteocalcin in the mid- to C-terminal region of the molecule. Pastoureau and Delmas[65] developed a radioimmunoassay for human osteocalcin using polyclonal anti-ovine osteocalcin antisera, which recognize only the intact molecule. Synthetic C- and N-terminal fragments were not recognized by the antiserum suggesting that either a mid-molecule or a conformational epitope was the target of the antiserum. When compared with a bovine assay, the ovine radioimmunoassay detected a significantly greater difference between osteoporotic patients and age- and sex-matched controls. Taylor and colleagues[66] developed a radioimmunoassay to human osteocalcin directed towards a mid-region epitope. In addition to intact osteocalcin, this assay also recognizes 'fragments' in serum and in urine.

Recently, several new assays for osteocalcin have been developed[69–73]. Hosoda and associates[70] reported a sandwich enzyme immunoassay using polyclonal antisera to synthetic C-terminal (7 residues) and N-terminal (20 residues) peptides of human osteocalcin. The assay detected only intact osteocalcin as compared to a commercially available kit which also recognized fragments. By comparing secondary structure with the cross-reactivity of the antisera of osteocalcin of different species with serum of these species it seemed likely that the epitopes for the antibodies are conformational. Deftos and colleagues[69] have reported two-site radioimmunometric assays using monoclonal antibodies to synthetic N-terminal (residues 1–12) and C-terminal (residues 38–49) peptides of human osteocalcin. Both assays employed the same antibody to the C-terminal peptide but different antibodies to the N-terminal peptide. Although serum concentrations of osteocalcin measured by each of these assays correlated well with each other ($r = 0.94$, $p < 0.01$), there was more than a twofold difference in absolute values. Similarly, results from both assays correlated well with results from a polyclonal radioimmunoassay for osteocalcin but the absolute values varied considerably. These differences probably result from the immunochemical heterogeneity of circulating osteocalcin, the structural basis for which is still unclear. The two-site radioimmunometric assay described by Garnero and colleagues[73] detects intact osteocalcin and a large N-terminal mid-region fragment. In normal subjects, this large fragment represents 50% of the total osteocalcin measured. Although there is a good correlation between levels of osteocalcin measured using this assay and measured using a conventional bovine radioimmunoassay, the absolute values are threefold higher. Preliminary results indicate that this assay may be more sensitive than bovine radioimmunoassay for investigation of metabolic bone disease.

The assays for osteocalcin vary in specificity especially with regard to the detection of fragments. A consequence of this is the large interlaboratory variation reported by Delmas and colleagues[74]. They suggested that all osteocalcin results be expressed as a percentage of the normal range for that laboratory.

Tracy and associates[68] have demonstrated that a number of osteocalcin assays are sensitive to hemolysis of the sample, which may reduce the apparent level of osteocalcin by up to 90%. This inhibition of the assay is not associated with red cell membranes nor with hemoglobin in the sample. Most of the osteocalcin in hemolysed plasma is converted to low molecular weight fragments, as shown by plasma electrophoresis. However, if hemolysis takes place in the presence of protease inhibitors, the effect is partially reduced. The inhibitory effect of hemolysis results from the action of soluble enzymes, in the red cell lysate, on the osteocalcin in the sample. Contrary to this, Jaouhari and colleagues[71] have reported that added hemoglobin (87 μmol/l), prepared from hemolysate, significantly decreases the measured osteocalcin concentration.

Some osteocalcin assays have been reported to be calcium-dependent[64,71,72]. Since calcium is required for the structural stability of the molecule it is probable that such assays employ antisera which are directed against conformational epitopes. This may be true even for epitopes which are not part of the calcium-binding region of the molecule[64]. Therefore, it is important to ensure that blood samples are not collected in EDTA tubes or tubes containing citrate, which complexes with calcium[71].

The effect of storage and repeated freeze–thaw cycles on serum osteocalcin is not absolutely clear and may depend on the assay being used to measure the osteocalcin. Power and Fottrell[67] suggest that it is stable for one freeze–thaw cycle, whereas Tracy and colleagues[68] reported up to a 10% loss of reactivity after three freeze–thaw cycles. Grundberg and colleagues[64] reported a variable 20–40% reduction in serum values after two freeze–thaw cycles. Storage at – 20 °C is acceptable for the short term, but for the long term storage at – 70 °C is required.

Osteocalcin in normal subjects

Serum concentrations of osteocalcin are higher throughout childhood than in adult life. Levels decline after the 1st year, but rise again during puberty before falling to adult levels[75,76]. Osteocalcin concentrations for girls during mid-puberty are five times those of normal adult women[77]. Most but not all studies show that men have slightly higher levels of osteocalcin than women[37,75,78,79] and that there is an age-dependent increase after the fifth decade, in women. Although Epstein and co-workers[80] confirmed the age-dependent increase in osteocalcin levels in men, he found that the levels were lower in men than in women. In women the age-related increase in serum osteocalcin concentration correlates significantly with bone formation rate as measured by bone histomorphometry[20] and inversely with bone mineral density at several sites[81]. Kelly and colleagues[82] suggest that this increase is not linear but peaks postmenopausally around the 6th or 7th decade and then declines, although not returning to premenopausal levels. This postmenopausal rise can be reversed by estrogen treatment[83].

Serum osteocalcin concentrations have been shown to exhibit seasonal variation of 23% with a zenith in February (winter) and a nadir in July (summer)[84]. However, this was not confirmed by Vanderschueren and colleagues[85]. Serum osteocalcin also varies during the menstrual cycle reaching a maximum level during the luteal phase[38]. A number of groups[40,86,87] have demonstrated a circadian rhythm in serum osteocalcin with a peak at 03.00.

Osteocalcin in metabolic bone disease

Osteoporosis Serum osteocalcin concentrations for patients with postmenopausal osteoporosis have been reported as higher[41], the same[61] or slightly lower[88] than those found in age-matched controls. However, in all studies there was considerable overlap of the values, when comparing the two groups. On an individual basis, serum osteocalcin concentration cannot be used diagnostically, although measurements of this marker could be useful in monitoring response to treatment[83,89], or possibly in the prediction of bone loss in postmenopausal women[90]. Similar results have been found in the less common condition of primary osteoporosis in men. There was no significant difference between serum osteocalcin concentrations of patients and age-matched controls[91].

Paget's disease Serum osteocalcin levels are increased in patients with untreated Paget's disease of bone but the magnitude of the increase is considerably smaller than for other markers of bone formation, such as serum bone alkaline phosphatase[37] (Figure 5). Torres and colleagues[92] have investigated the possibility that the difference in magnitude of increases in levels of osteocalcin and alkaline phosphatase is due to an alteration to the structure of the osteocalcin molecule, which enhances binding to the hydroxyapatite. However, the binding ability of osteocalcin from patients with Paget's disease was the same as that for normal subjects. The reason for the discrepancy is still unclear.

Osteomalacia Serum levels of osteocalcin are significantly elevated in osteomalacia and correlate with parameters of osteoid formation but not with parameters of mineralization or resorption[49]. Osteocalcin is normally incorporated into the bone after mineralization has started. In osteomalacia, where there is a defect in mineralization, the osteocalcin cannot be incorporated at the normal rate and so more 'leaks back' into the circulation.

Hypoparathyroidism and hyperparathyroidism Levels of circulating osteocalcin are significantly reduced in hypoparathyroidism whereas in hyperparathyroidism they are significantly increased[37] (Figure 4). Osteocalcin levels correlate better with levels of parathyroid hormone than do levels of serum alkaline phosphatase and urinary hydroxyproline/creatinine[43].

Metastatic bone disease Serum osteocalcin is decreased in patients with malignant hypercalcemia but is normal in patients with bone metastases without hypercalcemia[93] (Figure 5). This decrease in osteocalcin is reflected in the decrease of bone formation at the cellular level.

Multiple myeloma Carlson and colleagues[94] have shown that at the time of diagnosis osteocalcin levels were related to the stage of the disease; the more advanced the disease the lower the osteocalcin level. Furthermore, there was a significant positive correlation between serum osteocalcin levels and survival time.

Hyperthyroidism Several workers have reported increased levels of osteocalcin in patients with untreated hyperthyroidism, which is a well-known risk factor for osteoporosis[95,96]. These levels were considerably reduced after 6 months treatment, but still did not decrease to normal values. Serum osteocalcin correlated negatively with spinal bone density in untreated patients.

Procollagen Type I C-terminal propeptide (PICP)

PICP is a 100 kDa globular polypeptide released into the circulation during the conversion of procollagen to collagen (Figure 2a). The amount of PICP released is equimolar with the amount of collagen incorporated into the bone matrix[97]. It has been shown, in rats, that PICP is cleared by the mannose receptor of liver endothelial cells[98] and therefore serum PICP levels in patients with liver disease must be interpreted cautiously. Since type I collagen is also present in other tissues, in particular skin, it is possible that there is a contribution to the circulating PICP levels from non-osseous sources. Haukipuro and colleagues[99] have found that levels of PICP from interstitial fluid recovered from healing surgical wounds increased dramatically during the first week of healing. Parfitt and co-workers[100] demonstrated that although serum PICP concentration correlates with bone formation as measured by bone histomorphometry there was a positive intercept indicating that there is a contribution from other sources to the total serum PICP. However, it is thought that any non-osseous contribution is probably small and constant except in patients with liver disease[101].

Assay

PICP may be measured by radioimmunoassay. The first such assay was developed by Taubman and colleagues[102]. However, it has only become more widely available since it has been re-developed by Melkko and co-workers[97]. The antiserum was raised against PICP purified from culture medium of human skin fibroblasts. Serum PICP is stable at – 20 °C for at least several months and is unaffected by repeated freeze–thaw cycles (Table 2).

PICP in normal subjects

Melkko and colleagues[97] found that there was no change in the level of PICP with age in women aged 20–60 years. However, in men there was a significant decrease with age. Eastell and colleagues[103] reported that in women aged 50–85 years there is an increase in serum PICP with age. This was confirmed by Sharp and associates[104], who also reported that men have higher levels of PICP than women. PICP levels are at their highest in the 1st year of life and decline during childhood, rising again at puberty to a maximum at mid-puberty[105]. However, PICP is only three times the adult level at mid-puberty, unlike osteocalcin and urinary deoxypyridinoline which are up to ten times the adult level at mid-puberty[77]. This may be due to a specificity problem of the assay. PICP is 20% higher in postmenopausal women compared to premenopausal women. This increase is reversed by hormone replacement therapy[106]. Hassager and colleagues[107] demonstrated that PICP levels exhibit a circadian rhythm in healthy premenopausal women with a 20% increase at night.

PICP in metabolic bone disease

Osteoporosis PICP was not increased in patients with osteoporosis[108,109]. Hormone replacement therapy for 1 year reduced the levels of PICP significantly in parallel with other markers of bone turnover and with a concomitant rise in lumbar bone mineral content[108]. Parfitt and co-workers[100] reported no significant correlation

Table 2 *Effects of storage and sample conditions on measurement of serum biochemical markers of bone turnover*

*Marker**	*Recommended storage*	*Effect of freeze–thaw cycles*	*Effect of hemolysis*	*Comments*
BAP	– 20 °C	generally stable	moderate hemolysis has no significant effect	serum or heparinized plasma samples can be used. Avoid EDTA† and citrate
PICP	– 20 °C for several months	stable for 2–3 cycles	minimal effect	serum or plasma can be used
Osteocalcin	– 70 °C (– 20 °C acceptable for a very short period)	unstable	decreases apparent concentration	serum or heparinized plasma samples can be used. Avoid EDTA, oxalate and citrate
TRAP	– 70 °C (– 20 °C acceptable for a very short period)	unstable	increases apparent concentration	serum or plasma can be used. For serum minimize clotting time and freeze immediately

*BAP, bone-specific alkaline phosphatase; PICP, procollagen type I carboxyterminal propeptide; TRAP, tartrate-resistant acid phosphatase; †EDTA, ethylenediamine tetra-acetic acid

between bone formation rate measured by histomorphometry and PICP in patients with postmenopausal osteoporosis.

Paget's disease In Paget's disease PICP levels were found to be increased, with mean levels being approximately three times the mean for normal subjects. These elevated levels decrease within hours of an injection of salmon calcitonin and within weeks after oral dichloromethylene diphosphonate[110].

Hyperparathyroidism Saggese and co-workers[105] have shown in a small number of adults that PICP levels in hyperparathyroidism are in the upper part of the normal range.

Although PICP has potential as a marker of bone formation as yet it has not been shown to be as sensitive as other markers of bone formation such as osteocalcin and it requires further validation in different disease states.

Other markers of bone formation

Type I procollagen N-terminal propeptide (PINP)

Circulating PINP results from the cleavage of the N-terminal propeptide of type I procollagen during collagen synthesis (Figure 2). It is a 64–70 kDa, trimeric, globular protein, a proportion of which is incorporated into bone. Unlike PICP, PINP does not possess any interchain disulfide bridges and therefore may circulate as both intact molecule and fragments. It is cleared via the scavenger receptor of the endothelial cells[111]. Ebeling and colleagues[7] have developed an enzyme-linked immunosorbent assay for PINP. Serum concentrations of PINP were 100-fold higher than those for PICP and did not correlate with PICP although, theoretically, the two propeptides are released from procollagen in a stoichiometric ratio. The effects of age, sex and disease on serum concentrations of PINP were discordant with those found for PICP and other markers of bone formation. In contrast, PINP levels measured by a radioimmunoassay developed by Linkhart and associates[112] correlated strongly with PICP levels ($r = 0.92$) and changes in PINP with age were concordant with changes in PICP with age.

Urinary non-dialysable hydroxyproline

Ten per cent of urinary hydroxyproline is non-dialysable and comprises heterogeneous peptides of 5 kDa. Comparison of dialysable and non-dialysable hydroxyproline in metabolic bone disease, before and after treatment, suggests that non-dialysable hydroxyproline is associated with bone formation[113]. The N-terminal procollagen propeptide (PINP) released into the circulation during collagen synthesis has a short α-helical region which contains hydroxyproline residues[2]. Degradation products of this propeptide are the probable source of non-dialysable hydroxyproline. As a marker of bone formation, non-dialysable hydroxyproline lacks bone specificity and so is of limited use.

MARKERS OF RESORPTION

Urinary hydroxyproline

Hydroxyproline is a characteristic amino acid of collagen. The only other proteins which contain this amino acid are elastin, the C1q subcomponent of complement, and the tail structure of acetylcholinesterase. Hydroxyproline results from the post-translational hydroxylation of proline residues during procollagen synthesis (Figure 1). During bone resorption, hydroxyproline is released into the circulation and is not reincorporated into new collagen[2]. Circulating hydroxyproline exists either as free amino acid (90%), or as peptide-bound forms. The free hydroxyproline is filtered and almost entirely reabsorbed by the kidney and eventually completely oxidized in the liver and degraded by hydroxyproline oxidase to carbon dioxide and urea[113]. The peptide-bound hydroxyproline is filtered and excreted in the urine. Consequently urine contains three forms of hydroxyproline, in total accounting for only 10% of that released from collagen degradation. Approximately 5% is present as free amino acid, the remainder is peptide-bound, either as small dialysable peptides, or as larger non-dialysable peptides. This large non-dialysable form, which represents 10% of the total urinary hydroxyproline, is derived from the degradation of newly synthesized collagen and appears to be a marker of bone formation[113] (*see* above).

Not all urinary hydroxyproline is derived from bone. Deacon and colleagues[115] have shown that the intercept of the regression of hydroxyproline excretion on bone resorption rate, as measured by radioisotopic tracer methods, was significantly greater than zero (100 μmol/day). This indicates that a fraction of urinary hydroxyproline arises from non-osseous sources. It has also been established that absorption of hydroxyproline from the diet, e.g. gelatin, results in an increase in total urinary hydroxyproline excretion[116,117] and also increases the intraindividual variation of the measurement. Gasser and colleagues[116] reported that dietary restriction for 24 h was sufficient to achieve optimum precision and minimize the dietary contribution to total hydroxyproline.

Assay

Urinary hydroxyproline has usually been measured by colorimetric methods based on that of Lang[118], which involve oxidation of hydroxyproline to pyrrole, extraction of interfering substances, and reaction of the pyrrole with p-dimethylaminobenzaldehyde (Erlich's Reagent). Modifications of the method have been devised to remove interference of other chromophores[119]. Recently, several high pressure liquid chromatography methods have been devised which give a greater specificity, larger linear range and are faster than the colorimetric methods[120–122]. Measurements of urinary hydroxyproline can be made on 24-h, timed fasting, or 'spot' fasting urine samples and results are usually expressed as the ratio of hydroxyproline to creatinine. Podenphant and co-workers[123] have shown that a 1-h fasting urine provides a more reliable measurement of the hydroxyproline : creatinine ratio than a 24-h sample as the intraindividual variation for such samples is considerably lower than that for 24-h samples. Wilson and colleagues[124] also suggested that a fasting second void urine sample is adequate to give a reliable measurement of hydroxyproline. Hydroxyproline is known to be stable in urine for 6 months at − 20 °C and probably for much longer.

Hydroxyproline in normal subjects

Urinary excretion of hydroxyproline declines from high values in infancy towards lower adult levels with a peak during puberty[125]. Urinary hydroxyproline : creatinine ratio differs significantly between females and males. In males there is a small but steady age-related decline with a slight rise in the seventh and eighth decades. In females there is a significant rise in the sixth decade which then decreases[126]. Kelly and associates[82] however could not confirm this fall in the hydroxyproline : creatinine ratio in the seventh and eighth decades in females.

Mautalen[127] established that there is a circadian rhythm in the excretion of total hydroxyproline which peaks between 00.00 and 08.00 and is minimal between 12.00 and 20.00. This pattern did not vary significantly from day to day. There is no seasonal variation of hydroxyproline measured either as 24-h excretion or 2-h fasting hydroxyproline : creatinine ratio[85].

Hydroxyproline in metabolic bone disease

Osteoporosis Klein and colleagues[11] showed that there was a moderate reduction in 24-h urinary hydroxyproline in patients with osteoporosis.

Hyperparathyroidism Excretion of hydroxyproline was significantly increased in patients with hyperparathyroidism[43,126,128] and correlated with increased levels of osteocalcin ($r = 0.70$).

Paget's disease In Paget's disease the hydroxyproline : creatinine ratio is significantly higher than in normal controls[44] and decreases in response to treatment with antiresorptive drugs.

Urinary hydroxyproline lacks specifity as a marker of bone resorption due to the contributions from non-osseous sources. Levels are also sensitive to dietary hydroxyproline intake and therefore cannot be regarded as a particularly useful marker of resorption.

Tartrate-resistant acid phosphatase (TRAP)

The acid phosphatases are a group of enzymes which hydrolyse phosphate esters in an acid environment and are found in several tissues including bone, prostate, platelets, erythrocytes and spleen. There are at least six different isoforms, identified by their different electrophoretic mobility on polyacrylamide gel[129]. Acid phosphatase derived from bone migrates fastest, to Band 5. This so called 'Band 5' acid phosphatase is further distinguished from the other isoforms by its resistance to sodium tartrate (up to concentrations of 0.5 mol) which causes inhibition of activity in the other isoforms. Type 5 acid phosphatase has been further resolved to 5a and 5b[130]. Osteoclasts have been shown not only to contain TRAP activity but also to secrete this activity during *in vitro* bone resorption[131]. This osteoclast-derived TRAP has physical and biochemical properties which make it indistinguishable from Band 5b[132], making Band 5b TRAP potentially a good marker of bone resorption.

Assay

TRAP can be assayed in several ways, but is usually assayed by spectrophotometric methods[133,134] using a variety of substrates and buffers. Actual values for TRAP are dependent on the substrate used[130,135]. Lau and colleagues[136] reported a spectrophotometric method which may overcome some technical difficulties encountered using earlier methods. Erythrocytes have been shown to release enzyme activity during hemolysis; Lau and colleagues[136] found that this form of TRAP was heat sensitive and could be removed by routinely incubating the serum at 37 °C for 1 h before assay. However, the platelet-derived TRAP activity which causes a 5–10% increase in concentrations in serum as compared to plasma cannot be removed by heat. The platelet-derived TRAP activity increased with clotting time reaching a plateau between 4 and 12 h, so it is important to keep clotting time to a minimum. Up to three freeze–thaw cycles did not adversely affect TRAP activity using this method but it is preferable to thaw frozen serum only once (Table 2). Furthermore, Lau and colleagues[136] identified the presence of a mixed-type non-competitive inhibitor of TRAP in serum. Interference from this inhibitor can be minimized by diluting the serum with water before assay or increasing the substrate concentration. Using this method, storage of serum at − 70 °C has no significant effect on levels of TRAP for at least 105 days; at − 20 °C there is a significant decline in activity with length of storage. However, other workers using different assay methods[134,137] consider that it is important to assay the samples as soon as possible. TRAP can also be assessed qualitatively by polyacrylamide gel electrophoresis[130]. Although it was thought that TRAP was an osteoclast enzyme, it has recently been shown[138] that osteoblasts contain TRAP activity which means that the specificity and sensitivity of the spectrophotometric methods may not be adequate for clinical use of TRAP as a resorption marker. Kraenzlin and associates[139] have developed an enzyme-linked immunosorbent assay for human serum osteoclastic TRAP. The antiserum used in this assay is specific for hairy cell leukemia splenic TRAP, which resembles osteoclastic TRAP. The antibodies were shown to cross-react with acid phosphatases in osteoclasts and with commercial human serum Band 5b TRAP, and they did not react with extracts of osteoblast cell lines. Further validation of this assay will be needed but it is potentially a useful method of measuring osteoclast activity. TRAP has recently been purified from human bone[140] which may lead to the development of an immunoassay specific for skeletal, but not necessarily osteoclastic TRAP.

TRAP in normal subjects

TRAP levels are considerably higher in children (newborn to 12 years) than in adults[130] but there is no difference in levels between adult males and females[136,141]. Up to the age of 50 years, there is no age-related change in serum TRAP concentration. However, Scarnecchia[141] and Schiele[135] and their co-workers have shown that postmenopausal women have significantly higher levels of TRAP activity than menstruating women. In normal women, TRAP activity correlates negatively with bone mineral density of both the ultradistal radius and the lumbar spine ($r = -0.506$, $p < 0.01$) and ($r = -0.261$, $p < 0.05$) respectively[141]. Stepan and colleagues[142] have shown that surgically induced menopause causes serum TRAP to increase significantly, reaching a peak 2 years after oophorectomy, which coincides with the time of maximal rate of bone loss.

TRAP in metabolic bone disease

Osteoporosis Patients with clinically established postmenopausal osteoporosis have significantly higher levels of TRAP activity compared to normal controls[130,141].

Primary hyperparathyroidism In primary hyperparathyroidism there is a significant elevation in TRAP activity which correlates with other markers of bone turnover. This increase is reversed after surgery. The decrease in TRAP occurs before that of the formation marker, bone alkaline phosphatase, but after that of urinary hydroxyproline[141,143].

Paget's disease Several studies[136,137,141] have shown that serum levels of TRAP are significantly higher in patients with Paget's disease. These increased levels correlate well with urinary hydroxyproline levels and with levels of formation markers (serum osteocalcin and bone alkaline phosphatase). TRAP activity returns to the normal range in these patients after treatment with etidronate, an antiresorptive drug[136].

Pyridinium cross-links

Pyridinoline (Pyr) and deoxypyridinoline (Dpyr) are the non-reducible cross-links formed between the telopeptide regions of collagen molecules and specific residues in the helix region of neighboring collagen molecules during fibril formation (Figure 2b). Pyr is found in cartilage and bone, whereas Dpyr is found only in bone and dentin[144]. They are released from mature collagen during bone resorption and eventually excreted in the urine[145,146] without further degradation. The crosslinks are present in urine in two forms; free and peptide bound, in approximately equal amounts[8]. Although skin contains large amounts of Type 1 collagen, the major crosslink of Type 1 collagen in skin is thought to be hydroxyaldolhistidine[147]. Therefore, turnover of skin collagen does not contribute to urinary levels of pyridinium crosslinks. Pyr is the most abundant of the two cross-links, the ratio of Pyr to Dpyr in bone being 3.5 : 1[144]. Delmas and colleagues[148] showed that urinary Pyr and Dpyr are significantly correlated with bone formation (correlation coefficients ranging from 0.69 to 0.80, $p < 0.0001$) and resorption rates ($r = 0.35$, $p < 0.05$ for Pyr and $r = 0.46$, $p < 0.01$ for Dpyr) measured by bone histomorphometry of iliac crest biopsy of 36 elderly women with vertebral osteoporosis. The role of Pyr and Dpyr as markers of resorption is further supported by the work of Uebelhart and coworkers[149] who showed that intravenous treatment of patients with Paget's disease with aminopropylidene biphosphonate, a potent inhibitor of resorption, causes a 62% decrease in urinary excretion of Pyr and Dpyr in 4 days whereas urinary hydroxyproline decreased to a lesser extent and over a longer time course. Further confirmation that urinary cross-links are indeed markers of bone resorption comes from Eastell and co-workers[150] who showed a significant correlation ($r = 0.89$, $p < 0.001$) between resorption rate measured by radioisotopic measurement and daily urinary Dpyr output.

Assay

At present, the most commonly used method of measuring pyridinium cross-links is by high performance liquid chromatography (HPLC). The urine sample is first hydrolysed if total crosslinks are to be measured, and then prefractionated by partition chromatography. The appropriate fractions are then freeze-dried and subjected to HPLC. The pyridinium cross-links are then detected fluorimetrically[144,151]. Measurements are made on 24-h urine collections, 2-h fasting collections or spot collections. Results are usually expressed as a ratio to the urinary creatinine concentration (nmol/mmol creatinine) to allow for body size and therefore, indirectly, skeletal size. Ubelhart and colleagues[152] and Colwell and colleagues[116] have shown the correlations between concentrations of both cross-links in fasting and 24-h urine samples to be poor. The fasting urine concentration of cross-links was the better predictor of bone mineral loss at the radius. It may be preferable to express Dpyr excretion as nmol/day in diseases or treatments that affect muscle mass such as corticosteroids or anabolic steroids. When stored at – 20 °C cross-links in urine are stable for at least 1 year[153] and probably for longer. The disadvantage of this method is that it is very time consuming and technically complex. Improvements in the reproducibility of the assay have recently been made by the use of an internal standard. Colwell and colleagues[117] employed an elastin-derived material which has been tentatively identified as isodesmosine. Pratt and co-workers[154] used an acetyl derivative of pyridinoline as an internal standard and by replacing the drying step with an additional solvent step during sample preparation were able to automate the assay.

New methods have been developed to measure free and peptide bound crosslinks in both urine and serum. Seyedin and colleagues[155] have developed an enzyme-linked immunosorbent assay (ELISA) to measure free crosslinks in urine. The assay uses polyclonal antibodies to free Pyr which have 45% cross-reactivity with free Dpyr. Levels of crosslinks measured with this assay correlated strongly with levels of crosslinks measured by HPLC ($r > 0.9$). Robins and colleagues[156] have developed an ELISA which is specific for free Dpyr in urine. Levels of Dpyr measured using this assay correlated strongly with levels of total Dpyr measured by HPLC.

Hanson and colleagues[5] have developed an immunoassay to measure N terminal crosslinked telopeptide (NTx) in urine. This inhibition ELISA employs a monoclonal antibody to low molecular weight peptide-bound pyridinoline crosslinks of the N-telopeptide domain of type I collagen, isolated from the urine of adolescent men. NTx in normal subjects and patients with Paget's correlated significantly with total pyridinolines (Pyr + Dpyr) measured by HPLC ($r = 0.93$). An ELISA has also been developed to measure C terminal crosslinked telopeptide[157]. This assay employs an antibody to a synthetic peptide with an amino acid sequence specific for part of the C-telopeptide of the α_1 chain of Type I collagen. Urine levels of C-telopeptide cross-links in normal women correlated well with total pyridinolines (Pyr + Dpyr) measured by HPLC ($r = 0.73$).

Peptide bound crosslinks may be measured in serum. A preliminary report has described the measurement of C-telopeptide cross-links in serum[158]. A radioimmunoassay has also been developed to measure the C-terminal telopeptide of type I collagen in serum[107] (ICTP). This assay employs polyclonal antibodies to the C-terminal, pyridinoline crosslinked telopeptide domain of type I collagen extracted from human femoral bone. This method has been validated by calcium kinetics and bone histomorphometry[159,160]. However, changes in ICTP are not always in concordance with changes in other markers of bone resorption[161–163].

These newer methods of measuring free and peptide bound crosslinks still require full evaluation. Initial studies suggest that there are differences between free and peptide bound crosslinks in their response to antiresorptive treatment[164–166].

Pyridinium cross-links in normal subjects

Several groups[149,167] have shown that there is no significant difference between mean values of urinary Pyr and Dpyr in healthy males and females. Values for children are considerably higher than adult levels. During puberty levels of Pyr and Dpyr rise to a peak at mid-puberty, when they are seven times the adult level and then decrease towards adult levels, reflecting the pattern seen in other markers especially serum osteocalcin[77] (Figure 6). Postmenopausal women have levels of Pyr and Dpyr that are two to three times the levels of younger premenopausal women. The increase in Dpyr is greater than the increase in Pyr. Uebelhart and co-workers[168] also showed that, in an age-matched group of women, there is a significant rise in Pyr and Dpyr after the menopause. Hassager and colleagues[169] reported that the postmenopausal increase in Dpyr occurs within 6 months of the cessation of menstruation. This increase in cross-links in postmenopausal women can be reversed within 6 months by hormone replacement therapy[168,169].

There is a marked day-to-day variation of pyridinium excretion in adults[114]. Furthermore, Eastell[86] and Schlemmer[170] and their colleagues have shown that there is a circadian variation in urinary excretion of both Pyr and Dpyr with a peak at night and a nadir in the afternoon/evening (Figure 6). The night time increase represents a 28% difference of the mean daytime level. These large changes of Pyr and Dpyr excretion throughout the day must be borne in mind when timing urine collections. Colwell and co-workers[117] demonstrated that pyridinium cross-links are not affected by dietary gelatin, unlike urinary hydroxyproline.

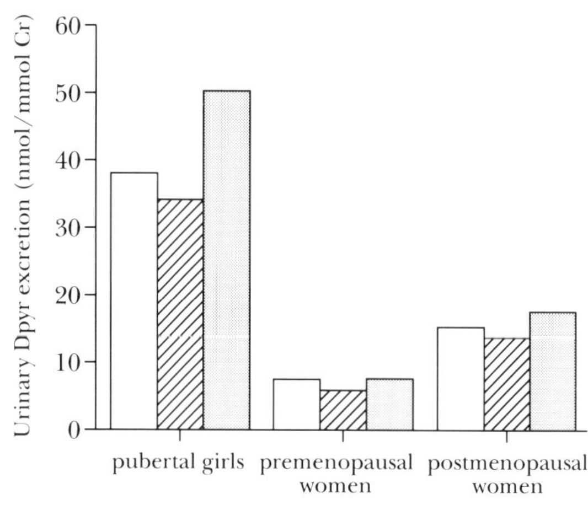

Figure 6 *Nyctohemeral variation in the urinary excretion of deoxypyridinoline (Dpyr) in pubertal girls, premenopausal women and postmenopausal women expressed as a ratio to creatinine (Cr) excretion; open blocks, 07.00–15.00; hatched blocks, 15.00–23.00; shaded blocks, 23.00–0.070; modified with permission from Eastell and colleagues*[86]

Pyridinium cross-links in metabolic bone disease

Osteoporosis Urinary excretion of Pyr and Dpyr is greater in women with vertebral osteoporosis compared to premenopausal women[148] or age-matched controls[171]. Eastell and colleagues reported a 40% increase in daily output of Dpyr in women with vertebral osteoporosis as compared with a group of age-matched controls[171]. Eastell and colleagues[172] have shown that the circadian rhythms of Pyr and Dpyr excretion in women with vertebral osteoporosis differ from those in age-matched controls. In normal women they are increased by 48% at night whereas in the osteoporotic women the increase was 62% and the increase persisted into the morning. This may be due to increased sensitivity of bone to parathyroid hormone.

Paget's disease In patients with Paget's disease there is a dramatic 12-fold increase in total urinary cross-links as compared to age-matched controls[149]. Free crosslinks (Pyr + Dpyr) are increased 4-fold[166] and free Dpyr are significantly increased[156]. Peptide bound crosslinks, urinary Crosslaps are also significantly increased (Z score + 4.4) in patients with Paget's disease[157].

Primary hyperparathyroidism Dpyr and Pyr are significantly higher in patients with primary hyperparathyroidism than in age- and sex-matched controls. Dpyr is twice as high and Pyr 1.5 times as high. Successful parathyroidectomy results in a fall of 47% Dpyr and 37% Pyr excretion[173]. Uebelhart and colleagues[149] reported even higher increases in cross-link excretion in hyperparathyroidism of three times the normal level. Free Dpyr and urinary C-telopeptide crosslinks are both significantly increased in patients with hyperparathyroidism[155,157].

Hyperthyroidism Patients with untreated hyperthyroidism have significantly elevated levels of urinary Pyr and Dpyr, both of which correlated (Pyr, $r = 0.61$: Dpyr, $r = 0.47$) with free triiodothyronine but not with age. In two groups of thyroxine-treated women, one group who were premenopausal and the other group who were postmenopausal, only the postmenopausal women had increased levels of Pyr and Dpyr excretion compared to age-matched controls[174]. Urinary C-telopeptide crosslinks are increased (Z-score + 6.7) in patients with hyperthyroidism[157].

Other markers of bone resorption

Free γ-carboxyglutamic acid (free Gla)

γ-Carboxyglutamic acid is formed by the vitamin K-dependent, post-translational carboxylation of glutamic acid. The majority of Gla is found in osteocalcin and matrix Gla-protein in bone. However, it is also present in a number of plasma proteins and coagulation factors[175]. Urinary excretion of free Gla has been proposed as a marker of bone resorption, and has been shown to be increased in postmenopausal osteoporosis[176]. Serum free Gla is significantly higher in patients, with diseases characterized by large changes in bone resorption, than in normal subjects[177]. There is no increase in serum free Gla in early postmenopausal women compared to age-matched premenopausal women. This is in contrast to the findings of Hassager and colleagues[169], who demonstrated a significant increase in urinary deoxypyridinoline, within 6 months of the menopause. Because of its lack of bone specificity, free Gla is probably only useful as a marker of bone resorption in assessing large changes in resorption.

Urinary hydroxylysyl glycosides

β-1-Galactosyl-*O*-hydroxylysine (Gal-Hyl) and β-1,2-glucosyl-galactosyl-O-hydroxylysine (Glu-Gal-Hyl) are excreted in the urine as a result of collagen degradation. These compounds are more tissue-specific than hydroxyproline. The ratio of Glu-Gal-Hyl : Gal-Hyl is 1.61 and 0.15 for human adult skin and bone, respectively, hence Gal-Hyl may be regarded as a fairly specific marker for bone collagen[178]. Urinary Gal-Hyl and Glu-Gal-Hyl can be measured by conversion of the amino groups of hydroxlysine into fluorescent dansyl derivatives prior to their separation by reverse-phase HPLC[179]. Urinary concentrations of Gal-Hyl are expressed as a ratio to urine creatinine (Gal-Hyl/Cr). Males and females between ages 30 and 49 years excrete similar amounts of Gal/Hyl, however after the age of 50 years there is an increase in urinary Gal-Hyl/Cr which is more marked in women than in men. In postmenopausal women Gal-Hyl/Cr is inversely correlated to bone mineral content ($r = -0.7$, $p < 0.001$)[180]. Bettica and coworkers[181], in a small comparative study, suggest that Gal-Hyl is comparable to urinary deoxypyridinoline and pyridinoline as a marker of bone resorption. Although Gal-Hyl is a promising marker further evaluation is required including comparison with direct measurements of bone resorption.

CONCLUSIONS

Biochemical markers of bone turnover have the following advantages:

(1) They allow non-invasive assessment of bone turnover;

(2) They allow for repeated measurements, so that study of short-term changes in bone turnover (circadian rhythms) and monitoring the effect of treatment are possible;

(3) They reflect changes in the entire skeleton; and

(4) They are relatively inexpensive compared to other techniques.

However, they also have the following disadvantages:

(1) They give no information about cellular activity compared to bone histomorphometry;

(2) They can be misleading, especially markers not specific to bone;

(3) They may be subject to idiosyncratic effects, e.g. osteocalcin and glucocorticoids; and

(4) It is difficult to compare bone formation (serum markers) with bone resorption (usually urine markers).

When we consider specific markers, there is no single marker of formation or resorption which is ideal. Where we are investigating large changes in bone turnover, such as in Paget's disease, markers which are not necessarily bone-specific, such as total serum alkaline phosphatase and urinary hydroxyproline, will adequately assess bone formation and resorption respectively and are used in clinical practice. However, when we consider conditions where changes in bone turnover are small and perhaps more subtle, as in osteoporosis much greater specificity is required.

At present the most suitable markers are serum osteocalcin and urinary deoxypyridinoline. Of the more recently developed markers, procollagen type I C-terminal propeptide (PICP) is theoretically the ideal marker of bone formation because it reflects production of the major protein of bone, collagen. Unfortunately it lacks specificity, which may be responsible for changes in PICP levels often being smaller than concomitant changes in other markers. Bone alkaline phosphatase is specific, but many of the assays used to measure it may, in certain circumstances, detect a proportion of the liver isoform. If the newer assays can overcome this problem satisfactorily it should prove to be a very useful marker. However, these assays still require extensive validation. The new methods for measuring pyridinium cross-links in urine and serum may be more convenient than the HPLC method but again they still require extensive validation. When trying to identify the best marker it should be remembered that different markers reflect different aspects of osteoblast and osteoclast activity so the most appropriate marker will vary with the disease being studied. Furthermore, in many situations there is much to be gained from measuring several markers in conjunction rather than relying on a single marker.

There are two major potential uses for these markers in metabolic bone disease. First, they could be used in prediction of change in bone mass. Hansen and colleagues[182] have used a combination of markers to predict bone loss in postmenopausal women over a 12-year period. However, before such use of markers can be generally accepted several problems associated with measurement of the markers and the mode of postmenopausal bone loss must be resolved[183].

The second potential use of biochemical markers is in monitoring of treatment of metabolic bone disease and hormone replacement therapy. Several markers have been shown to return to premenopausal levels after 6 months of hormone replacement therapy[89,108,168]. It is probable that these changes in markers are detectable much earlier, before any change in bone mineral density can be found, and could be used as early indicators of the efficacy of treatment.

Thus, there have been exciting developments in the assays for biochemical markers of bone turnover in the past few years. It is likely that they will prove of use in the investigation and management of osteoporosis in the near future.

ACKNOWLEDGEMENTS

We thank Mr Nicholas Gibbins for his technical assistance in the preparation of the illustrations. RAH is supported by Medical Research Council.

References

1. Burgeson RE. New collagens, new concepts [Review]. Annu Rev Cell Biol 1988; 4: 551–77.
2. Prockop DJ, Kivirikko KI, Tudermann L, Guzman NA. The biosynthesis of collagen and its disorders. N Engl J Med 1979; 301: 13–23.
3. Kivirikko KI, Myllylä R. Post translational processing of procollagens. Ann N Y Acad Sci 1985; 460: 187–201.

4. Kühn K. The classical collagens: types I, II, and III. In: Mayne R, Burgeson RE, eds. Biology of extracellular matrix: a series. 1987: 1–42.
5. Hanson DA, Weis MAE, Bollen A-M, Maslan SL, Singer FR, Eyre DR. A specific immunoassay for monitoring human bone resorption: quantitation of type I collagen cross-linked *N*-telopeptides in urine. J Clin Endocrinol Metab 1992; 7: 1251–8.
6. Krane SM, Neer RM. Connective tissue. In: Smith LH, Thier SO, eds. Pathophysiology. Philadelphia: W B Saunders Company, 1985: 611–53.
7. Ebeling PR, Peterson JM, Riggs BL. Utility of type I procollagen propeptide assays for assessing abnormalities in metabolic bone diseases. J Bone Min Res 1992; 7: 1243–50.
8. Robins SP, Duncan A, Reid DM, Paterson CR. Urinary hydroxy-pyridinium cross-links of collagen as markers of resorption in a range of metabolic bone diseases. Bone Miner 1989; 4: S397.
9. Segrest JP. Urinary metabolites of collagen. Methods Enzymol 1982; 82: 398–401.
10. Robinson R. The possible significance of hexosephosphoric esters in ossification. Biochem J 1923; 17: 286.
11. Klein, Lafferty FW, Pearson OH, Curtiss Jr PH. Correlation of urinary hydroxyproline, serum alkaline phosphatase and skeletal calcium turnover. Metabolism 1964; 13: 272–84.
12. Charles P, Poser JW, Mosekilde L, Jensen FT. Estimation of bone turnover evaluated by ^{47}Ca-kinetics. Efficiency of serum bone gamma-carboxyglutamic acid-containing protein, serum alkaline phosphatase, and urinary hydroxyproline excretion. J Clin Invest 1985; 76: 2254–8.
13. Delmas PD. Biochemical markers of bone turnover in osteoporosis. In Riggs BL, Melton III LJ eds. Osteoporosis: etiology, diagnosis, and management. New York Raven Press 1988; 297–316.
14. Fishman WH. Alkaline phosphatase isoenzymes: recent progress. Clin Biochem 1990; 23: 99–104.
15. Crofton PM. Biochemistry of alkaline phosphatase isoenzymes [Review]. Crit Rev Clin Lab Sci 1982; 16: 161–94.
16. Van Hoof VO, Hoylaerts MF, Geryl H, Van Mullem M, Lepoutre LG, De Broe ME. Age and sex distribution of alkaline phosphatase isoenzymes by agarose electrophoresis. Clin Chem 1990; 36: 875–8.
17. Moss DW. Alkaline phosphatase enzymes. Clin Chem 1982; 28: 2007–16.
18. Price CP. Multiple forms of human serum alkaline phosphatase: detection and quantitation. Ann Clin Biochem 1993; 30: 355–72.
19. Brixen K, Nielsen HK, Eriksen EF, Charles P, Losekilde L. Efficacy of wheat germ lectin-precipitated alkaline phosphatase in serum as an estimator of bone mineralization rate: comparison to serum total alkaline phosphatase and serum bone gla-protein. Calcif Tiss Int 1989; 44: 93–8.
20. Eastell R, Delmas PD, Hodgson SF, Eriksen EF, Mann KG, Riggs BL. Bone formation rate in older women: concurrent assessment with bone histomorphometry, calcium kinetics, and biochemical markers. J Clin Endocrinol Metab 1988; 67: 741–8.
21. Moss DW, Whitby LG. A simplified heat-inactivation method for investigating alkaline phosphatase isoenzyme in serum. Clin Chim Acta 1975; 61: 63–71.
22. Van Hoof VO, Lepoutre LG, Hoylaerts MF, Chevigne R, De Broe ME. Improved agarose electrophoretic methods for separating alkaline phosphatase isoenzymes in serum. Clin Chem 1988; 34: 1857–62.
23. Moss DW, Edwards RK. Improved electrophoretic resolution of bone and liver alkaline phosphatases resulting from partial digestion with neuraminidase. Clin Chim Acta 1984; 143: 177–82.
24. Ramasamy I. Affinity electrophoresis of alkaline phosphatase using polyacrylamide gels. Clin Chim Acta 1991; 199: 243–52.
25. Crofton PM. Wheat-germ lectin affinity electrophoresis for alkaline phosphatase isoforms in children: age-dependent reference ranges and changes in liver and bone disease. Clin Chem 1992; 38: 663–70.
26. Rosalki SB, Foo AY. Two new methods for separating and quantifying bone and liver phosphatase isoenzymes in plasma. Clin Chem 1984; 30: 1182–6.
27. Behr W, Barnert J. Quantification of bone alkaline phosphatase in serum by precipitation with wheat-germ lectin: a simplified method and its clinical plausibility. Clin Chem 1986; 32: 1960–6.
28. Sorensen S. Wheat-germ agglutinin method for measuring bone and liver isoenzymes of alkaline phosphatase assessed in postmenopausal osteoporosis. Clin Chem 1988; 34: 1635–40.
29. Day AP, Saward S, Royle CM, Mayne PD. Evaluation of two new methods for routine measurement of alkaline phosphatase isoenzymes. J Clin Pathol 1992; 45: 68–71.
30. Lawson GM, Katzman JA, Kimlinger TK, O'Brien JF. Isolation and preliminary characterisation of a monoclonal antibody that interacts preferentially with the liver isoenzyme of human alkaline phosphatase. Clin Chem 1985; 31: 381–5.
31. Seabrook RN, Bailyes EM, Price CP, Siddle K, Luzio JP. The distinction of bone and liver

isoenzymes of alkaline phosphatase in serum using a monoclonal antibody. Clin Chim Acta 1988; 172: 261–6.

32. Hill CS, Wolfert RL. The preparation of monoclonal antibodies which react preferentially with human bone alkaline phosphatase and not liver alkaline phosphatase. Clin Chim Acta 1989; 186: 315–20.
33. Garnero P, Delmas PD. Assessment of the serum levels of bone alkaline phosphatase with a new immunoradiometric assay in patients with metabolic bone disease. J Clin Endocrinol Metab 1993; 77: 1046–53.
34. Stepan JJ, Tesarova A, Havranek T, Jodl J, Formankova J, Pacovsky V. Age and sex dependency of the biochemical indices of bone remodelling. Clin Chim Acta 1985; 151: 273–83.
35. Krabbe S, Christiansen C, Rodbro P, Tranbol I. Pubertal growth as reflected by simultaneous changes in bone mineral content and serum alkaline phosphatase. Acta Paediatr Scand 1979; 69: 49–52.
36. Kuwana T, Sugita O, Yakata M. Reference limits of bone and liver alkaline phosphatase isoenzymes in the serum of healthy subjects according to age and sex as determined by wheat germ lectin affinity electrophoresis. Clin Chim Acta 1988; 273–80.
37. Duda RJ, O'Brien JF, Katzman JA, Peterson JM, Mann KG, Riggs BL. Concurrent assays of circulating bone gla-protein and bone alkaline phosphatase: effects of sex, age, and metabolic bone disease. J Clin Endocrinol Metab 1988; 66: 951–7.
38. Nielsen HK, Brixen K, Bouillon R, Mosekilde L. Changes in biochemical markers of osteoblastic activity during the menstrual cycle. J Clin Endocrinol Metab 1990; 70: 1431–7.
39. Nielsen HK, Brixen K, Mosekilde L. Diurnal rhythm in serum activity of wheat-germ lectin-precipitable alkaline phosphatase: temporal relationships with the diurnal rhythm of serum osteocalcin. Scand J Clin Lab Invest 1990; 50: 851–6.
40. Devgun MS, Paterson CR, Martin BT. Seasonal changes in the activity of serum alkaline phosphatase. Enzyme 1981; 26: 301–5.
41. Nielsen HK, Laurberg P, Brixen K, Mosekilde L. Relations between diurnal variations in serum osteocalcin, cortisol, parathyroid, and ionized calcium in normal individuals. Acta Endocrinol (Copenh) 1991; 124: 391–8.
42. Delmas PD, Wahner HW, Mann KG, Riggs BL. Assessment of bone turnover in postmenopausal osteoporosis by measurement of serum bone gla-protein. J Lab Clin Med 1983; 102: 470–6.
43. Minisola S, Scarnecchia L, Carnevale V, Bigi F, Romagnoli E, Pacitti MT, Rosso R. Clinical value of the measurement of bone remodelling in primary hyperparathyroidism. J Endocrinol Invest. 1989; 12: 537–42.
44. Torres, R, de la Piedra C, Rapado A. Osteocalcin and bone remodelling in Paget's disease of bone, primary hyperparathyroidism, hypercalcaemia of malignancy and involutional osteoporosis. Scand J Clin Lab Invest 1989; 49: 279–85.
45. Gonchoroff DG, Brabum EL, Cedel SL, Riggs BL, O'Brien JF. Clinical evaluation of high-performance affinity chromatography for the separation of bone and liver alkaline phosphatase isoenzymes. Clin Chim Acta 1991; 199: 43–50.
46. Broulik PD, Stepan JJ, Pascovsky V. Bone isoenzyme of serum alkaline phosphatase and urinary hydroxyproline excretion in thyrotoxicosis. Endocr Exper 1985; 19: 165–9.
47. Tibi L, Patrick AW, Leslie P, Toft AD, Smith AF. Alkaline phosphatase isoenzymes in plasma in hyperthyroidism. Clin Chem 1989; 35: 1427–30.
48. Nisbet JA, Eastwood JB, Colston KW, Ang L, Flanagan AM, Chambers TJ, Maxwell JD. Detection of osteomalacia in British Asians: comparison of clinical score with biochemical measurements. Clin Sci 1990; 78: 383–9.
49. Demiaux B, Arlot ME, Chapuy M-C, Meunier PJ, Delmas PD. Serum osteocalcin is increased in patients with osteomalacia: correlations with biochemical and histomorphometric findings. J Clin Endocrinol Metab 1992; 74: 1146–51.
50. Arnaud CD, Kolb FO. In: Greenspan FS, ed. Basic Clinical Endocrinology. Norwalk, Connecticut/San Mateo, California: Appleton and Lange, 1991; 303.
51. Deftos LJ, Wolfert RL, Hill CS. Bone alkaline phosphatase in Paget's disease. Horm Metab Res 1991; 23: 559–61.
52. Price PA, Otsuka AS, Poser JW, Kristaponis J, Raman N. Characterization of the γ-carboxyglutamic acid containing protein from bone. Proc Natl Acad Sci USA 1976; 73: 1447–51.
53. Hauchka PV, Carr SA. Calcium-dependent alpha helical structure in osteocalcin. Biochemistry 1982; 21: 2538–47.
54. Skjodt H, Gallagher JA, Beresford JN, Couch M, Poser JW, Russell RGG. Vitamin D metabolites regulate osteocalcin synthesis and proliferation of human bone cells *in vitro*. J Endocr 1985; 105: 391–6.
55. Price PA, Williamson MK, Lothringer JW. Origin of the vitamin K-dependent bone protein found in plasma and its clearance by kidney and bone. J Biol Chem 1981; 256: 12760–6.
56. Farrugia W, Melick RA. Metabolism of osteocalcin. Calcif Tiss Int 1986; 39: 234–8.
57. Taylor AK, Linkhart S, Mohan S, Christenson RA, Singer FR, Baylink DJ. Multiple osteocalcin

fragments in human urine and serum as detected by a midmolecule osteocalcin radioimmunoassay. J Clin Endocrinol Metab 1990; 70: 467–72.

58. Delmas PD, Wilson DM, Mann KG, Riggs BL. Effect of renal function on plasma levels of bone gla-protein. J Clin Endocrinol Metab 1983; 57: 1028–30.
59. Lian J, Roufosse A, Reit B, Glimcher M. Concentrations of osteocalcin and phosphoprotein as a function of mineral content and age in cortical bone. Calcif Tiss Int 1982; 34: S82.
60. Mundy G, Poser J. Chemotactic activity of g-carboxyglutamic acid containing protein in bone. Calcif Tiss Int 1983; 35: 164.
61. Brown JP, Delmas PD, Malaval L, Edouard C, Chapuy MC, Meunier PJ. Serum bone gla-protein: a specific marker for bone formation in postmenopausal osteoporosis. Lancet 1984; 1: 1091–3.
62. Delmas PD, Malaval L, Arlot ME, Meunier PJ. Serum bone gla-protein compared to histomorphometry in endocrine diseases. Bone 1985; 6: 339–41.
63. Price PA, Nishimoto SP. Radioimmunoassay for the vitamin K-dependent protein of bone and its discovery in plasma. Proc Natl Acad Sci USA 1980; 77: 2234–8.
64. Grunberg CM, Wilson PS, Gallop PM, Parfitt AM. Determination of osteocalcin in human serum: results with two kits compared with those by a well-characterised assay. Clin Chem 1985; 31: 1720–3.
65. Pastoureau P, Delmas PD. Measurement of serum bone gla-protein (BGP) in humans with an ovine bgp based radioimmunoassay. Clin Chem 1990; 36: 1620–4.
66. Taylor AK, Linkhadt SG, Mohan S, Baylink DJ. Development of a new RIA for human osteocalcin: evidence for a midmolecule epitope. Metabolism 1988; 37: 872–7.
67. Power MJ, Fottrell PF. Osteocalcin: diagnostic methods and clinical applications [Review]. Crit Rev Clin Lab Sci 1991; 28: 287–335
68. Tracy RP, Andrianorivo A, Riggs BL, Mann KG. Comparison of monoclonal and polyclonal antibody-based immunoassays for osteocalcin: a study of sources of variation in assay results. J Bone Min Res 1990; 5: 451–61.
69. Deftos LJ, Wolfert RL, Hill CS, Durton DW. Two-site assays of bone gla-protein (osteocalcin) demonstrate immunochemical heterogeneity of the intact molecule. Clin Chem 1992; 38: 2318–21.
70. Hosoda K, Eguchi H, Nakamoto T, Kubota T, Honda H, Jindai S, Hasegawa R, Kiyoki M, Yamaji T, Shiraki M. Sandwich immunoassay for intact human osteocalcin. Clin Chem 1992; 38: 2233–8.
71. Jaouhari J, Schiele F, Dragacci S, Tarallo P, Siest JP, Henny J, Siest G. Avidin-Biotin enzyme immunoassay of osteocalcin in serum or plasma. 1992; 38: 1968–74.
72. Bouillon R, Vanderschueren D, Van Herck E, Nielsen HK, Bex M, Heyns W, Van Baelen H. Homologous radioimmunoassay of human osteocalcin. Clin Chem 1992; 38: 2055–60.
73. Garnero P, Grimaux M, Demiaux B, Preaudat C, Seguin P, Delmas PD. Measurement of osteocalcin with a human-specific two-site immunoradiometric assay. J Bone Min Res 1992; 7: 1389–98.
74. Delmas PD, Christiansen C, Mann KG, Price PA. Bone Gla protein (osteocalcin) assay standardization report. J Bone Min Res 1990; 5: 5–11.
75. Gundberg CM, Lian JB, Gallop PM. Measurements of gamma-carboxyglutamate and circulating osteocalcin in normal children and adults. Clin Chem Acta 1983; 1128: 1–8.
76. Glastre C, Braillon P, David L, Cochat P, Meunier PJ, Delmas PD. Measurement of bone mineral content of the lumbar spine by dual energy X-ray absorptiometry in normal children: correlations with growth parameters. J Clin Endocrinol Metab 1990; 70: 1330–3.
77. Blumsohn A, Hannon RA, Wrate R, Barton J, Al-Dehaimi AW, Colwell A, Eastell R. Biochemical markers of bone turnover in girls during puberty. Clin Endocrinol 1994; 40: 663–70.
78. Vanderschueren D, Gevers G, Raymaekers G, Devos P, Dequeker J. Sex- and age-related changes in bone and serum osteocalcin. Calcif Tiss Int 1990; 46: 179–82.
79. Worsfold M, Sharp C, Davie MWJ. Serum osteocalcin and other indices of bone formation: an 8-decade population study in healthy men and women. Clin Chim Acta 988; 178: 225–36.
80. Epstein S, Poser J, McClintock R, Johnston CC, Bryce G, Hui S. Differences in serum bone gla-protein with age and sex. Lancet 1984; 1: 307–10.
81. Delmas PD, Stenner D, Waher HW, Mann KG. Increase in serum bone γ-carboxyglutamic acid protein with aging women. J Clin Invest 1983; 71: 1316–21.
82. Kelly PJ, Pocock NA, Sambrook PN, Eisman JA. Age and menopause-related changes in indices of bone turnover. J Clin Endocrinol Metab 1989; 69: 1160–5.
83. Johansen JS, Riis BJ, Delmas PD, Christiansen C. Plasma BGP: an indicator of spontaneous bone loss and of the effect of oestrogen treatment in postmenopausal women. Eur J Clin Invest 1988; 18: 191–5.
84. Thomsen K, Eriksen EF, Jorgensen JCR, Charles P, Mosekilde L. Seasonal variation of serum bone GLA protein. Scand J Clin Lab Invest 1989; 49: 605–11.

85. Vanderschueren D, Gevers G, Dequeker J, Geusens P, Nijs J, Devos P, De Roo M, Bouillon R. Seasonal variation in bone metabolism in young healthy subjects. Calcif Tiss Int 1991; 49: 84–9.
86. Eastell R, Simmons PS, Colwell A, Assiri AMA, Burritt MF, Russell RGG, Riggs BL. Nyctohemeral changes in bone turnover assessed by serum bone Gla-protein concentration and urinary deoxypyridinoline excretion: effects of growth and ageing. Clin Sci 1992; 83: 375–82.
87. Gundberg, CM, Markowitz ME, Mizruchi M, Rosen JF. Osteocalcin in human serum: a circadian rhythm. J Clin Endocrinol Metab 1985; 60: 736–9.
88. Ismail F, Epstein S, Pacifici R, Droke D, Thomas SB, Avioli LV. Serum bone gla protein (BGP) and other markers of bone mineral metabolism in postmenopausal osteoporosis. Calcif Tiss Int 1986; 39: 230–3.
89. Fuleihan GE-H, Brown EM, Curtis K, Berger MJ, Berger BM, Gleason R, Le Boff M. Effect of sequential and daily continuous hormone replacement therapy and indexes of mineral metabolism. Arch Intern Med 1992; 152: 1904–09.
90. Christiansen C, Riis BJ, Rodbro P. Screening procedure for women at risk of developing postmenopausal osteoporosis. Osteoporosis Int 1990; 1: 35–40.
91. Resch H, Pietschmann P, Woloszczuk W, Krexner E, Berneckner P, Willvonseder R. Bone mass and biochemical parameters of bone metabolism in men with spinal osteoporosis. Eur J Clin Invest 1992; 22: 542–5.
92. Torres R, de la Piedra C, Rapado A. Binding of serum osteocalcin to hydroxyapatite in Paget's disease of bone. Bone Min 1991; 14: 55–65.
93. Delmas PD, Demiaux B, Malaval L, Chapuy MC, Edouard C, Meunier PJ. Serum bone carboxyglutamic acid-containing protein in primary hyperparathyroidism and in malignant hypercalcemia. J Clin Invest 1986; 77: 985–91.
94. Carlson K, Ljunghall S, Simonsson B, Smedmyr B. Serum osteocalcin concentrations in patients with multiple myeloma – correlation with disease stage and survival. J Intern Med 1991; 231: 133–7.
95. Lee MS, Kim SY, Lee MC, Cho BY, Lee HK, Koh C-S, Min HK. Negative correlation between the change in bone mineral density and serum osteocalcin in patients with hyperthyroidism. J Clin Endocrinol Metab 1990; 70: 766–70.
96. Lukert BP, Higgins JC, Stoskopf MM. Serum osteocalcin is increased in patients with hyperthyroidism and decreased in patients receiving glucocorticoids. J Clin Endocrinol Metab 1986; 62: 1056–8.
97. Melkko J, Niemi S, Risteli L, Risteli J. Radioimmunoassay of the carboxyterminal propeptide of type I procollagen. Clin Chem 1990; 36: 1328–32.
98. Smedsrod B, Melkko J, Risteli L, Risteli J. Circulating C-terminal propeptide of type I procollagen is cleared via the mannose receptor in liver endothelial cells. Biochem J 1990; 271: 345–50.
99. Haukipuro K, Melkko J, Risteli L, Kairaluoma M, Risteli J. Synthesis of type I collagen in healing wounds in humans. Ann Surg 1991; 213: 75–80.
100. Parfitt AM, Simon LS, Villanueva AR, Krane SM. Procollagen type I carboxy-terminal extention peptide in serum as a marker of collagen biosynthesis in bone. Correlation with iliac bone formation rates and comparison with total alkaline phosphatase. J Bone Min Res 1987; 2: 427–36.
101. Risteli J, Melkko J, Niemi S, Risteli L. Use of a marker of collagen formation in osteoporosis studies. Calcif Tissue Int 1991; 49(Suppl.): S24–S25.
102. Taubman MB, Goldberg B, Sherr CJ. Radioimmunoassay for human procollagen. Science 1974; 186: 1115–17.
103. Eastell R, Peel NFA, Hannon RA, Blumsohn A, Price A, Colwell A, Russell RGG. Effect of age on bone collagen in older women. Bone 1992; 13: 275.
104. Sharp CA, Worsfold M, Davie MWT. Procollagen propeptide and other indices of bone turnover in healthy people and in untreated osteoporosis. In: Ring EFT, ed. Current Research in Osteoporosis and Bone Mineral Measurement II. London: British Institute of Radiology, 1992; 4.
105. Saggese G, Bertollini S, Baroncelli GI, Di Nero G. Serum levels of carboxyterminal propeptide of type I procollagen in healthy children from 1st year of life to adulthood and in metabolic bone diseases. Eur J Pediatr 1992; 151: 764–8.
106. Hassager C, Fabbri-Marbelli G, Christiansen C. The effect of the menopause and hormone replacement therapy on serum carboxyterminal propeptide of type I collagen. Osteoporosis Int 1993; 3: 50–52.
107. Hassager C, Risteli J, Risteli L, Jensen SB, Christiansen C. Diurnal variation in serum markers of type I collagen synthesis and degradation in healthy premenopausal women. J Bone Min Res 1992; 7: 1307–11.
108. Hassager C, Jensen LT, Johansen JS, Riis BJ, Melkko J, Podenphant J, Risteli L, Christiansen C, Risteli J. The carboxy-terminal propeptide of type I procollagen in serum as a marker of bone formation: the effect of nandrolone decanoate and female sex hormones. Metabolism 1991; 40: 205–8.
109. Hasling C, Eriksen EF, Melkko J, Risteli L, Charles P, Mosekilde L, Risteli J. Effects of a combined estrogen–gestagen regimen on serum levels of the carboxy-terminal propeptide of

human type I procollagen in osteoporosis. J Bone Min Res 1991; 6: 1295–300.
110. Simon LS, Krane SM, Wortman PD, Krane IM, Kovitz KL. Serum levels of type I and type III procollagen fragments in Paget's disease of bone. J Clin Endocrinol Metab 1984; 58: 110–20.
111. Melkko J, Hellevik T, Risteli L, Risteli J, Smedsrød B. Clearance of NH_2-terminal propeptides of types I and III proclooagenis a physiological function of the scavenger receptor in liver endothelial cells. J Exp Med 1994; 179; 405–12.
112. Linkhart SG, Linkhart TA, Taylor AK, Wergedal JE, Bettica P, Baylink DJ. Synthetic peptide-based immunoassay for amino-terminal propeptide of type I procollagen: application for evaluation of bone function. Clin Chem 1993; 39: 2254–8.
113. Haddad Jr JG, Cuoranz S, Avioli LV. Nondialysable urinary hydroxyproline as an index of bone collagen formation. J Clin Endocrinol 1970; 30: 282–7.
114. Kivirikko K. Excretion of urinary hydroxyproline peptides in the assessment of bone collagen deposition and resorption. In: Frame B, Potts JT, eds. Clinical disorders of bone and mineral metabolism. Amsterdam: Excerpta Medica, 1983: 105–7.
115. Deacon AC, Hulme P, Hesp R, Green JR, Tellez M, Reeve J. Estimation of whole body bone resorption rate: a comparison of urinary total hydroxyproline excretion with two radioisotopic tracer methods in osteoporosis. Clin Chim Acta 1987; 166: 297–306.
116. Gasser A, Celada A, Courvoisier B, Depierre D, Hulme PM, Rinsler M, Williams D, Wooton R. The clinical measurement of urinary total hydroxyproline excretion. Clin Chim Acta 1979; 95: 487–91.
117. Colwell A, Russell RGG, Eastell R. Factors affecting the assay of urinary 3-hydroxypyridinium cross-links of collagen as markers of bone resorption. Eur J Clin Invest 1993; 23: 341–9.
118. Lang K. Eine Micromethode zur Bestimmung des Prolines und des Oxyprolines. Z Physiol Chem 1933; 219: 148–54.
119. Podenphant J, Larsen N-E, Christiansen C. An easy and reliable method for determination of urinary hydroxyproline. Clin Chim Acta 1984; 142: 145–8.
120. Dawson CD, Jewell S, Driskell WJ. Liquid-chromatography of total hydroxyproline in urine. Clin Chem 1988; 34: 1572–4.
121. Lippincott S, Chesney RW, Friedman A, Pityer R, Barden H, Mazess RB. Rapid determination of total hydroxyproline (HYP) in human urine by HPLC analysis of the phenylisothiocyonate (PITC)-derivative. Bone 1989; 10: 265–8.
122. Paroni R, De Vecchi E, Fermo I, Arcelloni C, Diomede L, Magni F, Bonini PA. Total urinary hydroxyproline determined with rapid and simple high-performance liquid chromatography. Clin Chem 1992; 38: 407–11.
123. Podenphant J, Riis BJ, Larsen N-E, Christiansen C. Hydroxyproline/creatinine ratios as estimates of bone resorption in early postmenopausal women. Fasting and 24-h urine samples compared. Scand J Clin Lab Invest 1986; 46: 459–63.
124. Wilson PS, Kleerekoper M, Bone H, Parfitt AM. Urinary total hydroxyproline measured by HPLC: comparison of spot and timed collections. Clin Chem 1990; 36: 388–9.
125. Prockop DJ, Kivirikko KI. Relationship of hydroxyproline excretion in urine to collagen metabolism [Review]. Ann Int Med 1967; 66: 1243–66.
126. Hyldstrup L, McNair P, Jensen GF, Nielsen HR, Transbol I. Bone mass as referent for urinary hydroxyproline excretion: age and sex-related changes in 125 normals and in primary hyperparathyroidism. Calcif Tissue Int 1984; 36: 639–44.
127. Mautalen CA. Circadian rhythm of urinary total and free hydroxyproline excretion and its relation to creatinine excretion. J Lab Clin Med 1970; 75: 11–18.
128. de la Piedra C, Toural V, Rapado A. Osteocalcin and urinary hydroxyproline/creatinine ratio in the differential diagnosis of primary hyperparathyroidism and hypercalcemia of malignancy. Scand J Clin Lab Invest 1987; 47: 587–92.
129. Yam LT. Clinical significance of the human acid phosphatases [Review]. Am J Med 1974; 56: 604–16.
130. Lam W, Eastlund DT, Li C-Y, Yam LT. Biochemical properties of tartrate-resistant acid phosphatase in serum of adults and children. Clin Chem 1978; 24: 1105–8.
131. Minkin C. Bone acid phosphatase: tartrate-resistant phosphatase as a marker of osteoclast function. Calcif Tiss Int 1982; 34: 285–90.
132. Lam K-W, Lee P, Li C-Y, Yam LT. Immunological and biochemical evidence for identity of tartrate-resistant isoenzymes of acid phosphatases from human serum and tissues. Clin Chem 1980; 26: 420–2.
133. Hillman GZ. Fortlaufende photometrische Messung der Säuren Phosphatase-Aktivität. Klin Chem Klin Biochem 1971; 9: 273–4.
134. de la Piedra C, Torres R, Rapado A, Diaz Curiel M, Castro N. Serum tartrate-resistant acid phosphatase and bone mineral content in postmenopausal osteoporosis. Calcif Tiss Int 1989; 45: 58–60.
135. Schiele F, Artur Y, Floc'h AY, Siest G. Total, tartrate-resistant, and tartrate-inhibited acid phosphatases in serum: biological variations and reference limits. Clin Chem 1988; 34: 685–90.

136. Lau K-HW, Onishi T, Wergedal JE, Singer FR, Baylink DJ. Characterization and assay of tartrate-resistant acid phosphatase activity in serum: potential use to assess bone resorption. Clin Chem 1987; 33: 458–62.
137. Torres R, de la Piedra C, Rapado A. Clinical usefulness of serum tartrate-resistant acid phosphatase in Paget's disease of bone: correlation with other biochemical markers of bone remodelling. Calcif Tiss Int 1991; 49: 14–16.
138. Bianco P, Ballanti P, Bonucci E. Tartrate-resistant acid phosphatase activity in rat osteoblasts and osteocytes. Calcif Tiss Int 1988; 43: 167–71.
139. Kraenzlin ME, Lau K-HW, Liang L, Freeman TK, Singer FR, Stepan J, Baylink DJ. Development of an immunoassay for human serum osteoclastic tartrate-resistant acid phosphatase. J Clin Endocrinol Metab 1990; 71: 442–51.
140. Allen SH, Nuttleman PR, Ketchman CM, Roberts RM. Purification and characterization of human bone tartrate-resistant acid phosphatase. J Bone Min Res 1989; 4: 47–55.
141. Scarnecchia L, Minisola S, Pacitti MT, Carnevale V, Romaganoli E, Rosso R, Mazzuoli GF. Clinical usefulness of serum tartrate-resistant acid phosphatase activity determination to evaluate bone turnover. Scand J Clin Lab Invest 1991; 51: 517–24.
142. Stepan JJ, Pospichal J, Presl J, Pacovsky V. Bone loss and biochemical indices of bone remodelling in surgically induced postmenopausal women. Bone 1987; 8: 279–84.
143. Stepan JJ, Silinkova-Malkova E, Havranek T, Formankova J, Zichova M, Lachmanova J, Strakova M, Broulik P, Pacovsky V. Relationship of plasma tartrate-resistant acid phosphatase to the bone isoenzyme of serum alkaline phosphatase in hyperparathyroidism. Clin Chim Acta 1983; 133: 189–200.
144. Eyre DR, Koob TJ, Van Ness KP. Quantitation of hydroxypyridinium cross-links in collagen by high performance liquid chromatography. Anal Biochem 1984; 137: 380–8.
145. Gunja-Smith Z, Boucek RJ. Collagen crosslinking compounds in human urine. Biochem J 1981; 197: 759–62.
146. Fujimoto D, Suzuki M, Uchiyama A, Miayamoto S, Inoue T. Analysis of pyridinoline, a crosslinking compound of collagen fibres, in human urine. J Biochem 1983; 94: 1133–6.
147. Eyre DR. Crosslinking in collagen and elastin. Ann Rev Biochem 1984; 53: 717–48.
148. Delmas PD, Schlemmer A, Gineyts E, Riis B, Christiansen C. Urinary excretion of pyridinoline cross-links correlates with bone turnover measured on iliac crest biopsy in patients with vertebral osteoporosis. J Clin Endocrinol Metab 1991; 6: 639–44.
149. Uebelhart D, Gineyts E, Chapuy M-C, Delmas PD. Urinary excretion of pyridinium cross-links: a new marker of bone resorption in metabolic bone disease. Bone Min 1990; 8: 87–96.
150. Eastell R, Hampton L, Colwell A, Green JR, Assiri AMA, Hesp R, Russell RGG, Reeve J. Urinary collagen cross-links are highly correlated with radioisotopic measurements of bone resorption. In: Christiansen C, Overgaard K, eds. Osteoporosis 1990. Copenhagen: Osteopress Aps, 1990; 469–70.
151. Black D, Duncan A, Robins SP. Quantitative analysis of the pyridinium cross-links of collagen in urine using ion-paired reversed-phase high-performance liquid chromatography. Anal Biochem 1988; 169: 197–203.
152. Ubelhart D, Schlemmer A, Johansen JS, Gineyts E, Christiansen C, Delmas PD. Effect of menopause and hormone replacement therapy on the urinary excretion of pyridinium cross-links. J Clin Endocrinol Metab 1991; 72: 367–73.
153. Robins SP, Stewart P, Astbury C, Bird HA. Measurement of the cross linking compound, pyridinoline, in urine as an index of collagen degradation in joint disease. Ann Rheum Dis 1986; 45: 969–73.
154. Pratt DA, Daniloff Y, Duncan A, Robins SP. Automated analysis of the pyridinium cross-links of collagen in tissue and urine using solid-phase extraction and reversed-phase high-performance liquid chromatography. Ann Biochem 1992; 207: 168–75.
155. Seyedin S, Zuk R, Kung V, Danilov Y, Shepard K. An immunoassay to urinary collagen cross-links. Bone Min 1992; 17: S534.
156. Robins SP, Woitge H, Hesley R, Ju J, Seyedin S, Seibel M. Direct, enzyme-linked immunoassay for urinary deoxypyridinoline as a specific marker for measuring bone resorption. J Bone Miner Res 1994; 9: 1643–9.
157. Garnero P, Gineyts E, Riou JP, Delmas PD. Assessment of bone resorption with a new marker of collagen degradation in patients with metabolic bone disease. J Clin Endocrinol Metab 1994; 79: 780–5.
158. Bonde M, Qvist P, Fledelius C, Christiansen C. Crosslaps™ELISA PLUS – an immunoassay for the measurement of degradation products of type I collagen in serum. J Bone Miner Res 1994; 9 (Suppl. 1): S274.
159. Eriksen EF, Charles P, Mosekilde L, Risteli L, Risteli J. Cross-linked carboxyterminal telopeptide of type I collagen in serum (S-ICTP): a new bone resorption marker. J Bone Min Res 1991; 6 (Suppl. 1): S243.

160. Charles P, Mosekilde L, Risteli L, Risteli J, Eriksen EF. Assessment of bone remodeling using biochemical indicators of type I collagen synthesis and degradation: relation to calcium kinetics. Bone Miner 1994; 24: 81–94.
161. Hassager C, Jensen LT, Pødenphant, Thomsen K, Christiansen C. The carboxy-terminal pyridinoline cross-linked telopeptide of type I collagen in serum as a marker of bone resorption: the effect of nandrolone decanoate and hormone replacement therapy. Calcif Tissue Int 1994; 54: 30–3.
162. Prestwood KM, Pilbeam CC, Burleson JA, Woodiel FN, Delmas PD, Deftos LJ, Raisz LG. Short-term effects of conjugated estrogen on bone turnover in older women. J Clin Endocrinol Metab 1994; 79: 366–71.
163. Filipponi P, Pedetti M, Beghe F, Giovagnini B, Miam M, Cristallini S. Effects of two different bisphosphonates on Paget's disease of bone: ICTP assessed. Bone 1994; 15: 261–7.
164. Rosen HN, Dresner-Pollak R, Moses AC, Rosenblatt M, Zeind AJ, Clemens JD, Greenspan SL. Specificity of urinary excretion of cross-linked N-telopeptides of type I collagen as a marker of bone turnover. Calcif Tissue Int 1994; 54: 26–9.
165. Garnero P, Gineyts E, Arbault P, Christiansen C, Delmas PD. Different effects of bisphosphonate and estrogen therapy on the excretion of free and peptide-bound cross-links. J Bone Miner Res 1994; 9 (Suppl. 1): S154.
166. Delmas PD, Gineyts E, Bertholin A, Garnero P, Marchand F. Immunoassay of pyridinoline crosslink excretion in normal adults and in Paget's disease. J Bone Miner Res 1993; 8: 643–8.
167. Breadsworth LJ, Eyre DR, Dickson IR. Changes with age in the urinary excretion of lysyl- and hydroxylysylpyridinoline, two new markers of bone collagen turnover. J Bone Min Res; 5: 671–6.
168. Uebelhart D, Schlemmer A, Johansen JS, Gineyts E, Christiansen C, Delmas PD. Effect of menopause and hormone replacement therapy on the urinary excretion of pyridinium cross-links. J Clin Endocrinol Metab 1991; 72: 367–73.
169. Hassager C. Colwell A, Assiri AMA, Eastell R, Russell RGG, Christiansen C. Effect of menopause and hormone replacement therapy on urinary excretion of pyridinium cross-links: a longitudinal and cross-sectional study. Clin Endocrinol 1992; 37: 45–50.
170. Schlemmer A, Hassager C, Jensen SB, Christiansen C. Marked variation in urinary excretion of pyridinium cross-links in premenopausal women. J Clin Endocrinol Metab 1992; 74: 476–80.
171. Eastell R, Colwell A, Assiri AMA, Burritt MF, Calvo MS, Riggs BL, Russell RGG. Deoxypyridinoline as an improved marker for bone resorption in postmenopausal osteoporosis. Bone 1990; 11: 219.
172. Eastell R, Calvo M, Burritt M, Offord KP, Rossell RGG, Riggs BL. Abnormalities in circadian patterns of bone resorption and renal calcium conservation in type I osteoporosis. J Endocrinol Metab 1992; 74: 487–94.
173. Siebel MJ, Gartenberg F, Silverberg SJ, Ratcliffe A, Robins SP, Bilezikian JP. Urinary hydroxypyridinium cross-links of collagen in hyperparathyroidism. J Clin Endocrinol Metab 1991; 74: 481–6.
174. Harvey RD, McHardy KC, Reid IW, Paterson F, Bewsher PD, Duncan A, Robins SP. Measurement of bone collagen degradation in hyperparathyroidism and during thyroxine replacement therapy using pyridinium cross-links as specific urinary markers. J Clin Endocrinol Metab 1991; 72: 1189–94.
175. Johansen JS, Delmas PD, Riis BJ, Gineyts E, Christiansen C. Serum-free gamma carboxyglutamic acid (free gla) is a poor biochemical marker of bone resorption in early postmenopausal women. Bone 1991; 12: 257–60.
176. Gundberg CM, Lian JB, Gallop PM, Steinberg PM. Urinary carboxyglutamic acid and serum osteocalcin as bone markers: studies in osteoporosis and Paget's disease. J Clin Endocrinol Metab 1983; 57: 1221–5.
177. Fournier B, Gineyts E, Delmas PD. Measurement of free carboxyglutamic acid in serum: a new marker of bone turnover. J Bone Min Res 1988; 3 (Suppl. 1): S169.
178. Segrest JP. Urinary metabolites of collagen. Methods Enzymol 1982; 82: 398–410.
179. Moro L, Modricky C, Stagni N, Vittur F, de Bernard B. High-performance liquid chromatographic analysis of urinary hydroxylysyl glycosides as indicators of collagen turnover. Analyst 1984; 109: 1621–2.
180. Moro L, Mucelli RSP, Gazzarrini C, Modricky C, Marotti F, de Bernard B. Urinary β-1-galactosyl-*O*-hydroxylysine (GH) as a marker of turnover of bone. Calcif Tiss Int 1988; 42: 87–90.
181. Bettica P, Moro L, Robins SP, Taylor AK, Talbot J, Singer FR, Baylink DJ. Bone-resorption markers galactosyl hydroxylysine, pyridinium cross-links, and hydroxyproline compared. Clin Chem 1992; 38: 2313–18.
182. Hansen MA, Overgard K, Riis BJ, Christiansen C. Role of peak bone mass and bone loss in postmenopausal osteoporosis: 12-year study. Br Med J 1991; 303: 961–4.
183. Blumsohn A, Eastell R. Prediction of bone loss in postmenopausal women [Commentary]. Eur J Clin Invest 1992; 22: 764–6.

Biochemistry of calcium regulation

5

E. B. Mawer and J. L. Berry

INTRODUCTION

In this chapter the need to control the concentration of calcium in the extracellular fluid will be discussed, together with a brief consideration of the principal hormones involved in calcium homeostasis. Methods for the measurement of calcium in serum and urine and for serum parathyroid hormone (PTH, parathyrin) and vitamin D metabolites will be assessed. Methods for the assay of calcitonin are not included here since the physiological effect of this hormone on serum calcium concentration is not established, although when given in pharmacological doses it does play a role in lowering serum calcium by inhibiting osteoclastic bone resorption and promoting a calciuresis. Consideration will be given, however, to the recently described parathyroid hormone-related peptide (PTHrP) which contributes to hypercalcemia in some cases of malignancy, although it is believed to have no role in normal adult calcium homeostasis. The significance of assay results will be discussed in the light of their application to the differential diagnosis of problems of calcium metabolism.

CALCIUM

Metabolism

Calcium is the most abundant metallic element in the body, although less than 1% of the total is outside the skeleton and able to exchange readily with tissue and extracellular fluid pools. Of the total 25–35 mol (1–1.4 kg), only about 25 mmol (1 g) is present in the extracellular fluid and a further 25 mmol in soft tissues. Plasma calcium concentration is maintained within a narrow range, around 2.4 mmol/l, by means of complex homeostatic mechanisms. Inside cells the cytoplasmic calcium concentration may be as low as 0.1 μmol/l, though it can be concentrated at millimolar concentrations in intracellular organelles. Many fundamentally important cellular processes require calcium ions and it is the ionized fraction of the plasma and extracellular fluid calcium that controls these processes by a mechanism which is not fully understood[1].

Calcium is essential for the control of excitability of nerve and muscle cells, for muscular contraction, hormone secretion, blood clotting and intracellular signaling. The appropriate ionized calcium concentration for these processes is achieved both by non-hormonal mechanisms and by a series of hormonal loops which control fluxes of calcium between the extracellular fluid and the three major organs or tissues involved, namely, bone, intestine and kidney. The concept of a set-point for plasma calcium in an individual has been developed by Parfitt[2] to define the concentration of calcium achieved by the homeostatic processes at steady state, as determined from sequential measurements over a period of time. Compensation for chronic disturbances of calcium metabolism may result in homeostasis being achieved at a new set-point (*see* below). Parfitt distinguishes set-point from error correction in which minor deviations from the set-point are reversed by homeostatic mechanisms, though he considers these to be mainly rapid renal responses that do not depend on changes in secretion of calciotropic hormones[2].

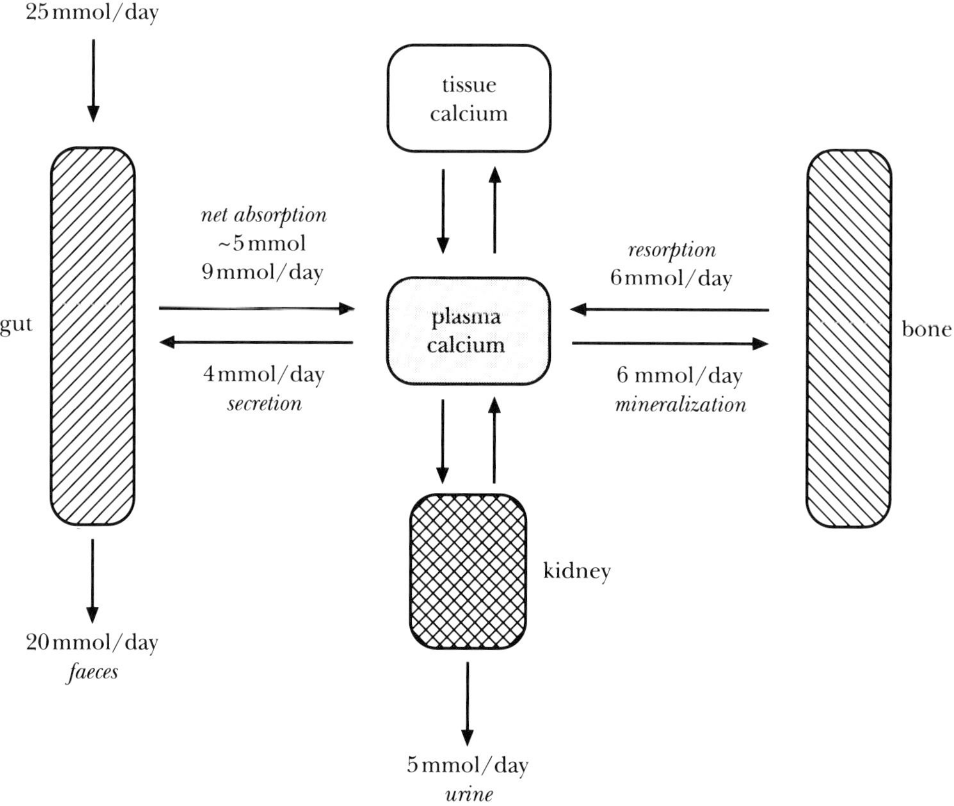

Figure 1 *Calcium equilibrium in a normal adult*

The components of the homeostatic system for calcium are summarized in Figure 1 showing representative values for an adult in a state of calcium equilibrium.

The processes governing calcium homeostasis are modulated by the actions of various hormones (Figure 2). Calcium enters the body from the intestinal lumen; a good dietary intake of calcium is about 25 mmol (1 g) of which perhaps 9 mmol may be absorbed, primarily by an active process in the small intestine, but most efficiently in the duodenum, promoted by the hormonal metabolite of vitamin D, 1,25-dihydroxyvitamin D (1,25$(OH)_2$D). Calcium enters the intestine in various secretions; this is not absorbed from the more distal parts of the gut and represents an obligatory loss of 3–4 mmol/day. In a person who is in calcium equilibrium, the daily net intestinal absorption of about 5 mmol is matched by excretion in the urine of the same amount. Urinary excretion is dependent partly on the filtered load (normally about 200 mmol), being increased when the load is large, and renal tubular reabsorption increasing when calcium needs to be conserved. The latter process is enhanced by PTH which promotes reabsorption in the distal tubule. Usually around 98% of the filtered load is reabsorbed but this can increase to nearly 100% if calcium is in short supply; some 65% is reabsorbed by an active mechanism linked to the reabsorption of sodium in the proximal tubule, 20–25% in the ascending limb of the loop of Henle and 10% in the distal convoluted tubules.

PTH further affects calcium metabolism through a renal mechanism in that it is the trophic hormone for the synthesis of 1,25 $(OH)_2$D in the cells of the proximal tubule. By this means PTH indirectly controls the absorption of calcium from the intestine; the role of 1,25$(OH)_2$D in the renal tubular reabsorption of calcium is not clearly established.

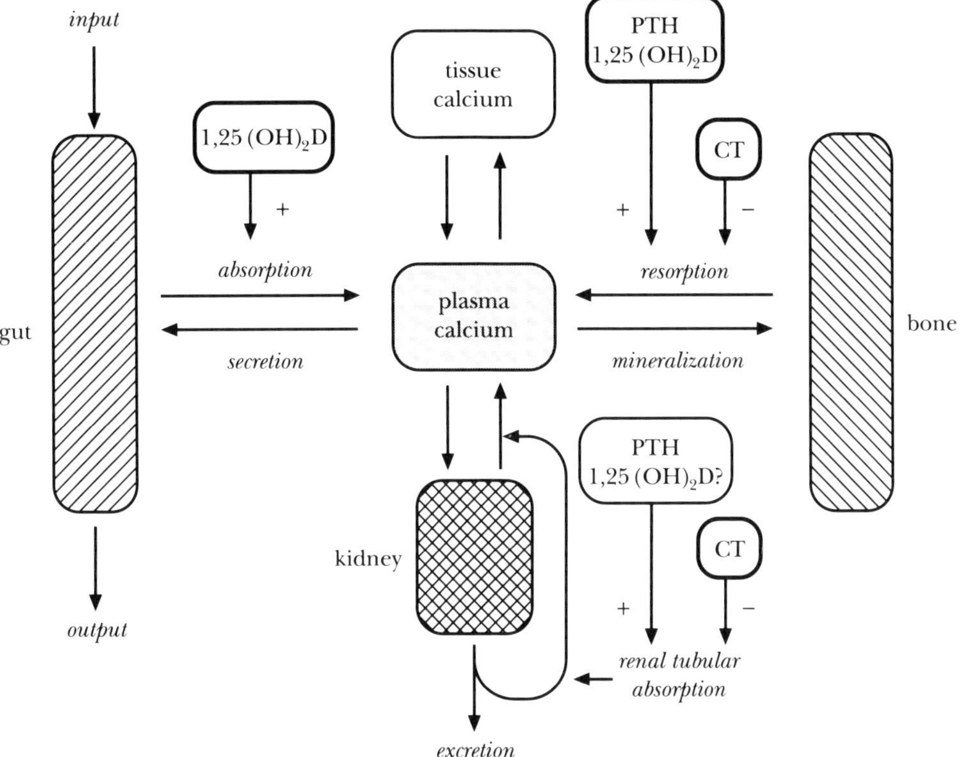

Figure 2 *The actions of various hormones on calcium homeostasis: 1,25(OH)$_2$D, 1,25-dihydroxyvitamin D; PTH, parathyroid hormone; CT, calcitonin*

Calcium is mobilized from the mineral phase in bone by the process in adults of remodeling. Under the influence of PTH and 1,25(OH)$_2$D bone matrix and mineral are removed by osteoclasts and replaced in a linked sequence by osteoblastic cells (see Chapter 2 by Selby). When the two processes are synchronized there will be no net gain or loss of calcium, but the opportunity for exchange with the plasma pool arises. The remodeling sequence, however, is too lengthy (measured in weeks) to be important in normal homeostasis, although net release of calcium may occur in certain pathological conditions. Probably more important in homeostasis and rapid correction is the exchange of calcium between the extracellular fluid and the bone lining and periosteal cells, across which a calcium flux has been demonstrated. A concept has been developed of a bone fluid, analogous to cerebrospinal fluid, enclosed by lining cells and able to exchange calcium between that on the mineralized surface of bone and the extracellular fluid. For a more detailed discussion of the concepts and mechanisms involved in calcium homeostasis, the reader is directed to the excellent book by Mundy[1].

Measurement of serum or plasma calcium

Total calcium

Serum is the fluid of choice for the measurement of calcium in blood, since some methods of collecting plasma involve the complexing of calcium to prevent clotting (see Table 4 below). Plasma can be used provided it has been prepared by a suitable method. The normal range for serum calcium varies slightly between laboratories but is usually within the range 2.15–2.65 mmol/l. Investigators should check the precise limits of normality with their local

Table 1 *Calcium fractions in the serum/plasma*

Total calcium	2.15–2.65 mmol/l
non-diffusible calcium (protein-bound)	46%
diffusible calcium	
free	47%
complexed (citrate, phosphate)	7%

laboratory. Most laboratories measure total calcium although it is the ionized fraction that is relevant physiologically. Just less than half the total calcium consists of a non-diffusible protein-bound fraction; this is in equilibrium with a diffusible fraction, largely ionized, but containing a small pool of complexed calcium (Table 1).

Total calcium is usually measured by autoanalyser by a direct colorimetric method using cresolphthalein complexone, but can also be estimated by atomic absorption spectrophotometry in which samples are diluted with lanthanum chloride and sprayed into an air–acetylene flame. Between-batch precision (0.01 mmol/l) is the same for both methods[3]. Values for serum calcium may be affected by changes in protein concentration caused by venous stasis while collecting the sample, although this has to be extreme to produce clinically relevant changes in serum calcium, and by changes in pH of the blood, the ionized fraction increasing with acidosis and decreasing with alkalosis.

It is possible to measure ionized calcium directly, see below, if this is needed for an experimental investigation, but this is not usually necessary on a routine basis. However, provided the concentrations of serum proteins are normal, a working assumption can be made that the ionized fraction will bear a fixed relationship to the total concentration. If serum protein concentrations are abnormal this relationship cannot be assumed and various methods have been developed to 'correct' the total calcium to a standard protein concentration (for example: corrected serum calcium (mmol/l) = measured serum calcium (mmol/l) + 0.02 [40 – serum albumin (g/l)]). This enables the ionized calcium concentration to be estimated.

Ionized calcium

The realization that ionized or free calcium was a more relevant index of biological activity than total calcium was prompted by experiments of McLean and Hastings in 1935[4] who showed that the contractile response of frog heart muscle was dependent on the ionized calcium concentration.

Ionized calcium is measured using an ion-selective electrode. One commonly used is the Radiometer electrode which employs a PVC membrane impregnated with Ca^{++}-bis-dioctylphenylphosphate, covered with a cellophane membrane to prevent interference by proteins. Aqueous samples, plasma or whole blood can be measured, but care must be exerted to ensure that the pH does not change during preparation or storage since this will affect the ionized concentration. The normal range for plasma ionized calcium concentration is about 1.15–1.30 mmol/l.

For routine clinical applications, once hypo- or hypercalcemia has been established, there may be little application for ionized calcium measurements in following the response of a patient[1]. Ionized calcium concentrations are of value particularly in conditions where protein metabolism is abnormal, e.g. in malignancy or liver disease, the fall in plasma albumin concentration may be so large that total calcium is extremely low and methods for calculating the corrected value are not valid. Conversely, in conditions such as myeloma excess secretion of globulin can result in increased calcium binding giving an apparently high circulating value.

Measurement of urine calcium

Either of the methods used for measuring total serum calcium may be applied to urine. Ideally a 24-h collection should be made in a vessel containing 10 ml concentrated hydrochloric acid as preservative. Urinary excretion should match net intestinal absorption in a person who is in calcium equilibrium, and in these circumstances the excretion is related to the dietary calcium intake. On an average diet, between 2.5 and 7.5 mmol/day may be excreted in urine[3].

Urinary excretion falls as the plasma calcium falls because of increased renal tubular reabsorption and may be as low as 0.5 mmol/day in severely hypocalcemic patients with secondary hyperparathyroidism; however, in hypoparathyroidism low serum calcium may be associated with a renal leak of calcium because PTH-driven reabsorption is absent. Conversely urinary excretion may be as high as 7.5–17.5 mmol/day if the plasma ionized calcium is high, as in primary hyperparathyroidism, despite the reabsorptive action of the hormone. Calcium excretion in urine is linked to protein intake and to sodium excretion, and shows diurnal variation linked to sodium output. Urinary calcium excretion after at least a 12-h fast is considered to represent net bone resorption[1].

Urine calcium is often related to creatinine, giving a calcium : creatinine ratio which permits comparisons of excretion to be made in circumstances where renal function may be altered. This type of correction has been refined by determining calcium excretion (Ca_E) at different serum calcium levels. Ca_E, defined as urinary calcium excretion in µmol/l glomerular filtrate, is derived from measurements of urinary calcium and creatinine expressed as a ratio and multiplied by serum creatinine.

$$Ca_E = \frac{\text{urine calcium (mmol/l)}}{\text{urine creatinine (mmol/l)}} \times \begin{array}{c}\text{serum}\\ \text{creatinine}\\ (\mu\text{mol/l})\end{array}$$

When Ca_E is plotted against serum calcium it is possible to assess the role of the renal tubule in determining serum calcium[5]. Thus, for example, in hypoparathyroidism where there is a renal tubular leak of calcium, Ca_E is high relative to serum calcium.

Hypocalcemia and hypercalcemia

Hypocalcemia is defined as a serum total calcium concentration of less than 2.20 or 2.15 mmol/l depending upon the established range of the assay used, or an ionized calcium concentration below 1.1 mmol/l. Below about 2.00 mmol/l serum total calcium concentration tetany may occur and neuronal hyperexcitability can be demonstrated (Trousseau and Chvostek signs). A fall in total serum calcium below 1.25 mmol/l leads to severe impairment of neuromuscular function and of basic cell processes and is considered to be life-threatening, although values as low as 0.95 mmol/l have been encountered[3]. Some of the main causes of hypocalcemia are listed in Table 2, and the more important ones, i.e. those related to a deficiency of PTH or vitamin D, will be discussed in detail under the appropriate headings later in this chapter.

Hypercalcemia, i.e. serum total calcium concentration above 2.60–2.65 mmol/l, is most commonly caused by hyperparathyroidism, with malignancy the second most frequent cause[6]. Symptoms, usually observed when serum calcium exceeds 3 mmol/l include thirst, polyuria, anorexia, nausea, constipation, lethargy, confusion, depression, with accompanying dehydration and impaired glomerular filtration and, sometimes, renal stones. Urinary calcium excretion is not necessarily increased. Table 3 summarizes the differential diagnosis of hypercalcemia. The involvement of PTH and vitamin

Table 2 *Principal causes of hypocalcemia*

Hypoparathyroidism/pseudohypoparathyroidism

Vitamin D deficiency
- nutritional or environmental
- acquired
  - renal failure
  - malabsorptive diseases
  - anticonvulsant treatment
- inherited
  - vitamin D-resistant/-dependent rickets (rare)

Magnesium deficiency

Acute pancreatitis

Table 3 *Principal causes of hypercalcemia*

Primary hyperparathyroidism
Malignant disease with/without metastases
Granulomatous disease
Vitamin D intoxication
Thyrotoxicosis
Familial hypocalciuric hypercalcemia
Idiopathic hypercalcemia of infancy
  (William's syndrome)
Milk alkali syndrome
Immobilization

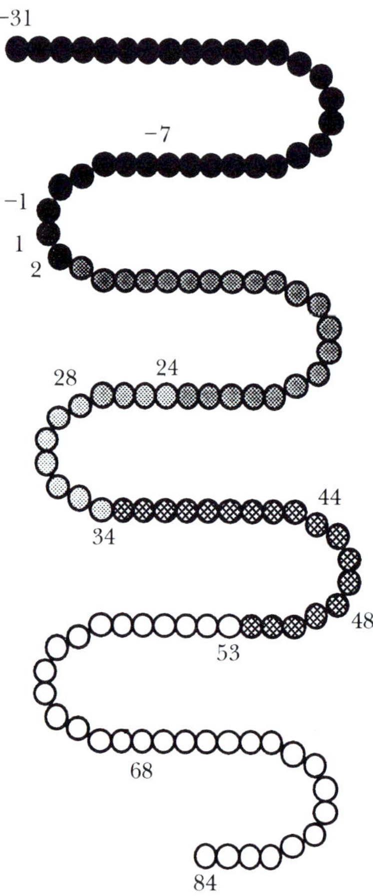

Figure 3 *Schematic map of the parathyroid hormone (PTH) molecule. Residues – 31 to – 7 and – 6 to – 1 represent the precursor and pro- sequences respectively; both are cleaved in the parathyroid gland before secretion. Amino acids 1–34 from the N terminus are required for optimal biological activity; residues 1 and 2 are essential for cAMP generation and the 24–34 region for receptor binding. The mid-region 34–53 contains cleavage sites; the C-terminal region 53–84 has no classical PTH activity*

D in hypercalcemia are discussed later in the chapter.

PARATHYROID HORMONE

Structure, secretion and functions

PTH is secreted as a straight chain of 84 amino acids by the four (in humans) parathyroid glands close to the thyroid. The gene is on chromosome 11 and encodes a longer molecule with pre- and pro- sequences which are cleaved before secretion (Figure 3). The secreted 1–84 form is often referred to as 'intact PTH' because it can undergo cleavage in liver and kidney as well as in the parathyroid gland yielding a series of fragments[7,8] which can be detected in the circulation. It will be necessary to consider briefly these fragments because recent studies suggest differential roles for different parts of the molecule[9], and also because it is important to know which portions of the molecule are recognized by particular assays.

The primary stimulus to PTH secretion is a fall in the concentration of plasma ionized calcium leading to a decrease in intracellular calcium within the gland causing rapid release of stored hormone and also stimulating synthesis *de novo*. Parathyroid cells have a calcium 'receptor' or sensor molecule on the surface, which has recently been isolated and cloned[10]. The plasma concentration of calcium is controlled by a series of hormonal loops involving primarily PTH and $1,25(OH)_2D$ in inter-related rapid and longer-term mechanisms. An example of the hormonal response to hypocalcemia is shown in Figure 4. The set-point for PTH release is defined as the concentration of plasma calcium at which half the maximal stimulation of PTH release occurs (Figure 5). Around this value very small changes in calcium concentration produce large changes in PTH secretion[11,12]. Calcium ions are, however, required for secretion of PTH and, paradoxically, in very profound hypocalcemia, such as might be caused by severe and prolonged vitamin D deficiency, PTH is not secreted until the calcium level has been raised by calcium and vitamin D treatment[13]. Synthesis and release of PTH are suppressed by high calcium concentrations, but a low level of plasma PTH is maintained under normocalcemic conditions.

Synthesis of PTH is modulated by $1,25(OH)_2D$, independently of the effects of this hormone on plasma calcium[14]. Vitamin D-response elements have been identified on the PTH gene; the effect is probably mediated through receptors for $1,25(OH)_2D$ which are present within parathyroid cells[15]. Magnesium ions are

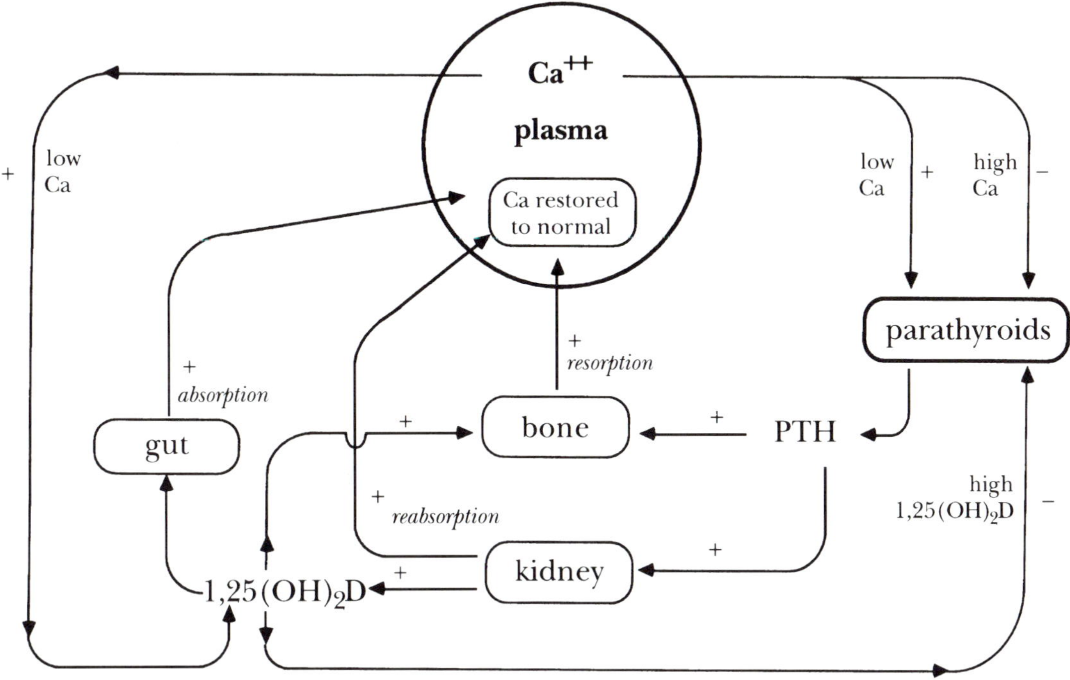

Figure 4 *The hormonal loops involved in the correction of hypocalcemia: PTH, parathyroid hormone; 1,25(OH)$_2$D, 1,25-dihydroxyvitamin D*

also necessary for PTH secretion and profound hypomagnesemia can give rise to functional hypoparathyroidism[16]. For further information on the regulation of synthesis and secretion of PTH see the recent review by Watson and Hanley[17].

The actions of PTH in its target tissues result from its interaction with cell-surface PTH receptors and all have the effect of increasing the supply of calcium to the extracellular fluid (Figure 4). The effect of PTH in the distal renal tubule is to control the fraction of the filtered load (about 10%) which can be actively reabsorbed. This action is accompanied by the generation of cyclic adenosine monophosphate (cAMP) which can be measured in urine[18]. PTH inhibits the renal tubular reabsorption of phosphate ion and of bicarbonate in the proximal tubule, which is also the site of PTH-stimulated synthesis of 1,25(OH)$_2$D. In bone, the overall effect of PTH is to stimulate osteoclast numbers and activity, although, to date, receptors for PTH have only been demonstrated convincingly in osteoblasts, and current hypotheses assume that there is intercellular signaling between the two cell types (see Chapter 2 by Selby).

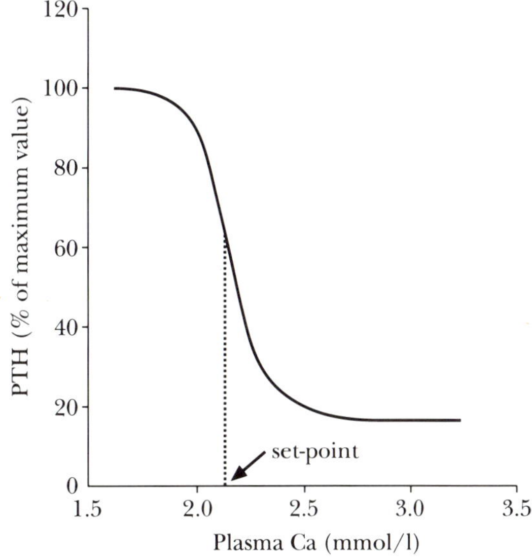

Figure 5 *The relationship between parathyroid hormone (PTH) secretion and plasma calcium; modified with permission from Boucher et al.[12] and the J Clin Endocrinol Metab*

PTH fragments, PTH receptors and biological activity

A fragment containing the first 34 amino acids can achieve all the classical biological effects (Figure 3) of the intact hormone. Fragments from the C terminus and the mid-molecule are biologically inert in this capacity but may be recognized by some assays. The clearance rate of the C-terminal fragment is less than that of the intact molecule or of the N-terminal moiety and so it is not only present in normal serum but accumulates to a high concentration in conditions such as renal failure; it is therefore critical to know the specificity of any assays used.

As mentioned above, target cells for PTH possess receptors on their membranes through which the biological actions are mediated. It was thought until recently that these actions were exclusively linked to the adenylate cyclase–protein kinase A pathway via specific G-proteins[19,20], but more recent evidence suggests that some major functions of PTH, such as regulation of calcium and phosphate concentrations by renal tubular cells, may be mediated by phosphoinositide breakdown and membrane-associated protein kinase C activity. The two different pathways appear to be linked to two classes of receptor with differing affinities for PTH and responsive to different circulating levels of the hormone[21,22]. The ability of PTH to activate two separate signaling pathways suggests that the hormone has both an adenylate cyclase activation and a protein kinase C activation domain.

The classical role of PTH in the renal reabsorption of calcium and stimulation of $1,25(OH)_2D$ synthesis, via the adenylate cyclase pathway, may be monitored by measuring the renally produced or 'nephrogenous' cAMP[18]. It is well known that the first two amino acids of PTH are essential for cAMP generation and the 24–34 region is needed for receptor binding, explaining why the whole 1–34 moiety is needed for optimal adenylate cyclase activation. This action of PTH is thought to be linked to low-affinity receptors which are activated when large amounts of hormone are secreted by the parathyroid gland in response to a fall in plasma calcium. High-affinity receptors, linked to the protein kinase C pathway, may be responsible for the continuous maintenance of normal plasma concentrations of calcium, phosphate and $1,25(OH)_2D$ at low concentrations of PTH. The effects of PTH on stimulating the proliferation of bone and cartilage cells also involve protein kinase C activation and can be achieved by the very short 28–34 fragment[21]. Although it is generally considered that the C-terminal fragments have no biological activity, high-affinity binding sites for the 53–84 region have been described in bone and renal cells[23] and stimulation of alkaline phosphatase activity has been reported in a cultured rat osteosarcoma cell line[24].

Measurement of PTH

It will be clear from the account above that because of the heterogeneity of the circulating forms of PTH, care needs to be taken to select an appropriate PTH assay for the purpose required[25]. Immunoassays are available for the intact 1–84 molecule as well as for the N- and C-terminal regions of the molecule and for the mid-region. In practice the most crucial decision is to distinguish whether hypercalcemia is due to primary hyperparathyroidism rather than to malignancy or sarcoidosis, so from this point of view, the touchstone of an assay is its ability to discriminate between these groups. C-terminal and mid-molecule assays can, in theory, discriminate best between normal subjects and patients with primary hyperparathyroidism, since these fragments circulate at higher concentrations and have longer half-lives than the intact hormone or N terminus, but caution needs to be exercised in interpretation when renal function is impaired. N-terminal assays are more reliable in this situation but do not always detect primary hyperparathyroidism[25] and are more difficult because of the extremely short half-life (about 1.5 min) of the 1–34 fragment[26] compared to that of the intact molecule (about 10 min). It is also important that PTH assays should be able to discriminate between the lower end of the normal range and hypoparathyroid samples, though many assays show some overlap. The ability to register very low or absent PTH in

Table 4 *Plasma/serum specimen requirements*

*Measurement**	*Type of specimen*	*Volume*† (ml)	*Storage*
Calcium (total)	serum or plasma‡	0.2	– 20 °C
Calcium (ionized)	serum or plasma‡ (pH must be maintained at 7.4)	0.2	– 20 °C (anaerobic)
PTH	serum or EDTA plasma (DO NOT FREEZE & THAW)	0.5	– 20 °C (4 months) – 70 °C (11 months)
PTHrP	EDTA plasma in tube with proteinase inhibitors; keep on ice, spin within 30 min	0.5	not yet established
25(OH)D	serum or plasma	0.5–2.0**	– 20 °C
1,25(OH)$_2$D	serum or plasma	1.0–2.0**	– 20 °C

* PTH, parathyroid hormone; PTHrP, parathyroid hormone-related peptide; 25(OH)D, 25-hydroxyvitamin D; 1,25(OH)$_2$D, 1,25-dihydroxyvitamin D; † volumes shown are the minimum for one determination in duplicate; ‡ serum is preferable; plasma may be used provided it has not been prepared with calcium-complexing agents such as EDTA, oxalate or citrate; ** depending on method used

Table 5 *Indications for plasma parathyroid hormone (PTH) assay*

Condition	*Cause*	*PTH assay result*
Differential diagnosis of hypercalcemia		
Primary hyperparathyroidism	excess PTH secreted by parathyroid adenoma	↑
Malignancy-associated hypercalcemia	cytokines and factors, e.g. PTHrP secreted by tumor	↓
Familial hypocalciuric hypercalcemia	increased tubular reabsorption of calcium	
Granulomatous disease, e.g. sarcoidosis	extrarenal synthesis of 1,25(OH)$_2$D	→ (↑)
Vitamin D intoxication	effects of ↑ 25(OH)D and ↑ 1,25(OH)$_2$D in intestine and bone	↓ ↓
Thyrotoxicosis	bone resorption by thyroid hormone	↓
Differential diagnosis of hypocalcemia		
Hypoparathyroidism	lack of PTH – surgical loss of tissue/autoimmune	↓
Pseudohypoparathyroidism	abnormality in G-proteins impairs PTH actions	↑
Vitamin D deficiency (secondary hyperparathyroidism)	lack of 1,25(OH)$_2$D impairs intestinal calcium absorption	↑
Magnesium deficiency	impaired PTH secretion	↓

PTHrP, parathyroid hormone-related protein; 1,25(OH)$_2$D, 1,25-dihydroxyvitamin D; 25(OH)D, 25-hydroxyvitamin D

hypoparathyroidism enables this condition to be distinguished from pseudohypoparathyroidism. In the latter condition there is also hypocalcemia, but it is associated with raised levels of PTH which is biologically ineffective because of defects in the G-proteins through which the hormone acts.

The requirements for the collection of samples are shown in Table 4 and the indications for measuring PTH are summarized in Table 5.

Biological assays

Sensitive bioassays have been developed which utilize the biological effects of PTH and more details of these are provided in the section on PTHrP below. Bioassays are too difficult and time-consuming to be used on a routine basis, but can act as a reference standard for other methods[27].

Immunoassays

Intact PTH (1–84) Originally, radioimmunoassays (RIAs) were developed for the intact molecule, but usually for heterologous forms such as the bovine or porcine hormones, and though able to detect serum PTH in most patients with primary hyperparathyroidism, these were too insensitive to measure normal or subnormal levels in the low picomolar range and too non-specific to exclude immunoreactive fragments[28]. These drawbacks have now been largely overcome by the development of immunoradiometric assays (IRMAs) using two antibodies raised to different parts of the molecule. In these assays, the 'capture' antibody is linked to a solid phase, and binds one part of the molecule to be assayed; the 'signal' or detection antibody binds to another part. Only molecules which can bridge the two antibodies will both be bound to the solid phase and bind the detection label. Various laboratories have developed such assays which are sensitive enough to detect low concentrations of circulating hormone and specific enough to avoid cross-reactivity with other molecular species[29–31]. The assay reported by Brown and co-workers[31] and a multisite assay recently described by Klee and co-workers[32] both use a chemiluminometric method of detection instead of radioiodine. The method of Klee and co-workers employs two capture antibodies, to human PTH 1–44 and 44–68, and acridinium-labeled anti-human PTH 1–34, so that both N-terminal fragments and the intact molecule will be detected, but not C-terminal fragments. Some IRMAs are now available as commercial kits; the best provide a robust but sensitive method employing antibodies which would not otherwise be available to the investigator. Reliable suppliers include the Nichols Institute and Incstar. Characteristics established for commercially available intact PTH assays have been reported[30]. The two-site immunoradiometric assays in current use give a normal range for PTH 1–84 of about 10–60 pg/ml or 1–6 pmol/l.

Mid-molecule assays The mid-region of the molecule is variably defined but usually includes residues 44–68 (Figure 3); the fragments measured do not have biological activity and are used as an index of the synthesis of intact PTH, because of their longer half-life. Schimdt-Gayk and co-workers[33] have reported a mid-region RIA using iodinated human PTH 44–68 as tracer, which has a normal range of 15–40 pmol/l with a detection limit of 15 pmol/l. Comparing results from this RIA with those of the same laboratory's intact PTH IRMA, the authors showed that only 2% of results from patients with primary hyperparathyroidism fell within the normal range of the IRMA whereas 11% were normal using the mid-region assay. The mid-region assay fared even worse in measuring serum from patients with hypercalcemia of malignancy with 68% assaying within the normal range compared to 5% using the intact PTH assay, but it was more useful in detecting raised values in patients with renal disease. Other workers, however, have reported a mid-regional assay in which some 95% of patients with primary hyperparathyroidism had elevated values[34].

N-terminal assays (PTH 1–34) N-terminal RIAs for PTH should, in theory, show the closest correlation with biological activity, since they should measure intact PTH together with N-terminal fragments. In fact the half-life of N-terminal fragments is believed to be so short that the assays probably only measure the intact molecule and, indeed, have largely been superseded by intact PTH IRMAs. However, an N-terminal PTH RIA, using guinea-pig antiserum 211, was in use in our laboratory for 15 years and discriminated well between hyperparathyroid patients and normals, although values were high by current standards[35]. A good correlation was obtained, though, between the results obtained with this assay and repeated assays of stored serum samples using a commercial kit IRMA. Another N-terminal RIA, with a sensitivity of 2 pg/ml (0.5 pmol/l) and using ^{125}I-labeled human PTH 1–34 as label, is available as a commercial kit from Nichols. More recently, a sensitive assay for PTH 1–34 (limit of detection 0.5 pmol/l) using a biotinylated peptide as tracer has been described[36]. In this assay, serum from five out of 43 patients with primary hyperparathyroidism gave values in the normal range. Finally, N-terminal assays have proved particularly useful in the investigation of patients with renal disease since the biologically active hormone can be measured even in the presence of high concentrations of inactive C-terminal fragments[37].

C-terminal assays Carboxy-terminal assays are designed to detect PTH 69–84[26]. They tend to give lower values than mid-region assays because they do not recognize the mid-molecule fragments that arise in the parathyroid glands. They are relatively insensitive and less useful than mid-region assays in the diagnosis of primary hyperparathyroidism, and are not reliable where renal function is impaired. Other types of assay are to be preferred.

Summary

Assays for PTH are useful in distinguishing the role of the hormone in disorders of calcium metabolism (Table 5). In addition they permit monitoring of patients with advancing renal disease, in whom one aim of management is the avoidance of secondary hyperparathyroidism and the development of renal osteodystrophy.

VITAMIN D AND ITS METABOLITES

Structure and function

A general account of vitamin D metabolism with reference to its role in health and disease can be found in a review by Reichel and co-authors[38]. 1,25(OH)$_2$D is the active metabolite responsible for the classical actions of vitamin D in calcium metabolism, namely regulation of intestinal calcium absorption and mineralization of bone. The parent compound, vitamin D, has no biological activity and the major circulating metabolite, 25-hydroxyvitamin D (25(OH)D), has none at normal concentrations[39].

Vitamin D may be present in one of two forms which differ in their side chain structure (Figure 6). Vitamin D$_3$ is supplied either physiologically by ultraviolet irradiation of a precursor in skin or may be obtained from the diet. Vitamin D$_2$ is only available in the diet, being formed by irradiation of the plant sterol ergosterol. This reaction is exploited commercially for the production of vitamin D$_2$ which is used both as a food additive and for pharmaceutical preparations. In measuring vitamin D metabolites, it may sometimes be useful to be able to distinguish between the two forms of the vitamin.

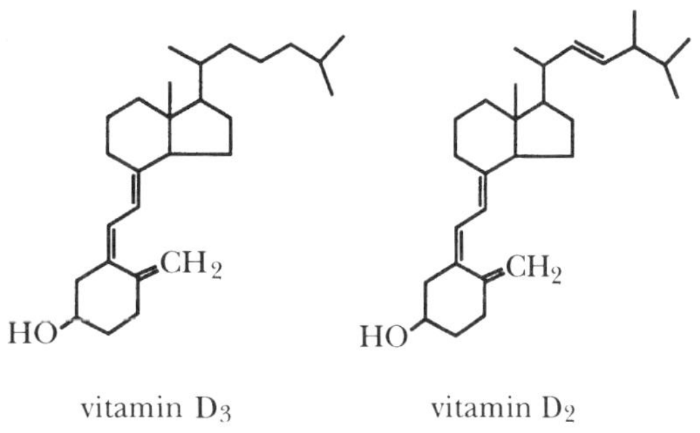

HO CH$_2$ vitamin D$_3$ HO CH$_2$ vitamin D$_2$

Figure 6 *Structures of vitamins D$_3$ and D$_2$*

Vitamin D, from whatever source, undergoes sequential cytochrome P$_{450}$-dependent hydroxylations to form 25(OH)D in the liver and then 1,25(OH)$_2$D and 24,25-dihydroxyvitamin D (24,25(OH)$_2$D) in the kidney (Figure 7) and metabolites may be present as D$_2$ or D$_3$ forms. The concentration of 25(OH)D (normal range around 25–100 nmol/l) is usually taken as an index of vitamin D status, vitamin D deficiency being identified with a circulating concentration of less than 12.5 nmol/l[40]. Both 25(OH)D and 24,25(OH)$_2$D (normal range around 2–10 nmol/l) are present in plasma at much higher concentrations than the hormonal metabolite 1,25(OH)$_2$D (around 100 pmol/l), but they have limited biological activity with respect to calcium homeostasis. The lipid-soluble vitamin D and its metabolites are transported in plasma by a vitamin D-binding protein[41].

Many of the actions of vitamin D are mediated through an intracellular receptor which has much higher affinity for 1,25(OH)$_2$D than for the other metabolites[42]. The receptor which is present in the target cells for vitamin D activity, e.g. intestinal mucosa and osteoblasts, is known as the vitamin D receptor, despite its lack of affinity for the parent vitamin. The receptor-bound hormone functions in a manner analogous to that of steroid hormones, and promotes binding of the receptor to nuclear chromatin resulting in the transcription of specific messenger RNAs. In intestinal mucosal cells, 1,25(OH)$_2$D controls the synthesis of proteins involved in calcium transport such as calbindin, and in osteoblasts it mediates the production of proteins associated with

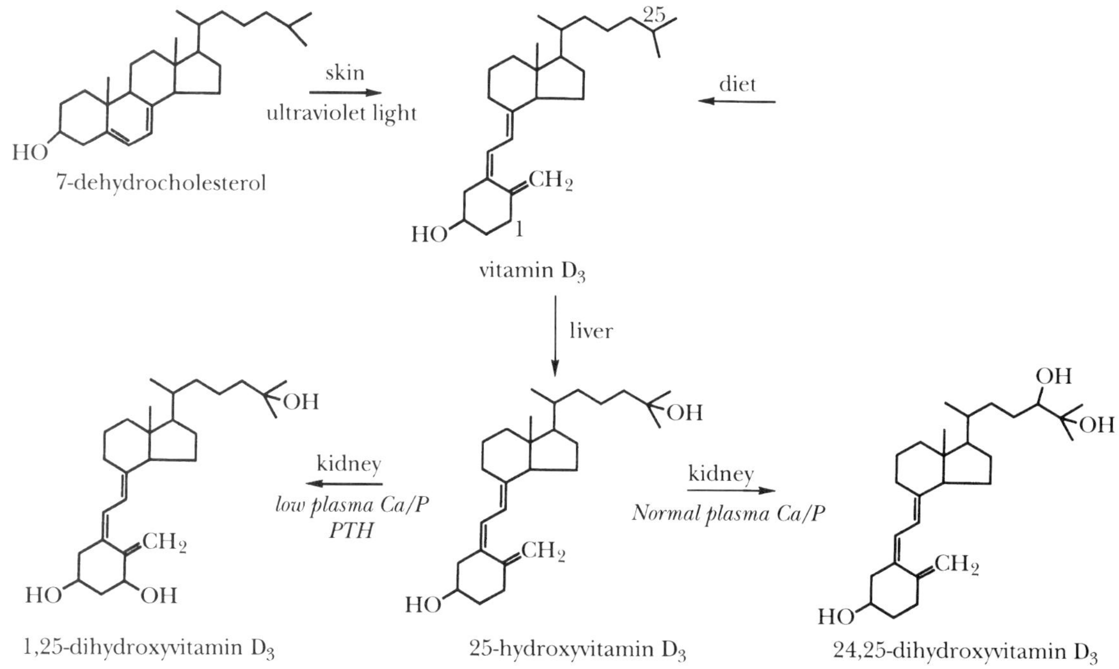

Figure 7 *Major pathways in the metabolism of vitamin D: PTH, parathyroid hormone; Ca/P, calcium/phosphate*

remodeling, like osteocalcin[43]. The symptoms of vitamin D deficiency arise when the supply of vitamin D is too low to provide adequate 1,25(OH)$_2$D for these processes, resulting in lack of calcium for bone mineralization.

The concentration of the hormonal metabolite 1,25(OH)$_2$D is tightly regulated, as part of the calcium homeostatic system, by complex feedback mechanisms involving plasma ionized calcium and inorganic phosphate, PTH and 1,25(OH)$_2$D itself. In a vitamin D-replete subject, plasma metabolite concentrations are in the ranges indicated above, and measurement of the activity of renal enzymes shows predominantly 24-hydroxylase with only minimal 1α-hydroxylase activity[35]. In vitamin D deficiency, plasma 24,25(OH)$_2$D concentrations are unmeasurable and only 1α-hydroxylase activity is detectable in renal preparations[44]. The stimulus to this increased 1α-hydroxylase activity in vitamin D deficiency is secondary hyperparathyroidism caused by the associated hypocalcemia; PTH enhances 1α-hydroxylase activity by the receptor-linked adenylate cyclase cascade described above. The 1,25(OH)$_2$D thus formed completes the control loop by promoting intestinal calcium transport and causing a flux in plasma ionized calcium which decreases the secretion of PTH (Figure 4). In addition, 1,25(OH)$_2$D down-regulates synthesis of preproPTH, probably by direct interaction with the PTH gene which contains a vitamin D-responsive element[14]. Within the renal cell 1,25(OH)$_2$D down-regulates the 1α-hydroxylase and up-regulates the 24-hydroxylase possibly by stimulation of a phosphokinase C-mediated pathway[45]. The renal origin of 1,25(OH)$_2$D means that the concentration of the hormone decreases with deteriorating renal function, leading to a condition of acquired vitamin D deficiency.

In some circumstances, synthesis of 1,25 (OH)$_2$D may take place outside the kidney. This may occur in activated macrophages in granulomatous diseases, such as sarcoidosis and tuberculosis, where excessive synthesis can lead to elevated plasma levels of 1,25(OH)$_2$D and to hypercalcemia[46]. Elevation of plasma calcium may occur in a similar way in some patients with lymphoma[47]. In these diseases the production of $1,25(OH)_2D$ is not regulated as in renal cells; the hypercalcemia characteristically occurs after exposure to sunlight, which causes a modest rise in plasma 25(OH)D. This increase in substrate leads to a large increase in $1,25(OH)_2D$, although the high calcium and concomitantly suppressed level of PTH are both factors which in renal cells would down-regulate 1α-hydroxylase activity. It is important to emphasize that under normal circumstances an increase in substrate 25(OH)D does not lead to increased concentrations of $1,25(OH)_2D$, which is maintained within narrow limits. Even in vitamin D intoxication, when levels of 25(OH)D may be increased as much as 40-fold, the rise in plasma $1,25(OH)_2D$ is small by comparison, and the hypercalcemia correlates with the 25(OH)D level[48].

Large increases in plasma $1,25(OH)_2D$ are seen, however, on correction of vitamin D deficiency. The previous lack of $1,25(OH)_2D$ gives rise to hypocalcemia, through failure to absorb dietary calcium and this promotes secondary hyperparathyroidism. This means that when substrate becomes available through treatment, the renal 1α-hydroxylase is up-regulated and 25(OH)D is rapidly turned over to $1,25(OH)_2D$[49]. The speed of this response has given rise to some misinterpretation of assay results in patients with osteomalacia. The bone disease and the biochemical abnormalities of vitamin D deficiency take much longer to resolve than does the restoration of vitamin D metabolite levels, so that samples taken soon after the start of treatment may show apparently normal vitamin D metabolites in association with hypocalcemia (Figure 8). The amount of vitamin D needed to initiate this response is so small (as little as 200 IU or 5 μg per day) that it may even be supplied by a hospital diet without formal treatment[40]. Vitamin D metabolism and vitamin D deficiency have been reviewed by Stanbury and Mawer[39].

Measurement of vitamin D metabolites

The most relevant metabolites to measure, in the majority of cases, are 25(OH)D and $1,25(OH)_2D$. 25(OH)D is usually assayed to investigate possible vitamin D deficiency or vitamin D intoxication. However, since vitamin D deficiency affects the concentration of $1,25(OH)_2D$, it is the practice in our laboratory always to assay 25(OH)D in any sample being assayed for $1,25(OH)_2D$. The indications for measuring these vitamin D metabolites are summarized in Table 6.

Requirements for sample collection are included in Table 4. It should be noted that vitamin D metabolites are extremely unstable chemically and whilst metabolites in serum are protected to a certain extent by binding to their carrier protein, standard solutions are very vulnerable to attack from heat, light or air. Serum samples should always be stored at – 20 °C and standard solutions kept at the same temperature under an inert gas. All methods for vitamin D metabolite analysis require extraction with lipid solvents and deproteinization. Most methods entail further preparation of the sample to eliminate non-specific interference from lipids; this usually takes the form of chromatography or of solid-phase extraction on mini-columns. This elaborate sample preparation necessitates the use of methods to monitor recovery, usually by the addition of the same metabolite labeled with tritium.

25-Hydroxyvitamin D assays

25(OH)D in serum may be measured routinely by RIA, by competitive protein binding assay (CBA) or by high performance liquid chromatography (HPLC) in which the absorbance of the molecule at 265 nm in the ultraviolet region is used to quantify the response. Other methods, theoretically more accurate, such as gas chromatography–mass spectrometry (GC/MS)[59], are not suitable for routine use. The latter technique is useful, however, in that it provides an absolute value which can be applied as a reference standard (see below). The concept of a normal range for 25(OH)D is not strictly applicable except at the extremes when related to vitamin D deficiency or excess. Provided levels are above about 12.5 nmol/l, the upper limit is of no significance up to a maximum of about 160 nmol/l, this being the highest level reported following con-

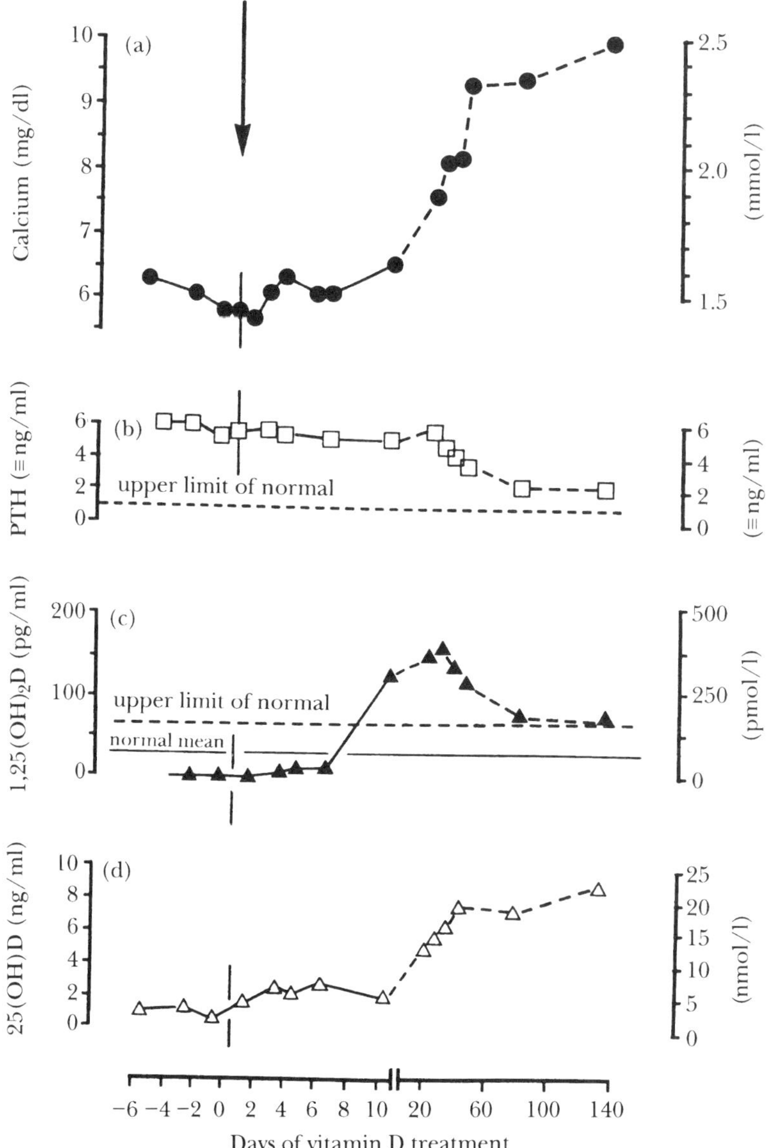

Figure 8 *The response to the treatment of vitamin D deficiency with small doses (200 IU (5 μg) per day) of vitamin D (a) serum calcium, (b) serum parathyroid hormone (PTH), (c) serum 1,25-dihydroxyvitamin D ($1,25(OH)_2D$) and (d) 25-hydroxyvitamin D (25(OH)D)*

tinuous exposure to natural sunlight[60]. Levels are subject to seasonal variation because they depend on exposure to sunlight[61]. Cutaneous vitamin D synthesis is strictly regulated and vitamin D excess arises only from oral overdose. In Britain and most European countries, the skin is the major source of circulating vitamin D as most diets do not supply sufficient to meet the daily requirement of about 400 IU (10 μg)[61].

Radioimmunoassays for 25-hydroxyvitamin D

Most RIA methods require chromatographic purification of the sample and do not recognize

Table 6 *Indications for 1,25-dihydroxyvitamin D (1,25(OH)$_2$D) assays*

Condition	*Effect on vitamin D metabolism*	*1,25(OH)$_2$D assay result*
Differential diagnosis of hypercalcemia		
Primary hyperparathyroidism	excess stimulation of 1,25(OH)$_2$D production*	↑ (→)
Malignancy-associated hypercalcemia (solid tumors)	Hypercalcemia suppresses 1,25(OH)$_2$D† ? inhibitory factor secreted by tumor	↓
Hematological malignancy, e.g. lymphoma (some)	extrarenal synthesis of 1,25(OH)$_2$D	↑
Sarcoidosis, tuberculosis[50]	extrarenal synthesis of 1,25(OH)$_2$D	↑
Vitamin D intoxication	massive increase in 25(OH)D	↑ (→)
Familial hypocalciuria[51]	no known effect	→
Differential diagnosis of hypocalcemia		
Vitamin D deficiency (dietary, lack of sunlight)	insufficient substrate to form 1,25(OH)$_2$D**	↓
Reversal of previous vitamin D deficiency	1,25(OH)$_2$D synthesis driven by ↓ Ca and ↑ PTH	↑ (→)
Renal failure	impaired synthesis of 1,25(OH)$_2$D	↓
Hypoparathyroidism	lack of PTH stimulus to 1,25(OH)$_2$D synthesis	↓ (→)
Pseudohypoparathyroidism	PTH ineffective because of receptor defect	↓ (→)
Oncogenous osteomalacia[52]	some, especially mesenchymal, tumors secrete factor which inhibits 1,25(OH)$_2$D synthesis	↓
X-linked hypophosphatemic rickets[53]	no known effect, but some overlap in diagnosis with oncogenous osteomalacia	→
Vitamin D-dependent rickets type I[54]	inherited defect in 1α-hydroxylase	↓
Vitamin D-dependent rickets type II[55]	inherited defect in vitamin D receptor	↑

NB: References are provided to some rare conditions not discussed in the text.
25(OH)D, 25-hydroxyvitamin D; PTH; parathyroid hormone; * PTH stimulation may be partly offset by raised calcium concentration[56]; † occasional cases have raised 1,25(OH)$_2$D concentration[57,58]; ** during development of vitamin D deficiency there may be a stage with raised 1,25(OH)$_2$D probably due to intermittent secondary hyperparathyroidism

25(OH)D$_2$[62]. One antiserum which does recognize 25(OH)D$_2$ also cross-reacts with vitamin D[63]. An improved RIA for 25(OH)D has recently been reported which employs an iodinated label instead of the tritium normally used[64]; the antiserum, however cross-reacted with most other metabolites. The small range of RIAs reported reflects the relative difficulty of producing good antibodies to the metabolite compared to the ready availability of the vitamin D-binding protein which forms the basis of most CBAs.

Competitive protein binding assays for 25-hydroxyvitamin D The source of the binding protein is usually the vitamin D-binding protein from human or rat serum which can be used at fairly high dilution, 1 : 10 000–1 : 50 000. The supernatant from rat kidney homogenates has also been used[60]. Samples require extraction and chromatographic purification to avoid both non-specific interference and interference from other metabolites (e.g. 24,25(OH)$_2$D, 25,26(OH)$_2$D). Bouillon and co-workers[62] have shown that omitting the chromatographic step increases values by about 20%, although this may not be important in a simple screen to distinguish between vitamin D deficiency and repletion. A few references are provided to the many CBA methods published[65–70] but these have been comprehensively reviewed[71] and details will not be given here. Normal mean 25(OH)D values for CBAs have been reported[72] and range from 8.2 to 100 nmol/l, but as explained above, this variation may relate more to the personal habits of the subjects and to season and latitude than to the characteristics of the method. There is, however, a problem in standardizing assays for vitamin D metabolites, and an evaluation made between different European laboratories has

Table 7 *25-hydroxyvitamin D (25(OH)D) Quality Assurance Scheme: types of assay and methoa-related means (CV%) (reproduced and adapted with the kind permission of Dr G. Carter, Charing Cross Hospital, London, UK)*

	Plasma pool‡			
	A	*B*	*C*	*D*
Type of assay†				
HPLC	16.0	16.0	59.0	50.0
	23.5	23.0	55.0	68.5
	20.0	8.0	28.0	73.0
CPB/RIA without chromatography				
CPB	22.0	55.0	52.0	102.0
[Kit]	*	*	*	–
[Kit]	43.0	78.0	69.0	*
RIA	22.0	55.0	43.0	92.0
	19.5	99.8	53.0	93.5
[Kit]	25.0	84.4	52.9	87.6
[Kit]	*	*	*	*
[Kit]	22.0	84.3	46.8	107.8
CPB/RIA with chromatography				
CPB	15.0	47.0	45.5	79.7
	11.8	10.8	29.0	46.5
	15.0	34.0	48.0	59.0
	12.0	67.0	33.0	61.0
	25.5	22.8	49.3	69.0
	17.0	23.0	45.0	89.0
	*	*	*	–
	9.0	8.0	19.0	38.0
	*	*	*	–
	19.0	20.0	39.0	64.0
	*	*	*	–
RIA	16.0	18.0	33.0	73.0
Method-related means (CV%)				
HPLC (n = 3)	19.8 (18.9)	15.7 (47.9)	47.3 (35.6)	63.8 (19.1)
CPB/RIA				
no chromatography (n = 6)	25.9 (33.6)	76.0 (23.5)	52.8 (16.8)	96.5 (8.4)
chromatography (n = 9)	15.6 (30.7)	27.8 (67.5)	37.9 (26.8)	64.4 (24.5)
Mean of all methods (n = 18)	18.8 (29.5)	40.4 (83.4)	44.5 (27.2)	73.9 (29.0)

HPLC, high pressure liquid chromatography; CPB, competitive protein binding; RIA, radioimmunoassay; †each entry represents a single laboratory, 25(OH)D units are in nmol/l, values greater than 3 SD units from the mean are shown by an asterisk; ‡ plasma pools A, C and D approximate to low, medium and high plasma concentrations of 25(OH)D, pool B is pool A spiked with 26.4 nmol/l of 24,25-dihydroxyvitamin D. (This is a supraphysiological amount but serves to highlight the poor specificity of some assays, particularly those performed without preparative chromatography)

shown widely differing results for the same samples[73,74]. A further comparison has been performed including three kit methods[75], in which accuracy was assessed by reference to GC/MS measurement. Two of the kits tested were very inaccurate by this criterion, as were the results from two service laboratories, although precision was acceptable. An unofficial external quality assessment scheme organized by the North West Thames Quality Assurance and Audit Working Party circulates samples to over 20 laboratories in Britain. An example of the results is given in Table 7 and shows the unsatisfactory performance of several commercial kits and of methods which do not include sample purification.

HPLC assays for 25-hydroxyvitamin D The use of HPLC with ultraviolet quantification provides the best method of measuring $25(OH)D_2$ and $25(OH)D_3$ directly[76,77]. These assays involve the use of a tritiated recovery standard, which means that a recovery correction has to be applied to the HPLC results. A novel method developed in our laboratory[78] overcomes this problem by the use of an ultraviolet-absorbing internal standard which is estimated on the same HPLC run as the samples, thus enabling an automatic correction to be made. HPLC-ultraviolet absorbance assays have the disadvantage of requiring a larger sample than RIA or CBA methods and may potentially suffer from interference by drugs or other compounds. The ability to measure $25(OH)D_2$ and $25(OH)D_3$ separately may on occasion be essential and outweigh these drawbacks. The only other way to achieve separate measurements is by using HPLC in a preparative mode to separate the two forms which can then be assayed individually by CBA.

1,25-Dihydroxyvitamin D assays

The problems posed by the assay of 25(OH)D pale into insignificance in comparison with those for $1,25(OH)_2D$, which is present in plasma at only picomolar concentrations. Methods fall into two categories, those using RIA which necessitates the use of preparative HPLC before performing the assay and those using naturally occurring receptors for $1,25(OH)_2D$. In the latter case, the greater specificity of the receptor, compared to most antisera, means that HPLC is not essential, though extensive sample purification is still required. Receptor methods have the additional advantage of equal cross-reactivity with $1,25(OH)_2D_2$ and $1,25(OH)_2D_3$, a feature shared by few antibodies. The use of C18-reversed-phase cartridges and 'phase-switching' cartridges[79,80] has greatly simplified sample preparation compared with earlier methods which required four chromatographic steps[81]. Normal ranges established with either receptor assays or RIAs are comparable at around 100 pmol/l[82]. Unlike 25(OH)D, values change little with season of the year and there is no established pattern of diurnal variation. The demonstration of changes in $1,25(OH)_2D$ levels depends upon the laboratory establishing sufficiently rigorous standards of precision and accuracy in this notoriously difficult assay[73,75]. Raised values may be expected in up to 50% of cases of primary hyperparathyroidism, or during the correction of vitamin D deficiency (Figure 8), and low values in severe vitamin D deficiency before treatment, in hypoparathyroidism and in renal disease, where $1,25(OH)_2D_3$ levels decrease in parallel with renal function. More details are given in Tables 6 and 8.

Receptor assays for 1,25-dihydroxyvitamin D The introduction of a novel method by Reinhardt

Table 8 *Conditions in which measurement of 25-hydroxyvitamin D (25(OH)D) is essential for interpretation of 1,25-dihydroxyvitamin D (1,25(OH)₂D) assay*

Correction of vitamin D deficiency	rapid increase in $1,25(OH)_2D$ on treatment may mask recognition of previous vitamin D-deficient state unless 25(OH)D is monitored simultaneously
Renal impairment	inability to synthesize $1,25(OH)_2D$ cannot be attributed to loss of renal function unless vitamin D deficiency has been excluded
Primary hyperparathyroidism with coincidental vitamin D deficiency (often normocalcemic)	apparently normal or even low levels of $1,25(OH)_2D$ may result from low concentrations of substrate 25(OH)D. If the condition is recognized then the risk of hypercalcemia can be anticipated when the vitamin D deficiency is corrected

and co-workers[80] has made radioreceptor assays for 1,25$(OH)_2D_3$ much more accessible. The innovation was the use of the receptor from calf thymus, instead of the previously used chick intestinal receptor[85]. The thymus receptor has such high affinity and specificity that interference from other metabolites is virtually eliminated, enabling a less rigorous sample preparation to be employed. Essentially, the method consists of protein precipitation of the serum sample by acetonitrile, an alkali wash to remove lipids and application to a C18 column. The vitamin D metabolites are eluted with acetonitrile and then applied to a silica column from which the 1,25$(OH)_2D$ is eluted for assay using the receptor. This method has been refined and modified in many other laboratories, notably in that of Hollis and Napoli[63] and forms the basis of the commercial kits that are now available. The receptor measures 1,25$(OH)_2D_2$ and 1,25$(OH)_2D_3$ equally, but the individual contributions of each form cannot be measured unless they are first separated by preparative HPLC. An assessment of commercial kits by one laboratory appeared to show poor performance by one manufacturer, but the number of samples examined was small[75]. In a more rigorous survey measuring 70 control samples and 28 pathological samples, the investigators concluded that all three kits tested compared well with the reference method which consisted of HPLC purification followed by thymus receptor assay[86]. Disadvantages of this method are that the receptor is less stable than an antibody and requires batch to batch standardization; purchase in the form of kits is extremely expensive. It is less convenient to combine the receptor assay for 1,25$(OH)_2D$ with a simultaneous measurement of 25(OH)D as can be done readily when HPLC preparation is used.

RIA methods for 1,25-dihydroxyvitamin D Despite the apparent advantages of the receptor assay, several laboratories prefer to use RIA, because of the better long-term reproducibility, the stability of antibodies compared to receptors and the possible interference from high concentrations of other metabolites if HPLC is not used; this may be particularly important for research investigations[82]. Various RIAs have been reported though most have used polyclonal antisera directed against 1,25$(OH)_2D_3$ and have not shown good cross-reactivity with 1,25$(OH)_2D_2$[82,87–91]. We have raised a monoclonal antibody in our laboratory which is sensitive and equipotent for 1,25$(OH)_2D_2$ and 1,25$(OH)_2D_3$, which now forms the basis of our routine assay[92]. This assay is as accurate and precise as most receptor assays with the advantage of a long-term supply of a stable reagent.

Summary

The relevant vitamin D metabolites to assay in serum are 25(OH)D and 1,25$(OH)_2D$. Various RIAs and protein- or receptor-binding assays are available, but all require extraction of the sample together with varying degrees of chromatographic purification.

PARATHYROID HORMONE-RELATED PEPTIDE (PTHrP)

Structure, secretion and functions

This polypeptide hormone was discovered through the systematic attempt by several laboratories to understand the hypercalcemia which, not infrequently, accompanies particular types of cancer. Hypercalcemia as a complication of malignant disease is believed to arise in most cases by one of two mechanisms; local osteolysis, following metastasis of the tumor to bone, or by the secretion by malignant cells of a humoral factor with bone-resorbing activity; in the latter case the condition is usually known as humoral hypercalcemia of malignancy[93]. The fascinating scientific detective work which led to the identification and molecular cloning of the PTH-like factor secreted by certain tumors and subsequently known as PTHrP is outside the scope of this chapter, but the course of this discovery, from the first suggestion by Fuller Albright in 1941[94] that a humoral factor might be involved, is well worth reading[1,93].

Measurement of PTHrP in biological fluids is rendered difficult by the numerous forms and fragments of the molecule which may be present; there is also uncertainty over their biological roles, so that it is not yet clear which molecular moieties should be measured. The tumor types associated classically with humoral hypercalcemia of malignancy are squamous cell carcinomas of skin, lung, head and neck as well as some breast and kidney cancers. Tumor tissue has been used experimentally as the source of messenger RNAs for PTHrP, enabling complementary DNAs to be cloned and the protein sequences deduced. The human gene for PTHrP is located on chromosome 12 and codes for three molecules, which differ in length and amino acid composition at the C terminus, as a result of alternative splicing (Figure 9). The number of molecular forms may also be increased by involving processes such as proteolysis, phosphorylation or *O*-glycosylation. A wide variety of tumor cells and cell lines have been shown to produce PTHrP but the precise relationship between the form of the molecule secreted by the tumor and the relationship with circulating forms is not yet clear[95,96].

In addition to its role in humoral hypercalcemia of malignancy, PTHrP is produced by some normal tissues including skin[97] and smooth muscle[98]. Various adult tissues express messenger RNAs for the hormone[99] and an important role for it has been revealed in maternal–fetal calcium homeostasis[100]. Large amounts are found in milk[101]. It is, however, in relation to humoral hypercalcemia of malignancy that most interest has been shown in measuring PTHrP.

The N terminus of PTHrP shows considerable homology with PTH (Figure 9); eight of the first 13 amino acids are common. PTHrP binds to the same receptors as PTH in classical target organs, stimulating the adenylate cyclase response. In cell systems *in vitro*, using the cyclase assay as an index, PTHrP is considerably less potent than PTH in renal cells, but is equipotent in bone cells[102]. Nevertheless, the renal actions of PTHrP are believed to contribute to the raised plasma calcium in humoral hypercalcemia of malignancy and evidence has been produced for increased renal tubular reabsorption of calcium[103]. Some investigators consider an elevated nephrogenous cAMP level[18] to be an important factor in the definition of humoral hypercalcemia of malignancy[104]. The major component of the increased plasma calcium, though, is that released from bone through enhanced osteoclastic resorption. This is effected in many cases by PTHrP, probably acting through PTH/PTHrP receptors on osteoblastic cells, which may then produce cytokines that promote osteoclastic activity. It should be noted that other bone-resorbing factors besides PTHrP have been identified in tumors and tumor cell lines[105]. The effects of PTHrP on the renal production of $1,25(OH)_2D$ are controversial. PTHrP might be predicted to stimulate synthesis in the same way as PTH, and there is some support for this in animal experiments and in tissue culture preparations. However, patients with humoral hypercalcemia of malignancy and raised levels of PTHrP tend to have suppressed plasma concentrations of $1,25(OH)_2D$. Possible explanations for this include the inhibitory effect of raised renal intracellular calcium on the 1α-hydroxylase (see below) or the specific secretion of a fragment of PTHrP which inhibits the enzyme[106]. The PTH-like actions of PTHrP are associated with the N-terminal region, i.e. residues 1–34, but different regions of the molecule appear to have other biological actions. Small peptides in the region 67–86 have been reported to promote placental transport of calcium[107] and a C-terminal fragment[107–111] appears to inhibit osteoclastic activity[108] (Figure 9).

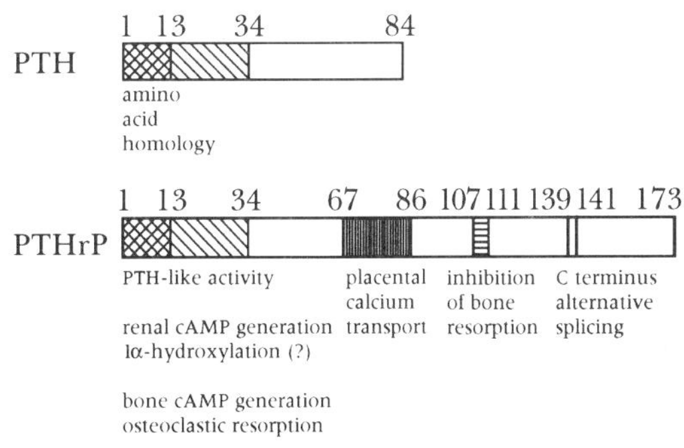

Figure 9 *Diagram of parathyroid hormone-related protein (PTHrP) showing regions of biological activity compared to parathyroid hormone (PTH)*

Measurement of PTHrP

Measurement of PTHrP in plasma may give additional information which is useful in the differential diagnosis of hypercalcemia. In practice, at the present time, measurement is difficult or expensive and sample collection requires careful preparation (see Table 4), so most assays are performed as part of research investigations rather than for routine diagnosis. In addition the range of assay systems is limited, so that only certain parts of the molecule can be measured. Interpretation of results is not straightforward, since this is a rapidly developing field, and concepts are changing as new information becomes available.

Bioassays

In theory PTHrP may be measured in various types of biological assay, many of them employing cells or tissue preparations *in vitro*, and assaying the generation of cAMP or glucose-6-phosphate dehydrogenase activity. Whilst these are useful for scientific investigation in particular laboratories, and indeed, played a seminal role in the discovery of PTHrP[109], they do not have general application.

Immunoassays

N-terminal assays The location of PTH-like biological activity at the N terminus of the PTHrP molecule led logically to the development of N-terminal assays, as being most relevant for understanding the role of the hormone in humoral hypercalcemia of malignancy. Several laboratories have described methods, both RIAs and IRMAs giving generally similar results, and two fairly robust commercial kits have been developed. In all assays for PTHrP it is essential to demonstrate that the antiserum used does not cross-react with PTH or its active fragments, otherwise it would not be possible to discriminate between the hypercalcemia of malignancy and hyperparathyroidism.

N-terminal radioimmunoassays The assay described by Budayr and co-workers[110] used a commercially available polyclonal antiserum to PTHrP 1–34 in an RIA, with ^{125}I-labeled PTHrP 1–34 amide as ligand. This assay had a detection limit of 1.7 pmol/l, normal controls had values below 3 pmol/l and 85% of patients with humoral hypercalcemia of malignancy had raised levels, with a mean of about 6 pmol/l. PTH 1–34 and PTH 1–84 were undetectable in this assay. The drawback was the need to extract the sample, using an affinity column, with the requirement for a 3 ml volume of serum. A non-extraction assay developed in Montreal by Henderson and co-workers[111] using an in-house antiserum to PTHrP 1–34 gave a sensitivity of 50 pmol/l, nevertheless distinction could be made between controls and patients although levels in both groups were elevated with concentrations at least an order of magnitude greater than in most other systems. A particular problem with this assay was the ability to detect considerable immunoactivity in patients with primary hyperparathyroidism despite validation studies showing that PTH 1–34 and PTH 1–84 did not displace bound PTHrP label. Two different RIAs for PTHrP 1–34 developed by Ratcliffe and co-workers[112], one employing extraction from 5 ml of plasma with a monoclonal antibody directed to the region 17–27, the other a directs assay, gave very different results. The direct RIA did not discriminate well between controls and humoral hypercalcemia of malignancy patients giving mean concentrations of 140 and 190 pmol/l respectively; the corresponding values for the extraction assay were 3 and 11 pmol/l. An explanation for the high results obtained in these non-extraction assays may not be found until further information is available on the structures of the different circulating fragments. An RIA reported by Grill and co-workers[113] employed a goat polyclonal antiserum against PTHrP 1–40, [^{125}I Tyr^{0}]-labeled PTHrP 1–34 and PTHrP 1–84 as standard. This assay did not require extraction, had a detection limit of 2 pmol/l with 37 out of 38 control plasmas giving undetectable concentrations and gave values for patients with humoral hypercalcemia of malignancy ranging between 2.8 and 51.2 pmol/l. Interestingly, using this assay, the authors found raised PTHrP levels in some hypercalcemic patients with breast cancer and bone metastases, suggesting that the two perceived mechanisms for hypercalcemia associated with malignant disease, namely local osteolysis and humoral secretion of an osteoclast-stimulating factor, may not be mutually exclusive. A commercial RIA using components very similar to the Grill assay is marketed by Incstar.

N-terminal immunoradiometric assays
Immunoradiometric assays which include the N-terminal end of the molecule are probably the method of choice until a better understanding has been achieved of the different molecular forms in circulation and their biological roles. Such assays have been reported by Burtis and co-workers[96] and Ratcliffe and co-workers[114]. The former uses a capture antibody against PTHrP 37–74 and a signal (labeled) antibody against PTHrP 1–36, whereas in the Ratcliffe assay it is the N-terminal antibody (against PTHrP 1–34) that is bound to a solid phase and used for capture, and 37–67 which is labeled with ^{125}I. Neither assay requires extraction of the sample. Burtis and co-workers found low or undetectable plasma PTHrP 1–74 in control subjects (mean 1.9 pmol/l) and a mean value of 21 pmol/l in patients with humoral hypercalcemia of malignancy, while Ratcliffe's group reported most control values below or close to the limit of detection of 0.23 pmol/l and a mean of 7.4 pmol/l in patients with humoral hypercalcemia of malignancy. Development of a commercially available modification of the Burtis IRMA has been reported by Pandian and co-workers[115] and the results of its application by Fraser and co-workers[116]. The IRMA kit used is supplied by the Nichols Institute.

Mid-region assays Various mid-region RIAs have been reported but results are difficult to interpret because of uncertainty about the nature of the epitope being measured. Ratcliffe and co-workers[112] used an antiserum to PTHrP 37–67 and produced an assay with a detection limit of 57 pmol/l, and values in normal controls of 320 pmol/l which did not differ significantly from those for patients with humoral hypercalcemia of malignancy. Blind's group[117] developed an assay using an antiserum directed against PTHrP 53–84 with 1–86 as standard and label. The limit of detection was 5 pmol/l with a normal range up to 21 pmol/l; 22 out of 27 patients had raised values, median 40 pmol/l. Comparing results from this assay with those for the same samples measured in the Nichols IRMA kit, Blind and co-workers[118] showed that only seven of 16 patients with humoral hypercalcemia of malignancy had raised levels of PTHrP in both assays, emphasizing the likelihood of multiple circulating forms of the hormone. An assay to a small mid-molecular fragment 63–77 has been reported from Sweden[119], but required the use either of immunoextraction or silica-cartridge purification to achieve clear differentiation of patients with humoral hypercalcemia of malignancy.

C-terminal assays Few assays have been developed to the C terminus of the molecule, but this region may well attract more interest in the future because of the reported antiosteoclastic activity of PTHrP 107–111[108]. The Burtis group[101] has developed an assay for PTHrP 109–138 in which control subjects had undetectable levels < 2 pmol/l, but patients with humoral hypercalcemia of malignancy had a mean value of 24 pmol/l and those with chronic renal failure also had elevated concentrations, suggesting that a C-terminal fragment is normally excreted by the kidneys.

Summary

At the present time, PTHrP is most reliably measured using an IRMA which forms a bridge between the N terminus and a mid-molecule region. Such assays produce low (< 2 pmol/l) or undetectable values in controls, and elevated levels in the majority of patients with proven humoral hypercalcemia of malignancy.

References

1. Mundy GR. In: Calcium Homeostasis: Hypercalcaemia and Hypocalcaemia. London: Martin Dunitz, 1990.
2. Parfitt AM. Bone and plasma calcium homeostasis. Bone 1987; 1: 51–8.
3. Varley H, Gowenlock AH, Bell M. Calcium, magnesium, phosphorus and phosphatases. In: Practical Clinical Biochemistry, vol. 1, 5th edn. London: William Heinemann Medical Books Ltd, 1980; 850–77.
4. McClean FC, Hastings AB. The state of calcium in the fluids of the body. J Biol Chem 1935; 108: 285–322.
5. Peacock M, Robertson WG, Nordin BEC. Relation between serum and urine calcium with particular reference to parathyroid activity. Lancet 1969; 1: 384–6.
6. Fisken RA, Heath DA, Somers S, Bold AM. Hypercalcaemia in hospital patients: clinical and diagnostic aspects. Lancet 1981; 1: 202–7.
7. Segre GV, D'Amour P, Hultman A, Potts JT Jr. Effects of hepatectomy, nephrectomy and nephrectomy/uremia on the metabolism of parathyroid hormone in the rat. J Clin Invest 1981; 67: 439–48.
8. Bringhurst FR, Stern AM, Yotts M, Mizrahi N, Segre GV, Potts JT Jr. Peripheral metabolism of parathyroid hormone: fate of biologically active amino-terminus *in vivo*. Am J Physiol 1988; 255: E886–93.
9. Mallette LE. The parathyroid polyhormones: new concepts in the spectrum of peptide hormone action. Endocr Rev 1991; 12: 110–17.
10. Brown EM, Gamba G, Ricardi D, Lombardi M, Butters R, Kifor O, Hediger M, Hebert SB. Cloning, expression and characterization of a G-protein coupled bovine parathyroid Ca^{2+} receptor. J Bone Min Res 1993; 8: S147.
11. Mayer GP, Hurst JG. Sigmoidal relationship between parathyroid hormone secretion rate and plasma calcium concentration in calves. Endocrinology 1978; 102: 1036–42.
12. Boucher A, D'Amour P, Hamel L, Fugère P, Gascon-Barré M, Lepage R, Ste-marie LG. Estrogen replacement decreases the set point of parathyroid hormone stimulation by calcium in normal postmenopausal women. J Clin Endocrinol Metab 1989; 68: 831–6.
13. Large DM, Mawer EB, Davies M. Case report: dystrophic calcification, cataracts and enamel hypoplasia due to long-standing, privational vitamin D deficiency. Metab Bone Dis Rel Res 1984; 5: 212–18.
14. Russell J, Lettieri D, Sherwood LM. Suppression by $1,25(OH)_2D_3$ of transcription of the parathyroid hormone gene. Endocrinology 1986; 119: 2864–6.
15. Demay M, DeLuca H, Kronenberg HM. Identification of sequences in the human parathyroid hormone gene that bind the 1,25 dihydroxyvitamin D_3 receptor. In: Norman AW, Bouillon R, Thomaset M, eds. Vitamin D: Gene Regulation, Structure-Function Analysis and Clinical Application. Berlin New York: Walter de Gruyter, 1991; 34–5.
16. Rude RK, Oldham SB, Singer FR. Functional hypoparathyroidism and parathyroid hormone end-organ resistance in human magnesium deficiency. Clin Endocrinol 1976; 5: 209–44.
17. Watson PH, Hanley DA. Parathyroid hormone: regulation of synthesis and secretion. Clin Invest Med 1993; 16: 58–77.
18. Chase LR, Aurbach GD. Parathyroid functions and the renal excretion of 3′, 5′-adenylic acid. Proc Natl Acad Sci USA 1967; 58: 518–25.
19. Habener JF, Rosenblatt M, Potts JT Jr. Parathyroid hormone: biochemical aspects of biosynthesis, secretion, action and metabolism. Physiol Rev 1984; 64: 985–1053.
20. Levine MA, Eil C, Downs RW Jr, Spiegel AM. Deficient guanine nucleotide regulatory unit activity in cultured fibroblast membranes from patients with pseudohypoparathyroidism type I: a cause of impaired synthesis of 3′,5′-cyclic AMP by intact and broken cells. J Clin Invest 1983; 72: 316–24.
21. Jouishomme H, Whitefield JF, Chakravarthy B, Durkin JP, Gagnon L, Isaacs RJ, MacLean S, Neugebauer W, Willick G, Rixon RH. The protein kinase-C activation domain of the parathyroid hormone. Endocrinology 1992; 130: 53–60.
22. Seitz PK, Nickols GA, Nickols MA, McPherson MB, Cooper CW. Radio-iodinated rat parathyroid hormone-(1–34) binds to its receptor on rat osteosarcoma cells in a manner consistent with two classes of binding site. J Bone Min Res 1990; 5: 353–9.
23. McKee MD, Murray TM. Binding of intact parathyroid hormone to chicken renal plasma membranes: evidence for a second binding site with carboxy-terminal specificity. Endocrinology 1985; 117: 1930–9.
24. Murray TM, Rao IG, Muzaffar SA, Ly H. Human parathyroid hormone carboxyterminal peptide (53–84) stimulates alkaline phosphatase activity in dexamethasone-treated rat osteosarcoma cells *in vitro*. Endocrinology 1989; 124: 1097–9.
25. Lufkin EG, Kao PC, Heath H III. Parathyroid hormone radioimmuno-assays in the differential diagnosis of hypercalcemia due to primary

hyperparathyroidism or malignancy. Ann Int Med 1987; 106: 559–60.
26. Manning RM, Adami S, Papapoulos SE, Gleed JH, Hendy GN, Rosenblatt M, O'Riordan JL. A carboxy-terminal specific assay for human parathyroid hormone. Clin Endocrinol 1981; 15: 439–49.
27. Goltzman D, Gomolin H, DeLean A, Wexler M, Meakins JL. Discordant disappearance of bioactive and immunoreactive parathyroid hormone after parathyroidectomy. J Clin Endocrinol Metab 1984; 58: 70–5.
28. Armitage EK. Parathyrin (parathyroid hormone): metabolism and methods or assay. Clin Chem 1986; 32: 418–24.
29. Blind E, Schmidt-Gayk H, Armbruster FP, Stadler A. Measurement of intact human parathyrin by an extracting two-site immunoradiometric assay. Clin Chem 1987; 33: 1376–81.
30. Nussbaum SR, Zahradnik RJ, Lavigne JR, Brennan GL, Nozawa-Ung K, Kim LY, Keutmann HT, Wang C, Potts JT Jr, Segre GV. Development of a highly sensitive two-site immunoradiometric assay for parathyroid hormone and its clinical utility in evaluation of patients with hypercalcaemia. Clin Chem 1987; 33: 1364–7.
31. Brown RC, Aston JP, Weeks I, Woodhead JS. Circulating intact parathyroid hormone measured by a two-site immunochemiluminometric assay. J Clin Endocrinol Metab 1987; 65: 407–14.
32. Klee GG, Preissner CM, Schryver PG, Taylor RL, Kao PC. Multisite immunochemiluminometric assay for simultaneously measuring whole-molecule and amino-terminal fragments of human parathyrin. Clin Chem 1992; 38: 628–35.
33. Schmidt-Gayk H, Schmitt-Fiebig M, Hitzler W, Armbruster FP, Mayer E. Two homologous radioimmunoassays for parathyrin compared and applied to disorders of calcium metabolism. Clin Chem 1986; 32: 57–62.
34. Mallette LE, Tuma SN, Berger RE, Kirkland J. Radioimmunoassay for the middle region of human parathyroid hormone using an homologous antiserum with a carboxy-terminal fragment of bovine PTH as radioligand. J Clin Endocrinol Metab 1982; 54: 1017–24.
35. Mawer EB, Backhouse J, Hill LF, Lumb GA, DeSilva P, Taylor CM, Stanbury SW. Vitamin D metabolism and parathyroid function in man. Clin Sci Mol Med 1975; 48: 349–65.
36. Stadler A. Homologous radioimmunoassay for human parathyroid hormone (residues 1–34) with biotinylated peptide as tracer. In: Schmidt-Gayk H, Armbruster FP, Bouillon R, eds. Calcium Regulating Hormones, Vitamin D Metabolites, and Cyclic AMP Assays and their Clinical Application. Berlin, Heidelberg, New York: Springer-Verlag, 1990; 137–50.
37. Andress DL, Endre DB, Maloney NA, Kopp JB, Coburn JW, Sherrard DJ. Comparison of parathyroid hormone assays with bone histomorphometry in renal osteodystrophy. J Clin Endocrinol Metab 1986; 63: 1163–9.
38. Reichel H, Koeffler HP, Norman AW. The role of vitamin D endocrine system in health and disease. N Engl J Med 1989; 320: 980–91.
39. Stanbury SW, Mawer EB. Metabolic disturbances in acquired osteomalacia. In: Cohen RD, ed. The Metabolic Basis of Acquired Disease. London: Balliere Tindall, 1990; 1717–82.
40. Mawer EB. Clinical implications of measurements of circulating vitamin D metabolites. In: Avioli LV, Raisz LG, eds. Clinics in Endocrinology and Metabolism. London, Philadelphia, Toronto: WB, Saunders Company Ltd, 9, 1980; Vol. 63–79.
41. Bouillon R, Van Baelen H. Transport of vitamin D: significance of free and total concentrations of the vitamin D metabolites. Calcif Tiss Int 1981; 33: 451–3.
42. Haussler MR, Terpening CM, Komm BS, Whitefield GK, Haussler CA. Vitamin D hormone receptors: structure, regulation and molecular function. In: Norman AW, Schaefer K, Grigoleit H-G, Herrath DV, eds. Vitamin D Molecular, Cellular and Clinical Endocrinology. Berlin, New York: Walter de Gruyter, 1988; 205–14.
43. Haussler MR, Terpening C, Haussler C, MacDonald P, Hsieh J, Jones B, Jurutka P, Meyer J, Komm B, Galligan M, Selznick S, Whitfield GK. A tale of two genes: regulation of rat osteocalcin (BGP) and chick calbindin-D28K by the vitamin D hormone and its nuclear receptor. In: Norman AW, Bouillon R, Thomaset M, eds. Vitamin D: Gene Regulation, Structure-Function Analysis and Clinical Application. Berlin, New York: Walter de Gruyter, 1991; 3–11.
44. Fraser DF. Regulation of the metabolism of vitamin D. Physiol Rev 1980; 60: 551–613
45. Henry HL, Dutta C, Cunningham N, Blanchard R, Penny R, Tang C, Marchetto G, Chou S-Y. The cellular and molecular regulation of $1,25(OH)_2D_3$ production. J Steroid Biochem 1992; 41: 401–7.
46. Adams JS, Singer FR, Gacad MA, Sharma OP, Hayes MJ, Vouros P, Holick MF. Isolation and structural identification of 1,25-dihydroxyvitamin D_3 produced by cultured alveolar macrophages in sarcoidosis. J Clin Endocrinol 1986; 60: 960–6.
47. Davies M, Mawer EB, Hayes ME, Lumb GA. Abnormal vitamin D metabolism in Hodgkin's lymphoma. Lancet 1985; 1: 1186–8.

48. Mawer EB, Hann JT, Berry JL, Davies M. Vitamin D metabolism in patients intoxicated with ergocalciferol. Clin Sci 1985; 68: 135–41.
49. Stanbury SW, Taylor CM, Lumb GA, Mawer EB, Berry JL, Hann J, Wallace J. Formation of vitamin D metabolites following correction of human vitamin D deficiency: observations in patients with nutritional osteomalacia. Min Electrolyte Metab 1981; 5: 212–27.
50. Gkonos PJ, London R, Hendler ED. Hypercalcemia and elevated 1,25-dihydroxyvitamin D levels in a patient with end stage renal disease and active tuberculosis. N Engl J Med 1984; 311: 1683–5.
51. Davies M, Adams PH, Berry JL, Lumb GA, Klimiuk PS, Mawer EB, Wain D. Familial hypocalciuric hypercalcaemia: observations on vitamin D metabolism and parathyroid function. Acta Endocrinol 1983; 104: 210–15.
52. Ryan EA, Reiss E. Oncogenous osteomalacia. Am J Med 1984; 77: 501–12.
53. Davies M, Stanbury SW. The rheumatic manifestations of metabolic bone disease. Clin Rheum Dis 1981; 7: 595–646.
54. Fox J, Maunder EMW, Ranall VA, Care AD. Vitamin D dependent rickets type I in pigs. Clin Sci 1985; 69: 541–8.
55. Marx SJ, Liberman UA, Eil C, Gamblin GT, DeGrange DA, Balsan S. Hereditary resistance to 1,25-dihydroxyvitamin D. Recent Proc Horm Res 1984; 40: 589–620.
56. Lalor BC, Mawer EB, Davies M, Lumb GA, Hunt L, Adams PH. Determinants of the serum concentration of 1,25-dihydroxyvitamin D in primary hyperparathyroidism. Clin Sci 1989; 76: 81–6.
57. Mawer EB, Still PE, Morton AR, Anderson DC. Effects of treatment with the bisphosphonate APD on 1,25-dihydroxyvitamin D in patients with malignant hypercalcaemia. In: Norman AW, Schaefer K, Grigoleit H-G, Herrath DV, eds. Vitamin D Molecular, Cellular and Clinical Endocrinology. Berlin, New York: Walter de Gruyter, 1988; 869–70.
58. Ralston SH, Cowan RA, Robertson AG, Gardiner MD, Boyle IT. Circulating vitamin D metabolites and hypercalcaemia of malignancy. Acta Endocrinol 1984; 106: 556–63.
59. Holmberg I, Kristiansen T, Sturen M. Determination of 25-hydroxyvitamin D in serum by high performance liquid chromatography and isotope dilution mass spectrometry. Scand J Clin Lab Invest 1984; 44: 275–82.
60. Haddad JG, Chyu KJ. Competitive protein binding assay for 25-hydroxycholecalciferol. J Clin Endocrinol Metab 1971; 33: 992–5.
61. Poskitt EME, Cole TJ, Lawson DEM. Diet sunlight and 25(OH)D in healthy children and adults. Br Med J 1979; 1: 221–3.
62. Bouillon R, Van Herck E, Jans I, Tan BK, Van Baelen H, De Moor P. Two direct (nonchromatographic) assays for 25-hydroxyvitamin D. Clin Chem 1984; 30: 1731–6.
63. Hollis BW, Napoli JL. Improved radioimmunoassay for vitamin D and its use in assessing vitamin D status. Clin Chem 1985; 31: 1815–19.
64. Hollis BW, Kamerud JQ, Selvaag SR, Lorenz JD, Napoli JL. Determination of vitamin D status by radioimmunoassay with an ^{125}I-labelled tracer. Clin Chem 1993; 39: 529–33.
65. Belsey R, DeLuca HF, Potts JT Jr. A rapid assay for 25-OH-vitamin D_3 without preparative chromatography. J Clin Endocrinol Metab 1974; 38: 1046–51.
66. Preece MA, O'Riordan JLH, Lawson DEM, Kodicek E. A competitive protein-binding assay for 25-hydroxyvitamin D. Clin Chim Acta 1974; 54: 235–42.
67. Bouillon R, Van Kerkhove P, DeMoor P. Measurement of 25-hydroxyvitamin D_3 in serum. Clin Chem 1976; 22: 364–8.
68. Garcia-Pasqual B, Peytremann A, Courvoisier B, Lawson DEM. A simplified protein-binding assay for 25-hydroxycholecalciferol. Clin Chim Acta 1976; 68: 99–105.
69. Morris JF, Peacock M. Assay of plasma 25-hydroxyvitamin D. Clin Chim Acta 1976; 72: 383–91.
70. Zeghoud F, Jardel A, Guillozo H, Nguyen TM, Garabedian M. Micromethod for the determination of 25-hydroxyvitamin D. In: Norman AW, Bouillon R, Thomaset M, eds. Vitamin D: Gene Regulation, Structure-Function Analysis and Clinical Application. Berlin, New York: Walter de Gruyter, 1991; 662–3
71. Porteous CE, Coldwell RD, Trafford DJH, Makin HLJ. Recent developments in the measurement of vitamin D and its metabolites in human body fluids. J Steroid Biochem 1987; 28: 785–801.
72. Bothe V, Schmidt-Gayk H. Competitive protein-binding assay for the diagnosis of hyper- and hypovitaminosis D. In: Schmidt-Gayk H, Armbruster FP, Bouillon R, eds. Calcium Regulating Hormones, Vitamin D Metabolites, and Cyclic AMP Assays and their Clinical Application. Berlin, Heidelberg, New York: Springer-Verlag, 1990; 258–79.
73. Jongen MJM, Van Ginkel FC, van der Vijgh WGF, Kuiper S, Netelenbos JC, Lips P. An international comparison of vitamin D metabolite measurements. Clin Chem 1984; 30: 399–403.
74. Mayer E. Interlaboratory comparison of calcidiol determination. In: Schmidt-Gayk H, Armbruster FP, Bouillon R, eds. Calcium Regulating Hormones, Vitamin D Metabolites, and Cyclic AMP Assays and their Clinical Application. Berlin Heidelberg, New York: Springer-Verlag, 1990; 286–99.

75. Makin HLJ, Coldwell RD, Trafford DJH. Assays for vitamin D and its metabolites: do we need to improve accuracy and precision? In: Norman AW, Bouillon R, Thomaset M, eds. Vitamin D: Gene Regulation, Structure-Function Analysis and Clinical Application. Berlin, New York: Walter de Gruyter, 1991; 34–5.
76. Jones G. Assay of vitamins D_2 and D_3 and 25-hydroxyvitamins D_2 and D_3 in human plasma by high-performance liquid chromatography. Clin Chem 1978; 24; 287–98.
77. Mayer E, Schmidt-Gayk H. Simultaneous determination of 25-hydroxyvitamin D_2 and 25-hydroxyvitamin D_3 by high performance liquid chromatography. In: Schmidt-Gayk H, Armbruster FP, Bouillon R, eds. Calcium regulating hormones, vitamin D Metabolites, and Cyclic AMP Assays and their Clinical Application. Berlin, Heidelberg, New York: Springer-Verlag, 1990; 247–57.
78. Mawer EB, Hann JT. Rapid automated high-performance liquid chromatographic assay for ercalcidiol and calcidiol (25-hydroxyvitamins D_2 and D_3) using trans-calcidiol as an ultraviolet-absorbing internal standard. J Chromatog Biomed Appl 1987; 415: 305–16.
79. Hollis BW. Assay of circulating 1,25-dihydroxyvitamin D involving a novel single-cartridge extraction and purification procedure. Clin Chem 1986; 32: 2060–3.
80. Reinhardt TA, Horst RL, Orf JW, Hollis BW. A microassay for 1,25-dihydroxyvitamin D not requiring high performance liquid chromatography: application to clinical studies. J Clin Endocrinol Metab 1984; 58: 91–8.
81. Haussler MR, Hughes MR, Pike JW, McCann TA. Radiological receptor assay for 1,25-dihydroxyvitamin D: biochemical, physiologic and clinical applications. In: Norman AW, ed. Vitamin D. Biochemical and Clinical Aspects Related to Calcium Metabolism. Berlin: Walter de Gruyter, 1977; 473–82.
82. Scharla S, Reichel H. A sensitive radioimmunoassay for 1,25-dihydroxyvitamin D_3 (calcitriol) after high-performance liquid chromatography of plasma or serum extracts. In: Schmidt-Gayk H, Armbruster FP, Bouillon R, eds. Calcium Regulating Hormones, Vitamin D Metabolites, and Cyclic AMP Assays and their Clinical Application. Berlin, Heidelberg, New York: Springer-Verlag, 1990; 300–17.
83. Mawer EB, Taylor CM, Backhouse J, Lumb GA, Stanbury SW. Failure of formation of 1,25-dihydroxycholecalciferol in chronic renal insufficiency. Lancet 1973; 1: 626–8.
84. Christiansen C, Christiansen MS, Melsen F, Rødbro P, DeLuca HF. Mineral metabolism in chronic renal failure with special reference to serum concentrations of $1,25(OH)_2D$ and $24,25(OH)_2D$. Clin Nephrol 1981; 15: 18–22.
85. Brumbaugh PF, Haussler DH, Bressler R, Haussler MR. Radioreceptor assay for 1α,25-dihydroxyvitamin D_3. Science 1974; 183: 1089–91.
86. Bertelloni S, Baroncelli GI, Benedetti U, Franchi G, Saggese G. Commercial kits for 1,25-dihydroxyvitamin D compared with a liquid-chromatographic assay. Clin Chem 1993; 39: 1086–8.
87. Bouillon R, De Moor P, Baggiolini EG, Uskokovic MC. A radioimmunoassay for 1,25-dihydroxycholecalciferol. Clin Chem 1980; 26: 562–7.
88. Fraher LJ, Adami S, Clemens TL, Jones G, O'Riordan JLH. Radioimmunoassay of 1,25-dihydroxyvitamin D_2 in man. Clin Endocrinol 1983; 19: 151–66.
89. Scharla S, Schmidt-Gayk H, Reichel H, Mayer E. A sensitive and simplified radioimmunoassay for 1,25-dihydroxyvitamin D_3. Clin Chim Acta 1984; 142: 325–38.
90. De Leenheer AP, Bauwens RM. Radioimmunoassay for 1,25-dihydroxyvitamin D in serum or plasma. Clin Chem 1985; 31: 142–6.
91. Gray TK, McAdoo T, Pool D, Lester GE, Williams ME, Jones G. A modified radioimmunoassay for 1,25-dihydroxycholecalciferol. Clin Chem 1989; 27: 458–63.
92. Mawer EB, Berry JL, Cundall JP, Still PE, White A. A sensitive radioimmunoassay using a monoclonal antibody that is equipotent for ercalcitriol and calcitriol (1,25-dihydroxy vitamin D_2 and D_3). Clin Chim Acta 1990; 190: 199–210.
93. Martin TJ. Parathyroid hormone-related protein [Editorial]. J Int Med 1993; 233: 1–4.
94. Albright F. Case records of the Massachusetts General Hospital (case 27641). N Engl J Med 1941; 225; 789–91.
95. Bowden SJ, Hughes SV, Ratcliffe, WA. Molecular forms of parathyroid hormone-related protein in tumours and biological fluids. Clin Endocrinol 1993; 38: 287–94.
96. Burtis WJ, Fodero JP, Gaich G, Debeyssey M, Stewart AF. Preliminary characterization of circulating amino- and carboxy-terminal fragments of parathyroid hormone-related peptide in humoral hypercalcaemia of malignancy. J Clin Endocrinol Metab 1992; 75: 1110–14.
97. Danks JA, Ebeling PR, Hayman J, Chou ST, Moseley JM, Dunlop J, Kemp BE, Martin TJ. Parathyroid hormone-related protein of cancer: immunohistochemical localization in cancers and in normal skin. J Bone Min Res 1989; 4: 273–8.
98. Kramer S, Reynolds FM, Castillo M, Valenzuela DM, Thorikay M, Sorvillo JM. Immunological identification and distribution of parathyroid hormone-like protein polypeptides in normal

and malignant tissues. Endocrinology 1991; 128: 1927–37.
99. Thiede MA. Expression and regulation of the parathyroid hormone-related protein gene in tumors and normal tissues. In: Halloran BP, Nissenson RA, eds. Parathyroid Hormone-Related Protein: Normal Physiology and Its Role in Cancer. Florida, Boca Raton: CRC Press, 1992; 57–91.
100. Rodda CP, Kubota M, Heath JA, Ebeling PR, Moseley JM, Care AD, Caple IW, Martin TJ. Evidence for a novel parathyroid hormone-related protein in fetal lamb parathyroid glands and sheep placenta: comparisons with a similar protein implicated in humoral hypercalcaemia of malignancy. J Endocrinol 1988; 117: 261–71.
101. Burtis WJ, Brady TG, Orloff JJ, Ersbak JB, Warrell RP, Olson BR, Wu TL, Mitnick ME, Broadus AE, Stewart AF. Immunochemical characterization of circulating parathyroid hormone-related protein in patients with humoral hypercalcaemia of cancer. N Engl J Med 1990; 322: 1106–12.
102. Orlof JJ, Wu TL, Stewart AF. Parathyroid-like proteins: biochemical responses and receptor interactions. Endocrinol Rev 1989; 10: 476–495.
103. Ralston SH, Fogelman I, Gardiner MD, Boyle IT. Relative contribution of humoral and metastatic factors to the pathogenesis of hypercalcaemia in malignancy. Br Med J 1984; 288: 1405–8.
104. Godsall JW, Burtis WL, Insogna KL, Broadus AE, Stewart AF. Nephrogenous cyclic AMP, adenylate cyclase-stimulating activity and the humoral hypercalcaemia of malignancy. In: Greep RO, ed. Recent Progress in Hormone Research, vol. 42. New York: Academic Press, 1986; 705–50.
105. Martin TJ, Ebeling RP, Rodda CP, Kemp BE. Humoral hypercalcaemia of malignancy: involvement of a novel hormone. Aust NZ J Med 1988; 18: 287–95.
106. Fukomoto S, Matsumoto T, Yamoto H, Kawashima H, Ueyama Y, Tamaoki N, Ogata E. Suppression of serum 1,25-dihydroxyvitamin D in humoral hypercalcaemia of malignancy is caused by elaboration of a factor that inhibits renal 1,25-dihydroxyvitamin D_3 production. Endocrinology 1989; 124: 2057–62.
107. Care AD, Abbas SK, Pickard DW, Barri M, Drinkhill M, Findlay JBC, White IR, Caple IW. Stimulation of ovine placental transport of calcium and magnesium by midmolecule fragments of human parathyroid hormone-related protein. J Expl Physiol 1990; 75: 605–8.
108. Fenton AJ, Kemp BE, Hammonds RG, Mitchellhill K, Moseley JM, Martin TJ, Nicholson GC. A potent inhibitor of osteoclastic bone resorption within a highly conserved pentapeptide region of parathyroid hormone-related protein; PTHrP [107–111]. Endocrinology 1991; 129: 3424–6.
109. Goltzman D, Stewart AF, Broadus AE. Malignancy associated hypercalcaemia: evaluation with a cytochemical bioassay for parathyroid hormone. J Clin Endocrinol Metab 1981; 53: 899–904.
110. Budayr AA, Nissenson RA, Klein RF, Pun KK, Clark OH, Diep D, Arnaud CD, Strewler GJ. Increased serum levels of a parathyroid hormone-like protein in malignancy-associated hypercalcemia. Ann Int Med 1989; 111: 807–12.
111. Henderson JE, Shustik C, Kremer R, Rabbani SA, Hendy GN, Goltzman D. Circulating concentrations of parathyroid hormone-like peptide in malignancy and in hyperparathyroidism. J Bone Min Res 1990; 5: 105–13.
112. Ratcliffe WA, Norbury S, Stott RA, Heath DA, Ratcliffe JG. Immunoreactivity of plasma parathyrin-related peptide: three region-specific radioimmunoassays and a two site immunoradiometric assay compared. Clin Chem 1991; 37: 1781–7.
113. Grill V, Ho P, Body JJ, Johanson N, Lee SC, Kukreja SC, Moseley JM, Martin TJ. Parathyroid hormone-related protein: elevated levels in both humoral hypercalcaemia of malignancy and hypercalcaemia complicating metastatic breast cancer. J Clin Endocrinol Metab 1991; 73: 1309–15.
114. Ratcliffe WA, Norbury S, Heath DA, Ratcliffe JG. Development and validation of an immunoradiometric assay of parathyrin-related protein in unextracted plasma. Clin Chem 1991; 37: 678–85.
115. Pandian MR, Morgan CH, Carlton E, Segre GV. Modified immunoradiometric assay of parathyroid hormone-related protein: clinical application in the differential diagnosis of hypercalcaemia. Clin Chem 1992; 38: 282–8.
116. Fraser WD, Robinson J, Lawton R, Durham B, Gallacher SJ, Boyle IT, Beastell GH, Logue FC. Clinical and laboratory studies of a new immunoradiometric assay of parathyroid hormone-related protein. Clin Chem 1993; 39: 414–19.
117. Blind E, Raue F, Götzmann J, Schmidt-Gayk H, Kohl B, Zeigler R. Circulating levels of midregional parathyroid hormone-related protein in hypercalcaemia of malignancy. Clin Endocrinol 1992; 37: 290–7.
118. Blind E, Raue F, Meinel T, Bucher M, Manegold C, Ebert W, Vogt-Moykopf I, Zeigler R. Levels of parathyroid hormone-related protein in hypercalcaemia of malignancy: comparison of midregional radioimmunoassay and two-site immunoradiometric assay. Clin Invest 1993; 71: 31–6.

119. Bucht E, Eklund A, Toss G, Lewensohn R, Granberg B, Sjöstedt U, Eddeland R, Tørring O. Parathyroid hormone-related peptide, measured by a midmolecule radioimmunoassay, in various hypercalcaemic and normocalcaemic conditions. Acta Endocrinol 1992; 127: 294–300.

Bone histomorphometry

6

A. J. Freemont

INTRODUCTION

As interest in bone and its diseases has increased, so too has the perceived need for the quantitation of skeletal elements[1]. The major aim of quantitation is to identify and enumerate changes in bone turnover that lead to, and characterize, disorders of the skeleton[2]. There are numerous ways in which quantitative data on bone can be obtained[3,4], but the increasing realization that bone is not just an inert matrix, but a dynamic structure controlled by complex cellular interactions has stressed the need to develop techniques capable of examining both matrix and cell function, ideally *in vivo*.

The only practical way of studying both cell function and matrix in a single exercise is by the examination of tissue sections of bone. Quantitative data derived in this way have given rise to the 'science' of bone histomorphometry.

Bone consists of two major components – a hard, calcified tissue in close association with a soft, variably cellular bone marrow. For accurate quantitation it is necessary to preserve this relationship. As a consequence, before it became practicable to study bone histomorphometrically, it proved necessary to develop new methods for processing and sectioning bone in its natural (undecalcified) state, new methods for obtaining bone samples and novel types of measuring systems[5,6]. In this chapter these aspects of bone histomorphometry and others will be discussed.

Bone biopsy

Most histomorphometry is performed on actively remodeling bone which, until recently, has meant that studies have concentrated largely on cancellous or trabecular bone[7]. For practical reasons of accessibility and patient safety, the ilium has become the preferred site of biopsy. It is possible to select biopsy sites because most of the diseases investigated histomorphometrically affect the whole skeleton. Comparative studies of postmortem samples taken from the iliac bone, rib, vertebral body and proximal tibial metaphysis have shown that the activity of cells in these different sites is very similar in these generalized (metabolic) bone diseases. The ilium is preferred because of its proximity to the surface, and therefore ease of biopsy, and because it is a relatively constantly loaded bone and is therefore not susceptible to changes in cellular activity and bone mass caused by altered weight bearing, one of the external factors known to influence bone[8].

As intellectual and technical sophistication have increased, so too has interest in Haversian cortical, periosteal and subcortical bone[9]. It is fortunate that for the study of these areas of bone the iliac crest has also proven to be a very suitable biopsy site.

The iliac crest biopsy is usually obtained with a trephine 5–10 mm in diameter[10] (Figure 1). Periosteal surfaces contain pain fibers and therefore taking a trephine biopsy could be very painful. By advancing a long needle percutaneously over the iliac crest the inner, or pelvic surface, of the ilium is anesthetized. The outer surface is then anesthetized and an incision made in the skin over the iliac crest 2 cm below and 2 cm behind the anterior superior spine. A trephine is used to obtain a core of bone incorporating both cortices and the intervening trabecular bone and marrow. A biopsy core of this size is usually removed painlessly and provides adequate amounts of tissue for histomorphometric analysis.

It is important to obtain the biopsy from a consistent site as differences in histomorphometric measurements of matrix have been obtained from different sites in the same ilium. Studies have shown that biopsies removed from identical positions in the two iliac bones are comparable histomorphometrically and the side from which the biopsy is taken is immaterial. It should be noted, however, that local disease such as osteoarthritis of the hip, and even a transiliac biopsy obtained within the preceding 5 years, can significantly alter histomorphometric values.

Section preparation

Various methods of preparing and staining histological sections of bone are available. As will be seen later, many histomorphometric parameters are absolute measurements or ratios of similar geometric features. At different stages in the processing of tissue from the unfixed state to the stained and mounted section, artefacts can be introduced which lead to shrinkage, expansion, compression and stretching which may alter the size and shape of structures within the biopsy. Histomorphometry requires that every effort is made to prevent this happening, and if it does to standardize the artefact (Figure 2).

Undecalcified sections are mandatory for accurate measurement. By leaving bone in its undecalcified state it is possible to assess how much of the matrix osteoid is mineralized and an extra dimension can be added to bone histomorphometry – that of dynamic measurements[11]. Dynamic parameters are assessed after the patient has been given a tetracyline-based fluorochrome at two intervals prior to biopsy[12,13].

Tetracycline labeling

Tetracycline has properties that make it a very valuable tool of the histomorphometrist. It binds to bone matrix, but only where osteoid is actively mineralizing; unbound tetracycline is cleared from the body fairly rapidly in the urine; finally it can be visualized by virtue of being a fluorochrome capable of converting ultraviolet energy into visible light in the yellow and yellow/green part of the spectrum. Thus, if a single dose of tetracycline is given to a patient prior to biopsy, an unstained section viewed in ultraviolet light will show the sites of active mineralization at the time the tetracycline was given as single yellow or yellow/green lines. If a second dose is given within a reasonable time the subsequent biopsy, when viewed in ultraviolet light will show, in some areas, two yellow lines in parallel. Knowing the interval between doses of tetracycline and measuring the distance between the lines allows the rate of mineralization to be determined and from this, other parameters can be derived (Figure 3).

To obtain the crispest lines and prevent the patient developing the nausea associated with

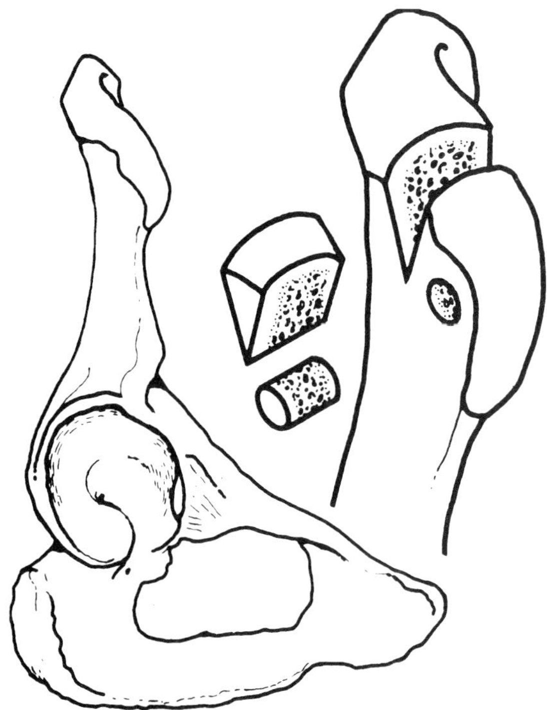

Figure 1 *Diagrammatic representation of the ilium and iliac crest showing the site of a wedge and transiliac core biopsy*

Note: Figures 2, 3, 4, 5, 8 and 9 appear on page 89

taking large doses of the drug, our patients, with normal renal function, receive a regimen of 10–15 mg/kg of tetracycline in two divided doses over the course of 24 h and a further dose regimen 10 days later. The second regimen is given 4 days before biopsy.

To interpret the staining patterns it is essential to know that the patient has absorbed the drug. Because tetracycline is excreted in the urine it will make the urine fluoresce. This can only happen if the drug has been taken, absorbed through the bowel and then excreted by the kidneys. We take a specimen of urine the morning after each dose regimen and examine it by ultraviolet fluorometry to identify the specific wavelength of tetracycline. This establishes that the tetracycline has been absorbed. We also take a specimen the morning before each dose regimen which eliminates the possibility that post-treatment fluorescence is due to another naturally occurring or ingested fluorochrome.

Fixation

Once the biopsy has been taken it is immersed in absolute ethanol. This fixative is used as it can be certain that it contains no acid with the potential of decalcifying the bone. In addition, because it is not aqueous any crystals present within the bone marrrow will be preserved.

Embedding and sectioning

Once the specimen has been received in the laboratory it is processed for sectioning in its undecalcified state. This requires embedding in a hard, relatively non-brittle medium[14]. We use a methylmethacrylate resin supplemented with polyethylene glycol distearate to improve its resilience. Others use different resins. Whatever the resin used, the principle is to achieve an unstressed polymer of the same 'hardness' as bone that will not distort the tissue or be so brittle that it shatters. It is also essential that the resin polymerization reaction does not spontaneously become exothermic. We achieve these objectives by polymerizing our resin at 60 °C in anoxic conditions at 3 atmospheres pressure. To minimize stress on the polymer as it forms, polymerization is carried out in a square-shaped container.

Accurate and reproducible sectioning of tissue embedded in this way requires the use of a powered microtome. Sections for staining are usually cut at 7–8 µm. The optimum thickness for viewing in ultraviolet light to detect tetracycline fluorescence is 15 µm.

Staining

Hematoxylin and eosin can be used for staining the sections. This combination of dyes is very good for detecting cytological detail; however, it is more usual to employ, as standard, stains that unlike hematoxylin and eosin can differentiate between mineralized and non-mineralized matrix, as well as showing good cellular detail. The most important matrix parameter is the state of mineralization. For this the gold standard is von Kossa's stain which detects mineralized matrix by demonstrating phosphate ions. It is usual to counterstain the von Kossa with either toluidine blue or neutral red to demonstrate non-mineralized matrix and cells. Toluidine blue on its own is another stain in regular use. For histomorphometry, trichrome techniques usually give the greatest color contrast between those elements of the tissue in which the histomorphometrist is most interested – osteoid, mineralized bone and cells – thus allowing the optimum use of automated computerized histomorphometric equipment. Of these, the most commonly employed is Goldner's modification of Masson's trichrome stain (Figure 4).

Tetracycline labeling is far superior to any *in vitro* method for the detection of bone mineralization. However, the toluidine blue stain made up in a solution containing ethylenediaminetetraacetic acid is said to give a deeper blue coloration at mineralizing interfaces between osteoid and mineralized bone (Figure 5). Solachrome cyanin and cobalt nitrate stains are also said to detect calcification fronts.

A closely related chemical to solachrome cyanin is solachrome azurine, a stain of great value in demonstrating aluminium in bone, a metal important in the genesis of bone disease in patients with renal failure[15]. Osteoclasts and osteoblasts can be identified by their morphology and relationship to bone surfaces. If it is necessary they can also be demonstrated by their staining reaction with acid and alkaline phosphatase, respectively.

Histomorphometric methodology

Stained tissue sections should be regarded as a single snapshot of cells and matrix at the time the biopsy was taken. As such, any measurements derived from them are 'static'. Tetracycline double-labeling can be used to derive 'dynamic' measurements which give information about the state of the bone during much of the 2 weeks prior to biopsy. A longer term dynamic assessment of the bone can only be made by taking serial biopsies at intervals.

Static measurements

Static measurements are number, length and area. The clinically useful static parameters define number and (as far as possible) activity of osteoblasts and osteoclasts, and the physical state of the matrix. There are many measured and derived static parameters. They do not, necessarily, all measure different aspects of cell activity or matrix structure, but by examining them as a group it is possible to piece together a picture of the bone and its cells. For instance, information on osteoclast function can be obtained by measuring the proportion of the surface of the bone that has been eroded by osteoclasts, the proportion of the surface covered by osteoclasts, the number of osteoclasts, or the depth of the Howship's lacunae the cells have resorbed. Each is important in isolation but taken together a clear overview of osteoclastic resorption can be obtained.

Measuring static parameters

Static measurements may be obtained either manually or automatically. The usual way of manually extracting histomorphometric information from a tissue section of bone is by using an eyepiece graticule, although other methods such as projecting an image of the tissue section onto a grid marked on a screen have been employed. The principle of the eyepiece graticule is that an etched piece of glass strategically positioned in the eyepiece of the microscope can be superimposed on the microscope image of the tissue section. The conventional graticule for bone histomorphometry has a standardized pattern of long parallel lines and much shorter intersecting lines etched on it. The lines and intersects can be used effectively to produce a statistical analysis of number, length and area within the section. One example of such a graticule is the Mertz graticule (Figure 6). This has six regularly spaced sinusoidal lines crossing a square that demarcates the edge of the usable component of the graticule. Each line is intersected by six much shorter lines forming 36 intersects within the area of the graticule. These 36 preconstructed intersects are used for measuring area. If, for instance, one wished to measure the area of the tissue section occupied by bone, the graticule would be placed so that the 36 intersects overlaid a part of the section. If, then, nine of the 36 were then found to lie over bone, as opposed to marrow, in that particular area of the section bone occupied 9/36 or 25% of the total area (Figure 7). By performing a large number of such observations the error of such a technique is diminished to a point where an accurate measurement of proportional area can be made. The same type of measurement can be performed using an automated image analyzer, except that now either the machine or an operator defines the reference area using a mouse or

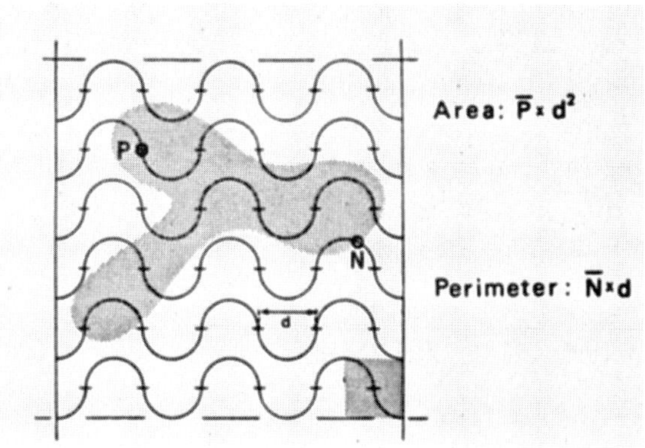

Figure 6 *Diagrammatic representation of a Mertz graticule*

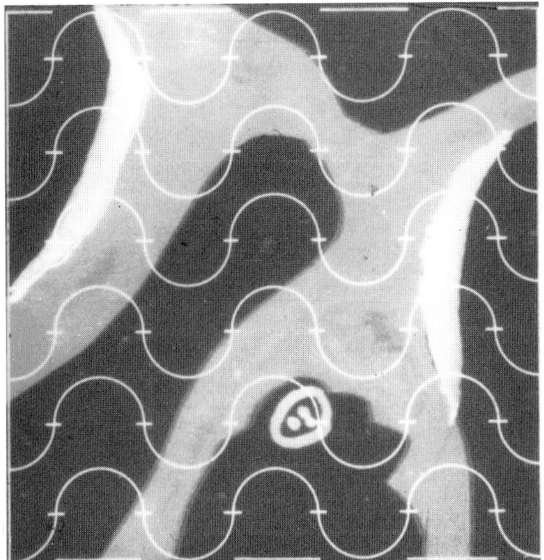

Figure 7 *A Mertz graticule overlying the representation of a tissue section*

a magic pen and then the object area, the proportion is usually calculated automatically. The advantage of the image analyzer is that it removes any errors that come from statistical analysis, and allows the data to be captured directly onto a database which has advantages when it comes to subsequent calculation, particularly of complex-derived functions.

One of the major features of bone histomorphometry is that measurements of area and length are rarely absolute, many being defined relative to another parameter. Microscope magnifications can therefore be selected to suit the user, and absolute calibration is not required. Length is readily measured using an image analyzer, and by storing data, proportional lengths are easily assessed. Because bone surfaces consist of intricately linked complex curves, graticules can only measure proportional length and do so using the same principle as that used in measuring proportional area. In the case of length, the number of times the long lines of the graticule intersect with a surface can be used to calculate proportional length.

Proportional measurements calculated in this way include assessments of the amount of osteoid and bone in the section and the length of surface covered in osteoid, being resorbed and bearing osteoblasts and osteoclasts. Some length measurements are straight lines, and are given in absolute units. They are usually defined between two points either using a calibrated eyepiece graticule or computer-derived two-point analysis. In both cases, it is necessary to calibrate the microscope. This type of measurement is used for measuring the thickness of osteoid, the thickness of a trabecula and the distance between trabeculae.

Two-point measurements are also used for defining the thickness of the individual packets of bone known as basic multicellular units (BMU)[16]. The BMU is a fundamental concept in the understanding of bone histomorphometry. One or more osteoclasts will erode a certain volume of bone. When they have completed their activities, the osteoclasts move away from the bone surface. As osteoclasts eat into bone they cut across the lamellae that characterize normal bone matrix. These are made up of rafts of collagen fibers within which the long axes of the collagen fibers run in the same direction. The lamella pattern comes from the interposition, between rafts with collagen fibers aligned in the same direction, of rafts with their long axes running at right angles. These alternating rafts can be recognized with the light microscope using polarization as alternating dark and light bands within the bone (Figure 8). Each band is a lamella. Polarizing microscopy therefore allows sites of erosion to be recognized as the lamellae, which are laid down with their long axis parallel to the surface, now lying at an angle to the surface, rather like exposed strata of sedimentary rocks at a cliff face. When the osteoclasts leave the bone surface, another as yet undefined cell deposits a thin layer of specialized matrix known as the cement or reversal line on the recently resorbed surface. Osteoblasts then start to deposit matrix, initially in the form of non-mineralized osteoid. When the osteoid 'seams' reach a certain thickness, mineralization is initiated by osteoblasts at the interface between the mineralized bone and osteoid. When the osteoblasts have finished depositing new bone matrix complete mineralization follows. It is this completed piece of new bone that is known as the BMU (Figure 9). Basic multicellular units of different ages are found at bone surfaces, but because of continuing erosive remodeling of bone the oldest usually disappear within a few years of their formation. By studying the size and shape of BMUs, however, it is possible to make some sort of statement about the nature of osteoclastic and osteoblastic activity in the medium-term past. The most important parameter to the histomorphometrist that can be derived from the BMU is the mean thickness of the BMU known as the mean wall thickness. In addition to these absolute linear measurements absolute numbers of osteoblasts and osteoclasts are usually measured.

Dynamic measurements

The last of the important parameters in histomorphometry are measured in tetracycline-labeled unstained sections. There are three and all are length measurements:

(1) The proportion of bone surfaces bearing one or more labels;

(2) The proportion of bone surfaces bearing two labels; and

(3) The mean distance between the two labels.

From these measurements dynamic parameters of bone histomorphometry are derived. They all constitute a measure of the osteoblasts' ability to mineralize bone. In most diseases the rate of mineralization of osteoid is equal to the rate at which osteoid is being formed; this is the principle that allows functions such as the bone formation rate to be calculated.

Normal values

The normal values for the parameters commonly measured are given in Tables 1, 2 and 3 and they are defined in Table 4. Since the report of Parfitt and colleagues[17,18] it has become customary to use a single histomorphometric nomenclature which requires that all data be expressed in three-dimensional terms (surface, volume, and so on). Data are, however, acquired in two-dimensional units (length, area, and so on) and must be converted. As most parameters are expressed as a ratio of the study parameter over a referenced parameter, providing sufficient sections can be examined, conversion of ratios of similar geometric indices (for example, length : length to surface : surface or area : area to volume : volume ratios) poses no problems. Complexity in conversion calculations arises in two circumstances. The first is when the ratios are not of similar geometric indices (i.e. when converting length : area ratios to surface : volume ratios[19]. The second is when the geometry becomes more complex than that of simple straight-sided figures, such as occurs with cylindrical or spherical geometry. There are several trabecular and cortical parameters which fall into this category. Osteoid volume measurement illustrates the problem well. Osteoid is generally deposited on the surface of a saucer-shaped depression, and its volume is best thought of (and calculated as) the difference between segmental portions of two parallel or overlapping spheres. For these more complex conversions mathematical equations are available to aid the numerically challenged, but they require an act of faith that some may find difficult to reconcile.

The most commonly voiced concern to those new to histomorphometry is the apparent complexity and somewhat contrived nature of some of the derived parameters. One example is the activation frequency which represents the rate at which new basic multicellular units are formed. Whilst conceptually simple, the equation from which it is derived is overwhelming:

$$[(1/[(ES/OS) \times (W.Th/Aj.AR)] + [W.Th/Aj.AR] + [(BS - \{ES + OS\} + OS)FP]]$$

where ES/OS = eroded surface/osteoid surface; W.Th = wall thickness; Aj.AR = adjusted apposition rate; BS = total bone surface; ES, eroded surface; OS, osteoid surface; FP, formation period.

Most histomorphometrists adopt a pragmatic approach, acknowledging the correctness of the formula, accepting the need to derive the measurement and understanding its significance.

The time-honored and widely used measured and derived parameters are listed in Table 4

Table 1 *Static trabecular histomorphometry of normal men and women*

		Age (years)						
Numbers of patients		*16–30* *M 3/F 4*	*31–40* *M 5/F 5*	*41–50* *M 6/F 8*	*51–60* *M 6/F 10*	*61–70* *M 5/F 10*	*71–80* *M 5/F 8*	*> 81* *M 3/F 6*
MARt (μm/day)	M	0.64 (0.12)	0.63 (0.34)	0.62 (0.19)	0.53 (0.19)	0.59 (0.20)	0.58 (0.12)	0.56 (0.19)
	F	0.63 (0.14)	0.63 (0.18)	0.61 (0.11)	0.57 (0.23)	0.56 (0.21)	0.49 (0.13)	0.52 (0.17)
MARc (μm/day)	M	0.74 (0.27)	0.76 (0.21)	0.74 (0.31)	0.73 (0.21)	0.71 (0.32)	0.68 (0.41)	0.67 (0.13)
	F	0.73 (0.19)	0.71 (0.18)	0.75 (0.28)	0.71 (0.23)	0.68 (0.12)	0.62 (0.21)	0.60 (0.13)
BFR/BV (% year) (dLs + ½sLs)	M	25.4 (8.9)	25.3 (14.9)	24.8 (17.6)	23.7 (9.9)	20.2 (16.5)	22.5 (12.4)	21.1 (7.9)
	F	25.3 (7.6)	26.1 (17.1)	25.2 (16.5)	22.5 (10.5)	18.3 (11.9)	17.9 (5.2)	16.9 (9.0)
BFR/BS ($\mu m^3/\mu\ m^2$/year) (dLs + ½sLs)	M	1.6 (0.4)	1.5 (1.0)	1.4 (0.6)	1.8 (0.6)	1.2 (0.6)	1.4 (0.3)	1.4 (0.5)
	F	1.6 (0.4)	1.6 (0.7)	1.8 (1.0)	1.3 (0.9)	1.5 (1.2)	1.1 (0.5)	0.9 (0.4)
BFR/TV (% year) (dLs + ½sLs)	M	3.7 (1.5)	4.0 (2.8)	3.6 (2.2)	2.9 (2.7)	3.3 (2.0)	3.1 (2.4)	2.8 (1.6)
	F	3.8 (0.9)	3.8 (1.5)	3.9 (2.3)	2.1 (2.6)	2.7 (2.5)	2.3 (1.9)	2.0 (1.8)
MS/BS (%) (dLs + ½sLs)	M	7.8 (1.9)	7.5 (3.6)	7.4 (3.8)	7.5 (2.1)	7.6 (3.7)	6.9 (1.8)	7.1 (2.9)
	F	7.2 (0.8)	7.4 (2.2)	7.4 (3.7)	7.7 (2.5)	7.2 (4.7)	6.8 (4.1)	6.1 (3.1)
MS/OS (sLs + dLs)	M	79.5 (4.8)	78.4 (12.9)	77.5 (13.4)	79.4 (11.1)	75.8 (15.3)	80.1 (9.2)	76.2 (5.1)
	F	78.0 (5.9)	81.0 (10.9)	79.9 (14.5)	80.1 (15.1)	78.3 (12.6)	77.5 (13.3)	77.0 (13.1)
MSd (dLs/tLs) × 100 (%)	M	62.4 (2.6)	62.5 (7.5)	59.3 (8.4)	57.5 (7.7)	55.4 (9.3)	54.3 (6.4)	52.5 (4.8)
	F	61.1 (2.3)	59.7 (7.6)	58.0 (10.1)	53.4 (11.1)	43.3 (7.4)	45.6 (9.6)	46.6 (6.8)
Aj.AR μm/day $\times 10^{-2}$ (dLs + ½sLs)	M	41.3 (12.4)	38.0 (31.1)	32.4 (26.5)	29.6 (5.5)	27.5 (20.6)	22.5 (13.4)	24.2 (9.8)
	F	34.7 (15.9)	36.2 (24.1)	30.0 (21.5)	27.5 (19.9)	26.6 (8.4)	22.4 (20.3)	22.1 (17.4)
FP (day) W.Th/Aj.AR	M	158.7 (107.5)	184.6 (122.3)	175.4 (86.4)	160.1 (91.8)	179.5 (87.2)	185.2 (83.6)	185.3 (134)
	F	161.7 (88.8)	158.9 (101.6)	190.3 (59.6)	146.2 (126)	168.8 (113)	173.9 (81.7)	191.4 (120)
Ac.f (day) 1 (EP + FP + QP)	M	6.9 (4.0)	6.2 (3.3)	7.4 (4.8)	7.8 (4.2)	7.9 (2.9)	8.3 (5.1)	8.6 (5.2)
	F	5.8 (3.4)	6.2 (3.0)	7.5 (3.6)	6.4 (2.1)	8.1 (4.9)	8.3 (5.1)	7.9 (4.6)
Mlt (day) O.Th/Aj.AR	M	17.6 (7.6)	18.4 (6.3)	17.3 (6.8)	18.9 (5.8)	17.8 (7.3)	19.4 (8.0)	18.0 (4.6)
	F	19.2 (5.7)	16.3 (9.1)	17.5 (7.3)	21.2 (6.8)	20.4 (8.1)	19.5 (6.4)	18.6 (7.3)
E.De (μm)	M	52.1 (28.4)	57.9 (30.6)	49.7 (23.4)	48.1 (15.8)	49.3 (12.6)	48.1 (18.8)	47.4 (26.9)
	F	61.0 (31.1)	56.2 (20.1)	59.3 (30.2)	54.3 (14.6)	50.2 (17.7)	48.6 (22.7)	47.3 (20.4)
ER (mm/year)	M	0.44 (0.19)	0.39 (0.23)	0.52 (0.16)	0.37 (0.21)	0.42 (0.18)	0.36 (0.21)	0.35 (0.17)
	F	0.54 (0.38)	0.38 (0.21)	0.42 (0.19)	0.48 (0.20)	0.40 (0.24)	0.33 (0.15)	0.36 (0.16)
EP (day) (a.ES/OS) × FP	M	134.6 (57.4)	121.7 (81.3)	140.5 (90.8)	118.9 (51.6)	130.6 (62.4)	129.4 (80.1)	101.9 (46.3)
	F	119.7 (65.8)	131.2 (61.1)	122.2 (59.6)	117.3 (53.4)	11.6 (51.8)	108.9 (41.6)	100.1 (70.0)

MARt, mineral apposition rate in trabecular bone; MARc, mineral apposition rate in cortical bone; BFR/BV, bone formation rate of bone volume; BFR/BS, bone formation rate at bone surface; BFR/TV, bone formation rate of tissue volume; MS/BS, mineralizing surface absolute (bone referent); MS/OS, mineralizing surface (osteoid referent); MSd, mineralizing surface (double); Aj.AR, adjusted apposition rate; FP, formation period; Ac.f, activation frequency, W.Th, wall thickness; EP, erosion period; QP, quiescent period; Mlt, mineralization lag time; O.Th, osteoid thickness; E.De, erosion depth; ER, erosion rate; a.ES, active eroded surface; OS, osteoid surface (absolute); dLs, double-labeled surface; sLs, single-labeled surface. Figures in parentheses are standard deviations

Table 2 *Dynamic trabecular histomorphometry of normal men and women*

		Age (years)								
Numbers of patients		*16–20 M 4, *1/ F 4, *1*	*21–30 M 9, *2/ F 10, *3*	*31–40 M 5, *5/ F 9, *5*	*41–50 M 8 *6/ F 14, *8*	*51–60 M 5, *6/ F 14, *10*	*61–70 M 10, *5/ F 20, *10*	*71–80 M 5, *5/ F 9, *8*	*81–90 M 8, *2/ F 6, *4*	*91–100 M 4, *1/ F4, *2*
BV/TV (%)	M	23.1 (4.5)	23.9 (5.0)	22.0 (3.9)	21.9 (5.3)	20.6 (5.2)	19.2 (5.0)	17.7 (4.7)	16.1 (4.6)	15.2 (3.4)
	F	24.1 (5.1)	23.8 (4.7)	22.6 (4.8)	19.9 (6.2)	17.5 (5.8)	16.0 (4.2)	14.6 (5.8)	13.2 (3.8)	11.9 (3.1)
W.Th (μm)	M	51.7 (5.6)	49.8 (5.8)	49.1 (7.3)	45.6 (4.9)	42.3 (5.3)	44.5 (3.7)	37.7 (3.7)	34.8 (2.8)	35.1 (5.9)
	F	52.6 (7.2)	53.2 (4.7)	52.9 (5.9)	48.9 (4.3)	39.7 (3.7)	34.3 (3.8)	32.8 (6.9)	31.3 (3.6)	30.6 (4.7)
OS/BS (%)	M	18.2 (5.7)	16.1 (5.3)	14.0 (4.6)	16.5 (5.4)	17.1 (6.1)	12.4 (4.2)	11.3 (3.3)	10.8 (2.7)	10.1 (3.0)
	F	16.1 (4.8)	16.2 (4.7)	15.3 (3.8)	14.4 (4.1)	12.6 (3.1)	13.1 (4.1)	11.1 (3.6)	11.3 (2.8)	9.2 (2.1)
OS/BV (%)	M	4.3 (2.1)	3.6 (1.9)	3.5 (1.9)	3.1 (1.2)	3.0 (1.6)	2.4 (1.1)	2.7 (1.0)	2.3 (0.7)	2.4 (1.2)
	F	3.0 (1.4)	3.0 (1.0)	3.1 (1.0)	2.9 (1.0)	2.4 (1.1)	1.5 (0.6)	1.7 (0.3)	2.2 (1.0)	2.2 (0.4)
O.Th (μm)	M	9.9 (2.5)	8.6 (3.2)	9.7 (4.6)	9.4 (3.9)	8.7 (2.0)	8.6 (2.5)	8.5 (2.2)	8.5 (1.9)	8.2 (4.4)
	F	9.0 (4.0)	8.7 (3.0)	8.7 (3.0)	8.4 (4.1)	8.2 (3.6)	8.2 (3.7)	8.0 (4.5)	7.6 (3.7)	7.5 (4.2)
ObS/BS (%)	M	5.6 (1.6)	5.4 (2.0)	6.0 (1.1)	5.2 (2.1)	4.6 (1.0)	4.7 (1.1)	4.2 (1.1)	4.5 (1.3)	4.2 (2.1)
	F	6.2 (2.2)	6.0 (2.2)	5.0 (1.6)	5.4 (2.0)	6.0 (1.8)	4.3 (1.8)	4.2 (1.0)	3.9 (0.8)	3.9 (2.1)
ES/BS (%)	M	3.7 (1.6)	3.7 (1.2)	4.5 (1.9)	4.1 (1.8)	3.6 (1.0)	3.5 (1.5)	3.8 (1.5)	3.9 (1.3)	3.5 (1.1)
	F	3.2 (0.8)	4.3 (1.6)	4.1 (1.2)	4.6 (1.8)	4.6 (1.6)	4.4 (2.0)	4.8 (2.0)	5.2 (2.1)	4.8 (2.8)
OcS/BS (%)	M	0.6 (0.3)	0.6 (0.3)	0.6 (0.4)	0.6 (0.2)	0.7 (0.3)	0.7 (0.3)	0.7 (0.5)	0.7 (0.4)	0.7 (0.3)
	F	0.5 (0.2)	0.6 (0.3)	0.5 (0.2)	0.6 (0.5)	0.7 (0.4)	0.8 (0.5)	0.8 (0.6)	0.8 (0.5)	0.8 (0.4)
NOc/TV (/mm^2)	M	5.9 (4.0–21)†	4.8 (0.1–18)†	4.5 (0.2–19)†	4.9 (0.3–20)†	5.3 (0.3–22)†	5.9 (0.4–22)†	5.5 (0.2–24)†	5.6 (0.3–22)†	5.7 (0.4–22)†
	F	5.3 (0.7–20)†	4.5 (0.1–19)†	4.3 (0.2–19)†	5.2 (0.7–21)†	6.1 (0.8–22)†	6.0 (0.8–23)†	6.5 (0.1–26)†	6.9 (1.3–35)†	6.8 (1.2–31)†
Tb.Th (μm)	M	140 (23)	141 (27)	138 (24)	136 (25)	137 (27)	138 (28)	136 (31)	135 (30)	135 (35)
	F	140 (23)	142 (22)	146 (19)	140 (23)	140 (40)	139 (38)	136 (35)	139 (35)	136 (34)
Tb.N (/mm)	M	1.7 (0.4)	1.7 (0.4)	1.7 (0.4)	1.7 (0.4)	1.6 (0.4)	1.5 (0.4)	1.5 (0.4)	1.4 (0.4)	1.4 (0.3)
	F	1.8 (0.5)	1.8 (0.4)	1.7 (0.4)	1.7 (0.4)	1.5 (0.4)	1.4 (0.4)	1.3 (0.3)	1.3 (0.2)	1.2 (0.2)
Tb.Sp (μm)	M	470 (76)	454 (53)	494 (82)	513 (102)	515 (113)	566 (126)	601 (109)	666 (100)	676 (123)
	F	481 (63)	468 (91)	505 (99)	529 (143)	557 (135)	602 (171)	652 (126)	709 (115)	713 (159)

BV/TV, bone volume/tissue volume; W.Th, wall thickness; OS/BS, osteoid surface/bone surface; OS/BV, osteoid surface (absolute)/bone volume; O.Th, osteoid thickness; ObS/BS, Osteoblast surface/bone surface; ES/BS, eroded surface/bone surface; OcS/BS, osteoclast surface/bone surface; NOc/TV, number of oesteoclasts/tissue volume; Tb.Th, trabecular thickness; Tb.N, trabecular number; Tb.Sp, trabecular separation

Table 3 *Static and dynamic cortical histomorphometry of normal men and women*

		Age (years)								
Number of cases		*16–20* *M 5/F 5*	*21–30* *M 11/F 13*	*31–40* *M 10/F 16*	*41–50* *M 14/F 22*	*51–60* *M 11/F 24*	*61–70* *M 15/F 30*	*71–80* *M 10/F 17*	*81–90* *M 10/F 10*	*90–100* *M 5/F 6*
NOc.s (/mm)	M	5.3 (1.2)	2.5 (1.3)	1.3 (0.4)	1.1 (0.5)	1.7 (0.4)	1.6 (0.6)	1.5 (0.7)	2.0 (0.8)	1.6 (0.4)
	F	6.1 (1.4)	2.0 (1.1)	1.6 (0.3)	1.7 (0.6)	1.9 (1.0)	2.1 (1.0)	2.2 (0.9)	3.5 (1.2)	3.1 (1.6)
C.Th (μm)	M	1245 (376)	1276 (434)	1136 (298)	1159 (297)	1303 (348)	1191 (110)	1078 (344)	1117 (398)	1096 (497)
	F	1264 (234)	1303 (348)	1151 (276)	1224 (397)	1151 (210)	1057 (401)	1003 (466)	894 (555)	893 (504)
CV (mm^3)	M	97.6 (2.8)	97.6 (3.1)	95.8 (3.6)	97.3 (2.7)	94.4 (1.0)	93.6 (0.9)	93.4 (4.8)	93.8 (3.6)	93.1 (5.9)
	F	95.4 (4.3)	97.1 (3.2)	96.5 (4.6)	94.4 (5.8)	91.8 (2.9)	89.3 (7.4)	86.5 (6.5)	85.0 (8.4)	83.3 (8.9)
NOc.c (/mm^2)	M	2.0 (0.4)	1.8 (0.6)	2.4 (0.7)	2.5 (1.3)	1.6 (0.9)	2.1 (1.0)	1.8 (0.7)	2.7 (0.9)	2.2 (1.8)
	F	2.5 (0.2)	1.6 (0.9)	2.2 (0.9)	2.7 (1.4)	3.2 (1.8)	3.0 (0.7)	3.2 (0.9)	4.2 (1.8)	3.8 (0.6)
W.Th.c (μm)	M	53.5 (7.0)	54.8 (6.3)	56.1 (8.5)	54.0 (9.9)	50.3 (3.2)	52.7 (10.8)	57.6 (6.5)	47.5 (9.7)	46.5 (9.4)
	F	56.2 (4.7)	55.5 (9.6)	55.7 (6.3)	53.5 (10.1)	50.6 (3.0)	43.5 (6.6)	42.2 (10.4)	47.9 (11.1)	41.1 (5.8)

NOc.s (/mm), number of cortical osteoclasts per mm length of subcortical bone; C.Th, mean cortical thickness from peristem to marrow; CV, volume of cortical bone/volume of total tissue in cortex, NOc.c (/mm^2), number of osteoclasts per square mm of cortical tissue; W.th.c, mean wall thickness of cortical bone packets

Table 4 *List of the parameters measured and derived during normal bone histomorphometry*

MAR = mineral apposition rate
dLs = double-labeled surface
sLs = single-labeled surface
Tb.N = trabecular number
Tb.Th = trabecular thickness
W.Th = wall thickness
TBV = trabecular bone volume
OS/BS = osteoid surface
MARt = mineral apposition rate in trabecular bone
BFR/BS bone formation rate at bone surface
BFR/BV bone formation rate of bone volume
Aj.AR = adjusted apposition rate
Mlt = mineralization lag time
FP = formation period
Ac.f = activation frequency
ES/BS = eroded surface/bone surface
OcS/BS = osteoclast surface
EP = erosion period
C.Th = cortical thickness
CV = cortical volume
W.Th.c = cortical wall thickness
MARc = mineral apposition rate in cortical bone
E.De = erosion depth
a.EP = active erosion period
ER = erosion rate
ES = eroded surface (absolute)
a.ES = active eroded surface
LP = label interval
iLs = interlabel distance
tLs = total label surface
MSc = mineralizing surface (corrected)
MSd = mineralizing surface (double)
MSt = mineralizing surface total (absolute)
MS/BS = mineralizing surface absolute (bone referent)
MS/OS = mineralizing surface (osteoid referent)
NOc.c = number of osteoclasts (cortical)
NOc.t = number of osteoclasts (trabecular)
NOc.s = number of osteoclasts (subcortical)
ObS = osteoblast surface
OcS = osteoclast surface
OS = osteoid surface (absolute)
OS/BS = osteoid surface (relative)
O.Th = osteoid thickness
O.Wi = osteoid width
OV = osteoid volume
QP = quiescent period
QS = quiescent surface
TN = trabecular number
TS = trabecular separation
TV = tissue volume

and are accepted as conveying information of value when considering diagnosis and changes in bone parameters with time and treatment.

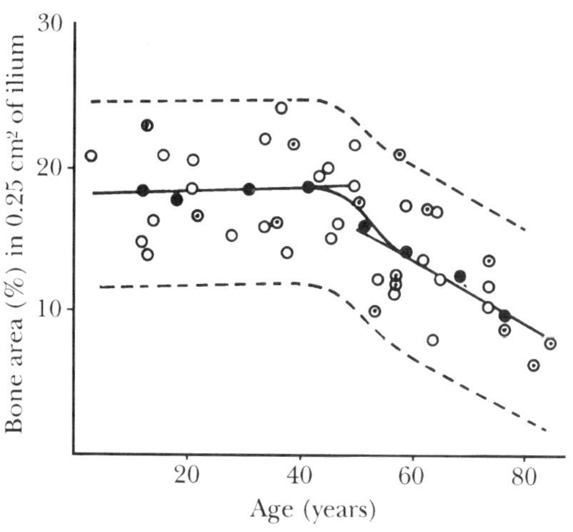

Figure 10 *Graph showing age-related changes in bone volume.* ○, *male;* ⊙, *female*

Normal data are derived from normal individuals but the question of who constitutes a normal person still engenders profound philosophical debate. Bone cells, and therefore their activity, are driven by systemic and local factors that themselves vary with age and sex. In women for instance, osteoblasts are exquisitely sensitive to the hormone estrogen. Osteoblastic activity therefore increases during puberty and falls off following the menopause. As osteoclasis is not affected in the same way, following the menopause an imbalance develops between bone formation and bone loss, with a nett loss of bone (Figure 10). In as much as the menopause is a physiological event, it is normal for women over the age of 50 years to lose bone[20]. Thus, if asymptomatic, apparently normal women are examined, their bone mass fluctuates until adulthood is reached, then plateaus (the peak bone mass[21]) until the perimenopausal years, and falls thereafter. If a woman lives sufficiently long, or if constitutively her bone mass falls unusually quickly, the apparently physiological loss of bone may lead to significant weakening of the bones and a very high risk of fracture. Under these circumstances a physiological change has led to a pathological phenomenon and it is around this argument that the debate on normality revolves. There is no simple answer and, as a consequence, bone histomorphometrists are divided into two camps. The first reports all parameters in relationship to those associated with the peak bone mass (i.e. the mean bone mass of women between 20 and 45 years of age). The second reports everything against age and sex matched controls. Fortunately, it is unnecessary to become embroiled in this argument, so long as the problem is recognized, and the data can be interpreted for what they are.

Quality control and audit

One of the major problems of bone histomorphometry is that, despite every effort, there are no objective ways of measuring many histomorphometric parameters, particularly osteoclast parameters. User definition of features within the biopsy, on the other hand, brings with it the possibility of the introduction of both inter- and intraobserver errors.

It is possible to check for interobserver errors using conventional double-blind tests. However, in many centers more than one histomorphometrist is a luxury that cannot be justified, and therefore bone histomorphometrists tend to work in isolation. Maintaining accuracy and objectivity becomes difficult under these circumstances. In our laboratory 'false' (previously reported) cases are introduced into the weekly reporting schedule. The reporter, ignorant of their nature, reports them subjectively in writing and numerically using bone histomorphometry. The original report and subsequent reports are compared and if the variance is greater than ± 5% the biopsy is painstakingly scrutinized to try to ascertain where a higher than expected variability has been introduced.

It is also our practice in the diagnostic setting that should a second or subsequent biopsy come from a patient previous biopsies will be reanalyzed at the time rather than relying on the numerical data alone. As a final safety measure, cases are discussed with the clinicians looking after the patient at regular intervals. This makes the histomorphometrist justify his/her data and review the data in the light of the clinical information.

Applications

An experienced pathologist is usually able to make diagnoses on bone biopsies on patients with metabolic bone disease without recourse to bone histomorphometry. Inexperienced individuals, however, find histomorphometric data of great value in diagnosis. The true value of bone histomorphometry, however, lies in two other areas. The first is in assessing the extent (rather than the nature) of a bone disorder or a defect in the function of a particular cell type. This is of particular value when deciding on when and how to intervene in the disorder. The second is in assessing changes in bone and bone cell function that occur with time, either as a consequence of disease progression or in assessing response to treatment. This is particularly important in very complex disorders such as the osteodystrophy seen in renal failure.

This is not an appropriate place, nor is there opportunity, for detailing how the various parameters change with disease states, although some are summarized in Table 1 in Chapter 9. As our understanding of metabolic bone disease increases so does the complexity of the patterns of cellular change found in each of the recognized disorders, and even the number and type of disorders themselves increases. To obtain a better understanding of these changes with disease requires accessing data from more detailed accounts than this[22–30].

There are, however, certain fundamental principles that underpin all histomorphometry. Histomorphometric data relate to similarities and differences in the function of two of the bone surface cells (osteoblasts and osteoclasts) and their influence on the nature and amount of bone matrix[31]. Thus, the histomorphometric data must identify whether the two histomorphometrically quantifiable functions of the osteoblast, osteoid formation and osteoid mineralization[32] are occurring and equal and whether osteoblast differentiation from the stem cell pool, crudely assessed by osteoblast number or proportion of the surface covered by osteoblasts, is normal, increased or decreased. Similarly, it must also specify whether osteoclast number and activity are normal, increased or decreased.

It is essential that the data allow an assessment of whether osteoblast and osteoclast activity is coupled. Finally, it is critical that the amount and nature of bone matrix is detailed.

The principles can be illustrated by specific examples. In osteoporosis, bone volume is often very low, osteoblastic activity is generally decreased whilst osteoclastic activity is either normal or increased and clearly bone cell coupling no longer exists[33]. In osteomalacia osteoblastic osteoid formation is usually normal or increased, but mineralization is reduced. Osteoclastic activity is either normal or increased and is coupled with osteoblastic activity. In primary hyperparathyroidism both osteoclastic and osteoblastic activity are increased and coupling is usually present.

Primary hyperparathyroidism is an interesting disorder in this respect in that it occurs primarily in elderly women who may also have an estrogen deficiency. Thus, many patients with primary hyperparathyroidism also have osteoporosis. Although bone loss may be sufficient to cause symptomatic osteopenia in these women with primary hyperparathyroidism, if the cause is analyzed carefully the reduction in bone mass is seen to be as a consequence of the postmenopausal state, not the hyperparathyroidism. This degree of complexity is now being seen in iatrogenic disorders such as the renal osteodystrophies[34–36] and it is in these very complex situations that it becomes so important to detail the disturbances in cell function and matrix structure rather than trying to assign a totally inadequate single term diagnosis to the condition.

The future

Philosophically, bone histomorphometry is flawed. The purpose of the technique is to better understand the changes that underlie bone disease. Many of the parameters are derived from a study of the matrix and yet the primary changes affect bone cells. Matrix changes occur, but are secondary, and often follow the underlying cellular defect by many months or years. A much better way of studying defects of bone cell function would be to examine the cells themselves. Recognition of the cellular defect would facilitate earlier diagnosis and thus more satisfactory intervention. With the advent of *in situ* hybridization[37,38] and quantitative immunohistochemistry, the possibility of examining cells, rather than their effects on the matrix, is now becoming a viable possibility. The introduction of these techniques to the study and diagnosis of bone disease heralds the next, and most exciting, development of the histopathologist's role in the diagnosis and management of metabolic bone disease.

References

1. Rodahl K, Nicholson JT, Brown EM. Bone as a Tissue. New York: McGraw-Hill, 1960.
2. Melson F, Moskilde L. The role of bone biopsy in the diagnosis of metabolic bone disease. Orthoped Clin N Am 1981; 12: 571–602.
3. Engatrom A, Wegstedt L. Equipment for microradiography with soft Roentgen rays. Acta Radiologica 1951; 35: 345–55.
4. Genant HK, Block JE, Steiger P. Appropriate use of bone densitometry. Radiology 1989; 170: 817–22.
5. Weibel ER. Principles and methods for the morphometric study of the lung and other organs Labor Invest 1963; 12: 131–42.
6. Frost HM. Bone histomorphometry: techniques and interpretation. In: Recker RR, ed. Metabolic Bone Disease. Florida: CRS Press Inc, 1983; 109–132.
7. Erikson EF, Hodgson SF, Eastell R, Cedal SL, O'Fallon WM, Riggs BL. Cancellous bone remodelling in type I (postmenopausal) osteoporosis: quantitative assessment of rates of formation, resorption and bone loss at tissue and cellular levels. J Bone Min Res 1990; 5: 311–19.
8. Rubin CT, Lanyon LE. Osteoregulatory nature of mechanical stimuli. Function as a determinant of adaptive remodelling in bone. J Orthopaed Res 1987; 5: 300–10.

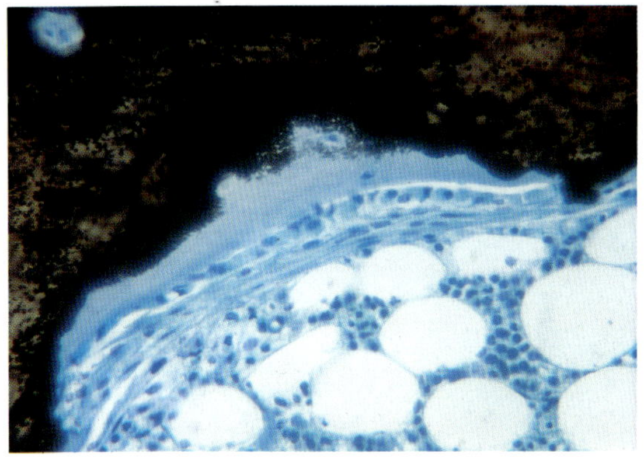

Figure 2 *Von Kossa-stained undecalcified tissue section showing mineralized matrix (black), non-mineralized osteoid (blue) and bone marrow in close aposition*

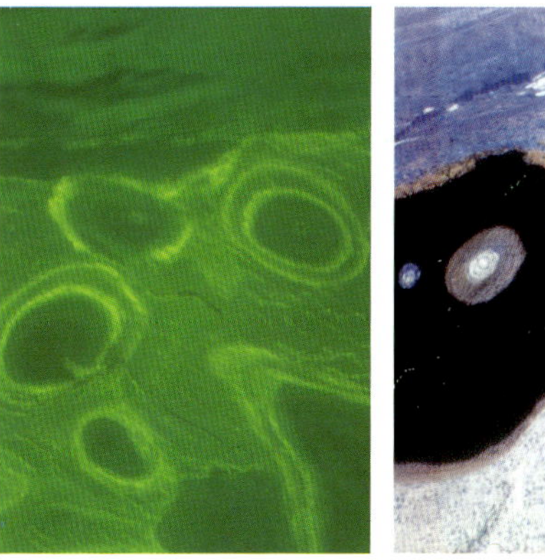

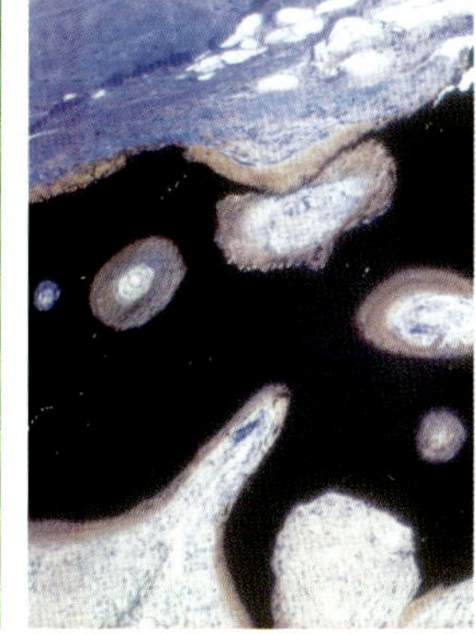

Figure 3 *Two serial sections of bone, one stained with Von Kossa's stain and the other showing double-tetracycline label*

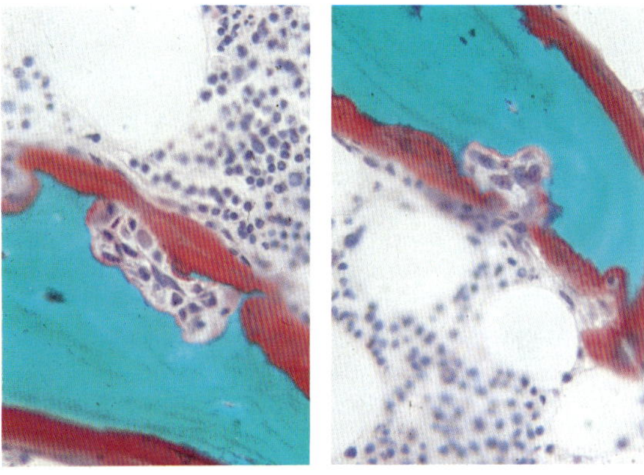

Figure 4 *Goldner's stain. Mineralized bone is green and osteoid red*

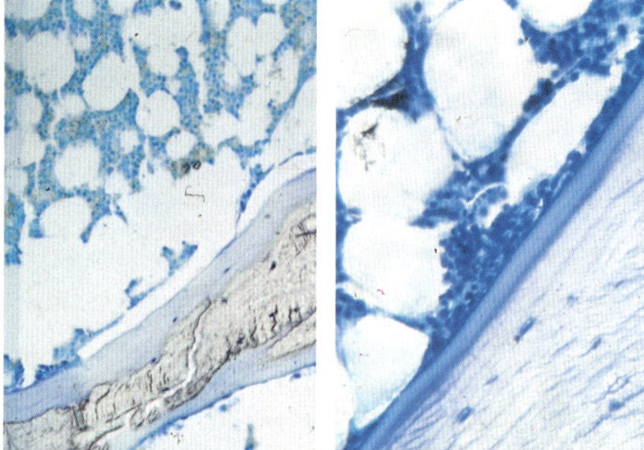

Figure 5 *Two toluidine blue-stained sections. One is from normal bone and shows a dark blue line at the interface between mineralized bone and osteoid. The other is from a patient with vitamin D deficiency in which no such line is visible*

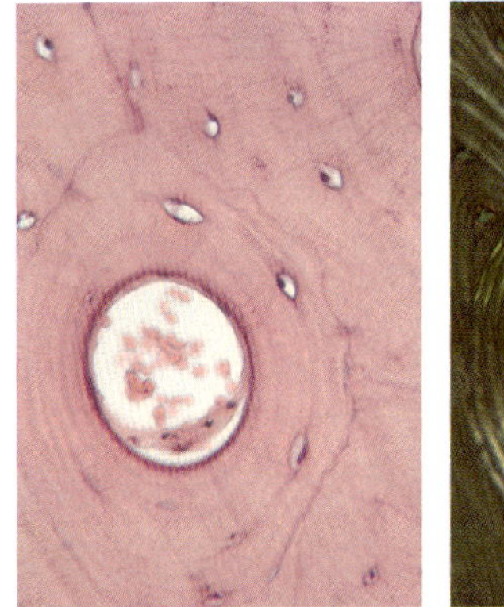

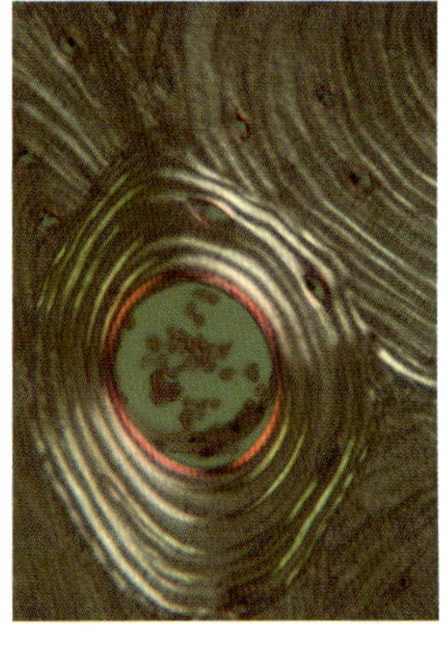

Figure 8 *An Haversian canal stained with hematoxylin and eosin. The lamellar structure of bone is seen using polarizing microscopy*

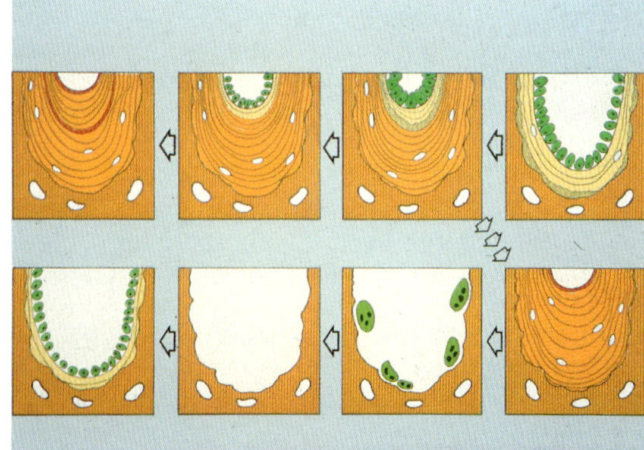

Figure 9 *Diagrammatic representation of the formation of a basic multicellular unit*

9. Christiansen P, Steinech T, Brockstedt H, Mosekilde L, Hessove I, Melsen F. Primary hyperparathyroidism: iliac crest cortical thickness, structure and remodelling evaluated by histomorphometric methods. Bone 1993; 14: 755–62.
10. Lalor B, Freemont AJ, Carlile S. An improved transilial bone biopsy drill for quantitative histomorphometry. Bone 1986; 7: 273–6.
11. Melsen F, Mosekilde L. Dynamic studies of trabecular bone formation and osteoid maturation in normal and certain pathological conditions. Met Bone Dis Rel Res 1978; 1: 45–8.
12. Mosekilde L, Melsen F. A tetracycline based histomorphometric evaluation of bone resorption and turnover in hyperthyroidism and hyperparathyroidism. Acta Med Scand 1978; 204: 97–102.
13. Frost FM. Tetracycline-based histological analysis of bone remodelling. Calc Tiss Res 1969; 3: 211–37.
14. Arnold JS. A method for embedding undecalcified bone for histological sectioning and its application in autoradiography. Science 1951; 114: 178–80.
15. Denton J, Freemont AJ, Ball J. The detection and distribution of aluminium in bone. J Clin Pathol 1984; 37: 136–42.
16. Lips P, Coupron P, Meunier PJ. Mean wall thickness of trabecular bone packets in the human iliac crest: changes with age. Calc Tiss Res 1978; 26: 13–17.
17. Parfitt AM. Bone histomorphometry; proposed system for standardisation of nomenclature, symbols and units. Calc Tiss Int 1988; 42: 284–6.
18. Parfitt AM, Drezner MK, Glorieux FH *et al.* Bone histomorphometry: standardisation of nomenclature, symbols and units. Report of the ASBMR histomorphometry nomenclature committee. J Bone Min Res 1987; 2: 595–610
19. Chalkley HW, Cornfield J, Park H. A method for estimating surface to volume ratios. Science 1949; 110: 295–7.
20. Coupron P, Lepire P, Arlot M, Meunier PJ. Mechanisms underlying the reduction of the mean wall thickness of trabecular bone basic structure unit (BSU) of human iliac bone. In: Jee WS, Parfitt AM, eds. Bone Histomorphometry, 3rd International Workshop. Met Bone Dis Rel Res 1980; 2 (Suppl. 1): 131–46.
21. Burckhardt P, Michel C. The peak bone mass concept. Clin Rheumatol 1989; 8 (Suppl. 2): 16–21.
22. Byers PD, Smith R. Quantitative histology of bone in hyperparathyroidism. Its relation to clinical features, X-ray and biochemistry. Quart J Med 1971; 40: 471–6.
23. Malluche HH, Ritz E, Lange HP, Kutschera J, Hodgson M, Seiffert U, Schoppe W. Bone histology in incipient and advanced renal failure. Kid Int 1976; 9: 355–62.
24. Ellis HA, Pierides AM, Feest TG, Ward MK, Kerr DNS. Histopathology of renal osteodystrophy with particular reference to the effects of 1a-hydroxyvitamin D_3 in patients treated by long-term haemodialysis. Clin Endocrin 1977; 7 (Suppl. 3): 31S–38S.
25. Long RG, Meinhard E, Skinner RK, Varghese Z, Wills MR, Sherlock S. Clinical, biochemical and histological studies of osteomalacia, osteoporosis, and parathyroid function in chronic liver disease. Gut 1978; 19: 85–90.
26. Singer FR, Schiller AL, Pyle EB, Krane SM. Paget's disease of bone. In: Avioli LV, Krane SM, eds. Metabolic Bone Diseases, Vol II. New York: Academic Press, 1978; 489–575.
27. Frame B, Parfitt AM. Osteomalacia: current concepts. Ann Inter Med 1978; 89: 966–82.
28. Davies M, Mawer EB, Freemont AJ. The osteodystrophy of hypervitaminosis D – a metabolic study. Quart J Med 1986; 61: 911–19.
29. Anderson DC, Richardson PJ, Freemont AJ, Cantrill JC. Paget's disease and its treatment with intravenous APD. Adv Endocrinol 1989; 6: 156–64.
30. Rehman MTA, Hoyland JA, Denton J, Freemont AJ. Histomorphometric classification of postmenopausal osteoporosis: implications for the management of osteoporosis. J Clin Pathol 1995; 48: 229–35.
31. Rasmussen H, Bordier P. The Physiological and Cellular Basis of Metabolic Bone Disease. Baltimore: Williams and Williams, 1974;
32. Ellis HA, Peart KM. Quantitative observations on mineralised and non-mineralised bone in the iliac crest. J Clin Pathol 1972; 25: 277–86.
33. Compston JE, Croucher PI. Histomorphometric analysis of trabecular bone remodelling in osteoporosis. Bone Mineral 1991; 14: 91–102.
34. Ellis HA, Peart KM. Azotaemic renal osteodystrophy: a quantitative study on iliac bone. J Clin Pathol 1973; 26: 83–101.
35. Hutchinson AJ, Freemont AJ, Lumb GA, Gokal R. Renal osteodystrophy in CAPD. Adv Periton Dial 1991; 7: 237–9.
36. Hutchinson AJ, Whitehouse RW, Boulton HF, Adams JE, Mawer EB, Freemont AJ, Gokal R. Correlation of bone histology with parathyroid hormone, vitamin D_3 and radiology in end-stage renal disease. Kid Int 1993; 44: 1071–7.
37. Hoyland JA, Hopkinson I, Odedra R, Freemont AJ. Detection of type I collagen mRNA in routine bone biopsies. Matrix 1990; 10: 241–2.
38. Walsh L, Freemont AJ, Hoyland JA. The effect of tissue decalcification on mRNA retention within bone for *in situ* hybridisation studies. Int J Exper Pathol 1993; 74: 237–41.

Radiographic morphometry and photodensitometry

7

F. I. Tovey

Radiographic morphometry although largely historical, in certain situations may still have a useful place in the measurement of bone mass. It has the advantage of its universal application without sophisticated equipment, particularly in places where resources are limited. It has the additional advantage of cheapness, of low radiation doses and of easy availability. The measurements may be qualitative or quantitative.

QUALITATIVE MORPHOMETRY

This depends on the subjective assessment of radiographs taken under standard conditions and has been applied largely to the spine and upper end of the femur. The measurement is relatively insensitive. Andran[1] has shown that 30% of bone has to be lost before radiological changes are apparent and others have given larger percentages[2,3].

Spine

Vertebral density may be assessed from a non-deformed vertebra on a lateral film of the lumbar spine. L_2 is preferred, but L_1 or L_3 may be used. In osteoporosis the horizontal and longitudinal trabeculae are absorbed, but there is compensatory thickening of some of the longitudinal trabeculae giving rise to vertical striation.

These changes can be graded, the highest grade representing normal density.

Grade IV Homogeneously opaque vertebral body, the end plates and cortical shell almost indistinguishable from the body;

Grade III Central portion of the body no longer homogeneous with a faint vertical trabecular pattern and cortical shell clearly seen;

Grade II Relatively translucent vertebral body with marked vertical trabecular pattern; and

Grade I Radiotranslucent vertebral body without any trabecular pattern and ghost-like cortical outline.

When using this grading method it is helpful to have a set of radiographs representing each grade for comparison. It is of particular value to radiologists when assessing a radiograph with a single crushed vertebral body, to know whether it is the result of trauma alone or localized pathology or whether there is an underlying generalized osteopenia.

Other techniques involve an assessment of vertebral deformity. Barnett and Nordin[4] incorporate a spinal score as part of their index. This involves measurement of the middle and the anterior border of the body of the best centered vertebra, usually L_3 (Figure 1).

$$\text{Spinal score} = \frac{\text{Vertical height of middle of vertebral body}}{\text{Vertical height of anterior border}} \times 100$$

If the end plate shows a double contour a tomographic film is clearer for measurement.

Raymakers and co-workers[5] have developed a mathematical model requiring a computer program based on the anterior, central and post-

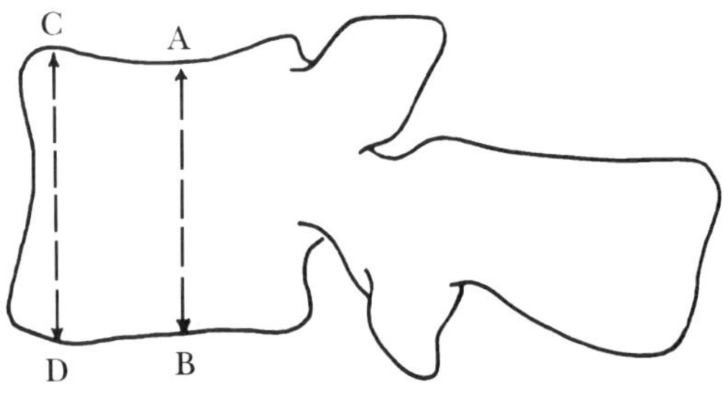

$$\frac{AB}{CD} \times 100 = \text{lumbar spine score}$$

Figure 1 *Barnett and Nordin Index: diagrammatic representation of the measurement and calculation of the spinal score; reproduced with permission from reference 4*

erior heights of the vertebral bodies from T_4 to L_5. The model follows a simple sinusoidal function, from which they obtain a Spine Fracture Index, Vertebral Deforming Events and a Vertebral Deformity Score. These results correlate with estimates of lumbar bone mineral content obtained by dual photon absorptiometry.

The criticism of measurements of vertebral deformity is that central vertebral collapse (codfish deformity) depends on degrees of stress as well as softness of bone[6]. Virtama and colleagues[7] found no relationship between the shape of a vertebral body and the amount of trabecular bone it contained.

Femoral neck

The trabeculae in the upper end of the femur are arranged along lines of compression and tension stresses produced during weight bearing. The trabeculae fall into four major groups according to Singh[8,9] (*see also* Chapter 8).

(1) Principal compressive group: extending from the medial cortex of the shaft in curved radial lines to the upper portion of the head of the femur;

(2) Secondary compressive group: arising from the medial cortex below the above group and curving laterally and upwards towards the greater trochanter and the upper portion of the neck;

(3) Principal tensile group: springing from the lateral cortex below the greater trochanter, curving upwards and inwards across the neck of the femur to the inferior portion of the femoral head; and

(4) Secondary tensile group: arising from the lateral cortex below the principal tensile group, running upwards and medially ending irregularly after crossing the midline.

These enclose an area of thin, loosely arranged trabeculae called Ward's triangle.

Using standard anterior/posterior X-rays of the hip taken with 15° internal rotation Singh describes the following six grades (Figure 2).

Grade 6	All the normal trabecular groups are visible and the upper end of the femur seems completely occupied by cancellous bone;
Grade 5	Accentuation of the principal compressive and tensile trabeculae, Ward's triangle prominent;
Grade 4	Principal tensile trabeculae reduced in number but still visible;
Grade 3	Break in continuity of the principal tensile trabeculae opposite the greater trochanter;
Grade 2	Only the principal compressive trabeculae prominent, the others have been resorbed more or less completely; and
Grade 1	Even the principal compressive trabeculae are markedly reduced in number and no longer prominent.

Grades 1–3 signify osteoporosis.

Singh and co-workers[10] found that the index correlated with axial osteoporosis, but Dequeker and colleagues[11,12] did not find such good correlation, taking vertebral collapse as their index. They also found that external rotation of the hip masked the principal tensile group of trabeculae.

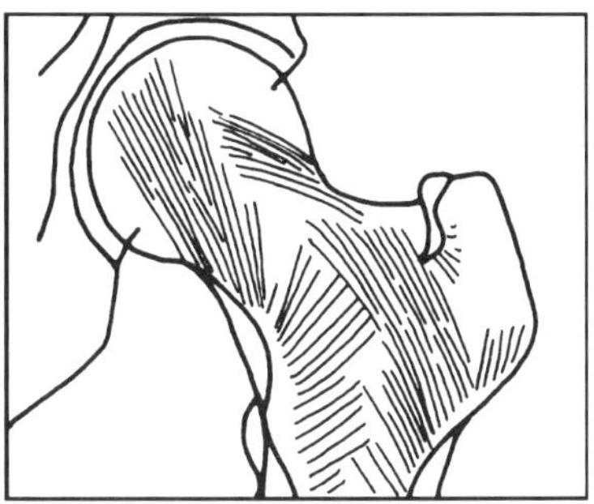

Grade 6
All the normal trabecular groups are visible and the upper end of the femur seems to be completely filled by cancellous bone.

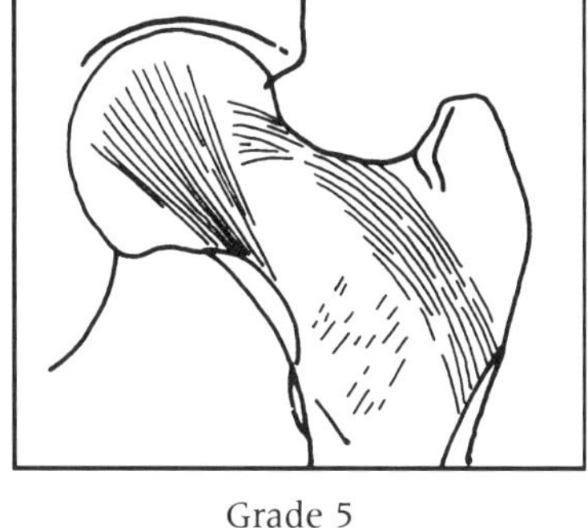

Grade 5
The structure of the principal tensile and compressive trabeculae is accentuated. Ward's triangle appears to be prominent.

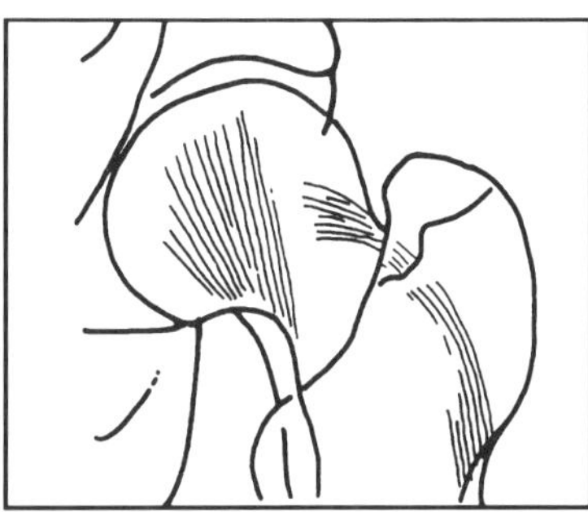

Grade 4
Principal trabeculae are markedly reduced in the number but can still be traced from the lateral cortex to the upper femoral neck.

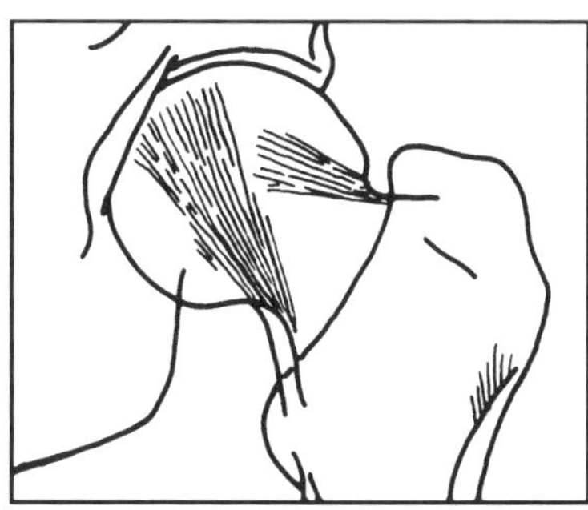

Grade 3
There is a break in the continuity of the principal trabeculae opposite the greater trochanter. This indicates osteoporosis.

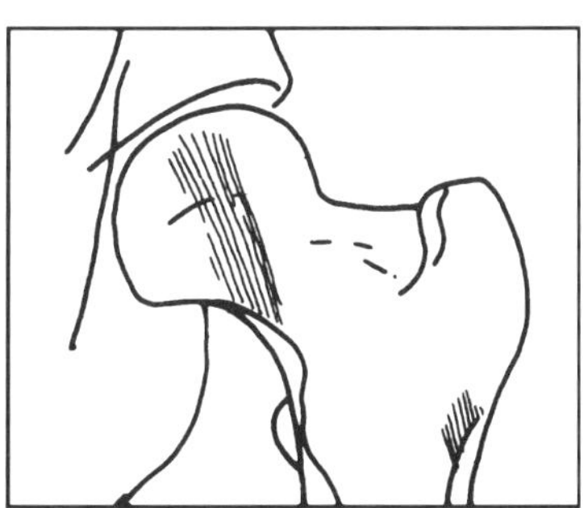

Grade 2
Only the principal compressive trabeculae stand out prominently; the others have been more or less completely resorbed.

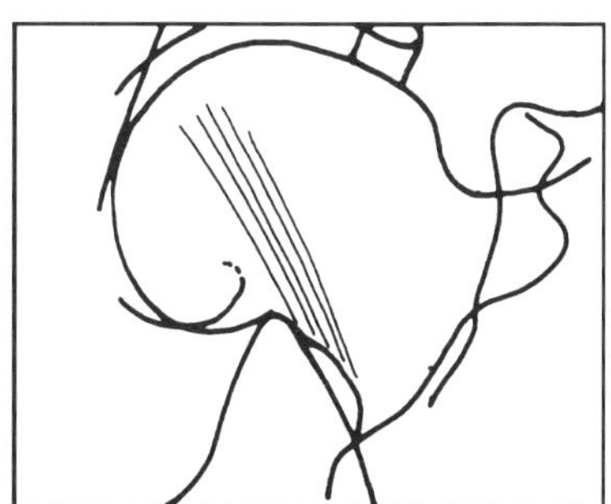

Grade 1
Even the principal compressive trabeculae are markedly reduced in number and no longer prominent.

Figure 2 *The Singh Index shows the relationship of the principal trabecular structures to the degree of osteoporosis; reproduced with permission from reference 8 and Reed Healthcare Communications*[45]

QUANTITATIVE MORPHOMETRY (RADIOGRAMMETRY)

These methods involve the measurement of the cortical bone thickness of various long bones. The bones most frequently used are the metacarpals, particularly the second, but some workers have used the clavicle, the radius, the humerus, the femur and the tibia. Osteoporotic changes develop more slowly in the weight-bearing bones of the lower limb and consequently these are rarely used.

Several indices have been developed based on the assumption that the portion of bone being used for the measurements is circular. Different indices have to be used for the tibia which is triangular in cross-section.

The various indices for cylindrical bones are best illustrated by considering measurements of the second metacarpal.

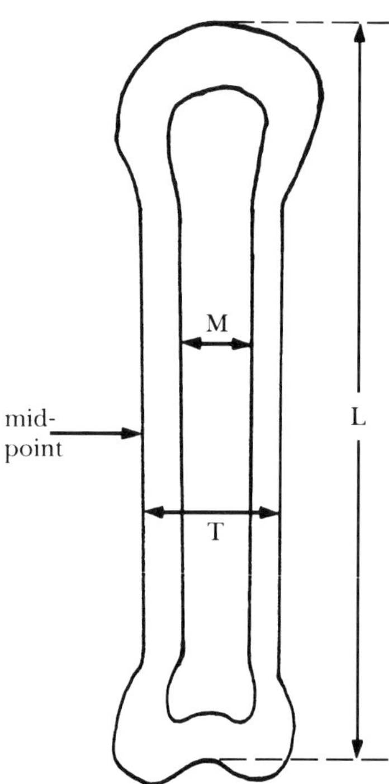

Figure 3 *Measurements for the second metacarpal on the right hand: L = bone length; T = bone thickness; M = medullary width*

The second metacarpal

Technique

Usually the right or dominant hand is used[13], as the measurements of total and medullary width may be greater than with the non-dominant hand. The hand is placed palm down on a cassette containing a fine-grain, non-screen film[14]. The exposure depends on the operator, a typical one being 52 kVp for 0.04 s at a tube current of 500 mA and a tube distance of 1 m[15]. The film is processed using a standard automatic processor. Measurements are made with the film on a horizontal viewing box.

The length of the metacarpal (L) from the apical point of the proximal concavity to the apical point of the distal convexity as shown in Figure 3 is measured with a ruler, and a line is drawn across the bone at right angles to the mid-point. The thickness of the bone (T) and the medullary thickness (M) are measured using a needle point Vernier caliper measuring down to 0.05 mm. An alternative is to use a transparent millimeter rule. Morgan and co-workers[16] maintained that this was as good as a caliper because of the irregularity of the endosteal border which allows an accuracy of only 0.5 mm. Adams and colleagues used a rule with a magnifying eyepiece and 0.1 mm scale, but the magnification may only increase the difficulty of defining the border of the endosteal surface (see later)[13].

Calculations

From the measurements of T and M the following indices can be obtained:

(1) Cortical thickness (C)
$$C = T - M$$

(2) Metacarpal Index (MI)
$$MI = \frac{T - M}{T}$$

(3) The percentage cortical thickness or hand score (HS)
$$HS = MI \times 100$$
(The Barnett & Nordin Index)[4]

(4) The cortical area (CA) (i.e. the cross-section of the walls of a cylinder)
$$CA = \frac{\pi}{4}(T^2 - M^2)$$

(5) The percentage cortical area (%CA)

$$\frac{T^2 - M^2}{T^2} \times 100$$

(6) The Garn Index[17–19]

$$\frac{T^2 - M^2}{T^2}$$

(7) The cortical area/surface area (CA/SA)

$$CA/SA = \frac{CA}{\pi \times T \times L} \text{ or } CA/SA = \frac{T^2 - M^2}{4L \times T}$$

(8) The Exton-Smith Index[20,21]

(a variation in CA/SA) $\frac{T^2 - M^2}{TL}$

The Metacarpal Index (MI) and the Barnett & Nordin Index (HS) are based on the concept that C varies directly with T, and this concept is supported by Adams and co-workers[13]. Morgan and co-workers[16], however, deny this correlation and maintain that C alone is an adequate measurement. By using the squares of T and M the errors due to the difficulty in measuring M are reduced, however a small increase in T may negate a larger increase in M. Cortical area measurements are more sensitive to endosteal resorption and Exton-Smith and colleagues[20,21] found that they gave good correlation with measurements of bone ash. The Cortical Area/Surface Area Index or the Exton-Smith Index aim at correlating for variations in C related to skeletal size. This compensates only partly however for differences in bone size due to skeletal build, gender and ethnic differences (Figure 4). It assumes that the ratio of compact bone/total bone remains the same for different sizes of bone[22], but in fact less compact bone/total bone is required to maintain resistance to flexion in larger bones. Hence, while C, Cortical Area and Cortical Area/Surface Area increase, %Cortical Area decreases with increasing outside diameter. Dequeker[23] found that Cortical Area gave the best correlation with outside diameter when data were divided into strata of skeletal size.

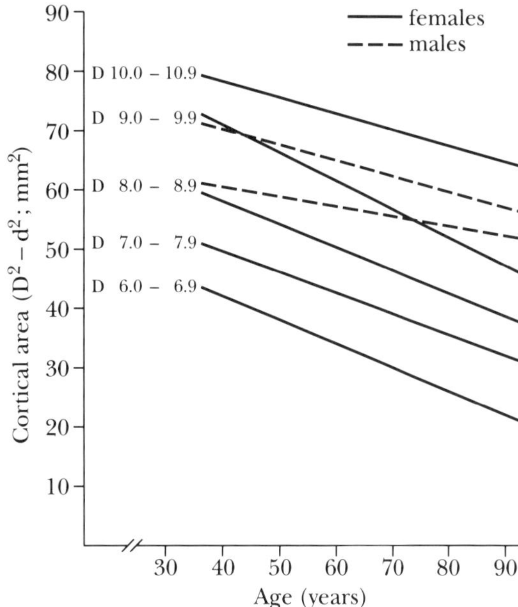

Figure 4 *Regression of cortical area on age according to skeletal size as shown by the bone thickness at the mid-point of the second metacarpal (Belgian women and men): D = bone thickness, d = medullary width; reproduced with permission from reference 22*

Reproducibility

The main difficulty lies in the identification of the endosteal border. This is often irregular and indefinite due to areas of bone resorption. These areas of bone resorption should be ignored and solid cortex only should be measured. Individual observers adopt their own criteria for defining the border which must be adhered to consistently to obtain reproducibility.

According to Garn[19] the measuring error using a caliper is between ± 0.10 and 0.15 mm, which means that only changes of ± 0.30 mm are meaningful. The error is greater in the measurement of M. When the bone is small, this may amount to 10%, and for an average sized bone with a medullary width of 3–5 mm it is 2–5%.

Adams and co-workers[13] gave the error for T as 2–4% and for M as 8–11% in a series of measurements in elderly women. Comparing one and two observers Naor and co-workers[15] found that the range of accuracy for measurements of Cortical Index was 10% in the former and 6% in the latter.

Dequeker and Johnston[24] give an overall coefficient of variation (SD/Average mean) in cortical thickness measurements of the second metacarpel of 3%, requiring a difference in readings of 6% to be meaningful. Their intraobserver coefficient for T and M was 1.2% and 4.8% respectively and for interobserver variation was 1.5% and 6.4%[25]. Interobserver error tends to be larger than intraobserver error, but this becomes less with experience and agreement with regards to criteria in the identification of the endosteal border. Adams and co-workers gave the figures as follows: C, 8–11% and 8–10%; T, 2–4% and 2–4% and the Barnett & Nordin Index (C/T × 100), 8–11% and 8–10% for interobserver error and intraobserver error respectively.

In conclusion, if the average overall measuring error for cortical thickness is taken as 8% and the average annual rate of bone loss between 40 and 80 years of age is taken as 0.9% for women and 0.4% for men, then many years would be required in a longitudinal study to detect individual changes[22].

Multiple metacarpal measurements

Horsman and Simpson[14] showed that the coefficient of variation could be reduced to 1.3% by taking the mean of the cortical width measurements of the second, third and fourth metacarpals of both hands. The fifth metacarpal was omitted because its endosteal surface tends to be irregular. The method is unsuitable for patients with brachydactyly or an XO syndrome. Both hands are X-rayed on the same film. To minimize error the mid-points of the metacarpals, taking the halfway point between the metaphyses, were marked on the first films in the series and subsequent films were superimposed to ensure identical points for measurement.

Table 1 from Dequeker[25] compares the coefficients of variation in the observations of one observer in measurements of a single (second) metacarpal and of six metacarpals using three films of the same hands taken on the same day in six postmenopausal women.

Other bones

The radius

Measurements are made of the proximal end of the radius just distal to the tuberosity. Radiographs may be taken with the hand supinated and a vertical beam, or using a horizontal beam with the hand supinated and with the arm in an L-shaped wooden frame which supports the cassette on the lateral side in a vertical position. The latter has the advantage of a reduced radius/film distance (Figure 5). The cortices are measured at a site where the periosteal and endosteal lines become parallel.

Meema and Meema[26] used the minimum combined cortical thickness as a means of correction for skeletal size (Figure 6). The diameter (d) of the head of the radius is measured and a site 2.5 × d distal to the capitulum humeri is chosen on the radiograph. From this point pro-

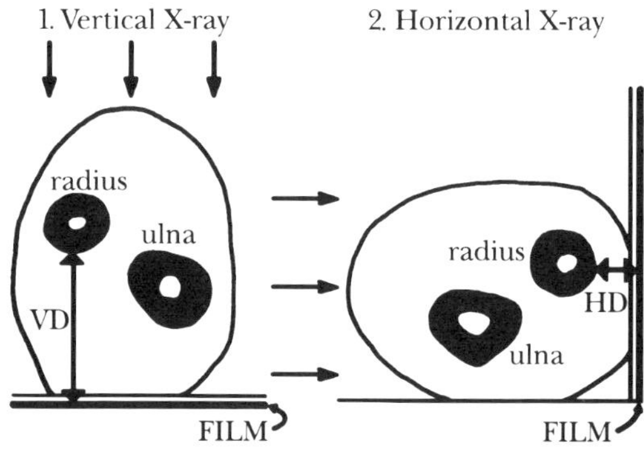

Figure 5 *Lateral projections of supinated forearm showing distance of the proximal radius from the X-ray film is greater with a vertical beam (VD) than with a horizontal beam (HD); reproduced with permission from reference 34*

Table 1 *Comparison of coefficients of variation between measurements obtained at one metacarpal (second) and in six metacarpals; reproduced with permission from reference 25*

	Second metacarpal	*Six metacarpals*
Periosteal diameter (D)	1.68 ± 0.60	0.82 ± 0.37
Endosteal diameter (d)	3.77 ± 2.16	2.23 ± 1.27
Cortical thickness (D – d)	3.09 ± 1.65	1.29 ± 0.40
% cortical thickness (D – d/D)	2.23 ± 1.03	0.91 ± 0.14

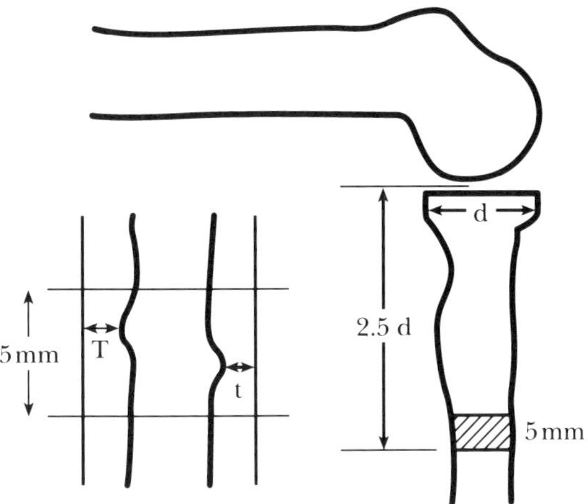

T + t = minimal cortical thickness of radius

Figure 6 *The site of measurement of the minimum combined cortical thickness of the radius and the measurement of the minimum combined cortical thickness of the radius when intracortical resorption is visible*[26]

ximally a zone 5 mm long is marked on the radiograph. The smallest cortical thickness within the zone is measured on each side. Where bone resorption is present only solid cortex is measured. The minimum combined cortical thickness is the sum of the two measurements. They have found this to be the most sensitive parameter of bone loss in both sexes.

Early bone loss may occur first in either the second metacarpal or the radius and Meema and Meema[27] accordingly recommend combining both measurements.

Humerus

The lower end of the humerus can be included and measured at the same time if the horizontal X-ray beam technique is used for the radius. The cortical thickness is again measured where the outlines of the bone become parallel. The measurement of cortical thickness is combined with that of the radius to give the combined cortical thickness (Figure 7).

Clavicle

This has the advantage that measurements of the mid-shaft can be made on routine posterior/anterior chest radiographs. These have been tabulated for a normal Finnish population[28,29].

Femur

An anterior/posterior film is used avoiding superimposition of the linea aspera on the cortex. Osteoporotic changes occur later in weight-bearing bones and for this reason many avoid using the femur. Barnett and Nordin measured C and the external width (T) at the mid-shaft and expressed the results as a score: $(C/T) \times 100$.

Tibia

At mid-shaft this is triangular in cross-section and the formula for cortical area is $[\sqrt{3}(T^2 - M^2)]/4$ or $0.43\,(T^2 - M^2)$ which for per cent cortical area is simplified to $100[(T^2 - M^2)/T^2]$.

Normal ranges

Normal ranges need to take into account variations due to age, sex, race and skeletal size. Virtama and Helelä[28] have prepared extensive tables (215 pages in number) from Finland of measurements of cortical thickness of the clavicle, of the right and left proximal and distal humerus, the radius, ulna, second, third and fourth metacarpals and proximal phalanges, femur, tibia, fibula and the second and third metatarsals between the ages of 1 and 90 years.

Garn[19] and co-workers[30] have prepared tables of the measurements of the second metacarpals for American Black and White males and females and for Mexican Americans of both sexes. They have also broken down the latter into populations from Guatemala, El Salvador, Honduras, Nicaragua, Costa Rica and Panama.

Meema[31] published a table of the mean combined cortical thickness of the upper end of the radius for a population of Canadian women (Figure 8). Meema and Meema also prepared graphs showing the corresponding cortical thicknesses of the upper radius and lower humerus[26] (Figure 9) for men and women.

One of the most useful graphs is that of the Exton-Smith Index $[(T^2 - M^2)/TL]$ showing the values of the different percentiles for sex and

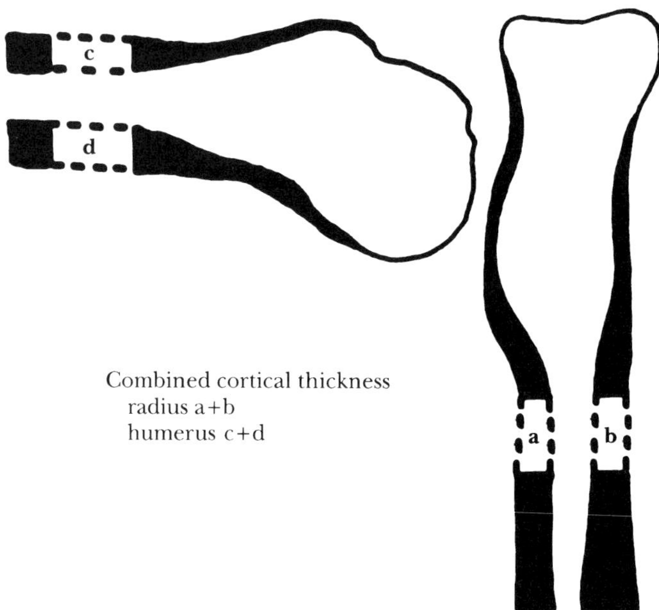

Figure 7 *Sites of measurement of the cortical thickness in the proximal radius (a and b) and distal humerus (c and d). Normal ranges in males and females of 21–45 years are 5–10 mm and 5–8 mm for radius and 7–15 mm and 7–12 mm for the humerus, respectively; reproduced with permission from references 27 and 34*

age. Figures 10a and b are taken from actual graphs personally used by Exton-Smith in 1969. Between the ages of 50 and 80 there is an average bone loss of 7% for women and of 5% for men per decade[32].

The Barnett and Nordin Combined Score

Barnett and Nordin[4] combined the Femoral and Hand Score Indices ([T – M)/T] 100) with the Spinal Score (*vide supra*) obtained from measurements of lateral film of the lumbar spine centered on L3. They regarded the following as evidence of osteoporosis: Spinal Score ≤ 80; Femoral Score + Hand Score (Peripheral Score) ≤ 88; and Total Score ≤ 168.

Later, Nordin and co-workers[33] reported that biconcavity did not increase in postmenopausal women correspondingly with loss of vertebral density thus questioning the value of the combined score.

MAGNIFICATION RADIOGRAMMETRY

For the estimation of intracortical Haversian absorption a magnification technique is required because of the small width of the normal resorption spaces (200 – 400 μm). It is also suitable for measuring subperiosteal resorption. Two methods are available: optical and radiographic[34].

Optical

This requires a fine-grain radiographic film permitting magnifications of × 4–5 or higher. These films are slow and require longer exposure times, so the method is only suitable for small parts such as the hands or feet. Different techniques can be used:

(1) Photographic magnification on film or paper; this is time-consuming and expensive and is used mostly for demonstration purposes;

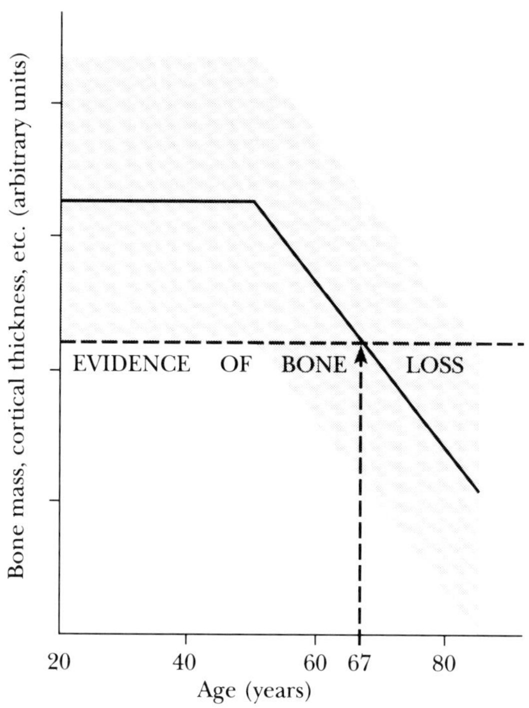

Figure 8 *Pattern of age-dependent bone loss in the proximal radial shaft in normal women; shaded area indicates ± 2 SD. Similar patterns have been described for the metacarpal and humeral shafts; reproduced with permission from reference 46*

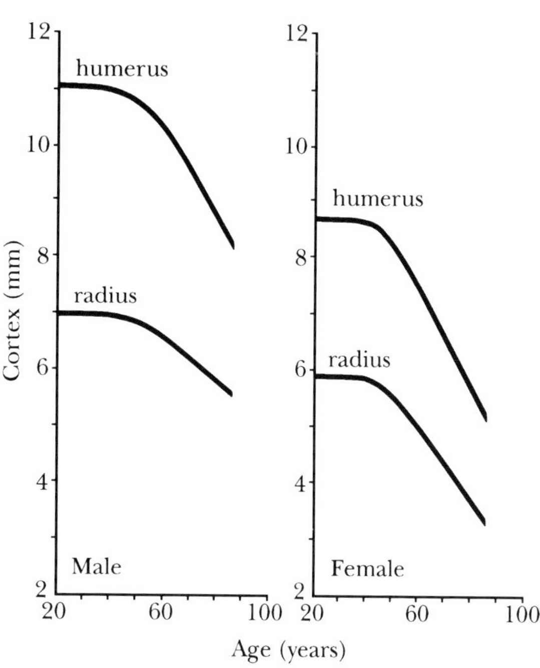

Figure 9 *Comparison of four mean curves for the normal combined cortical thickness, of the humerus and radius; reproduced with permission from reference 27*

(2) Projection magnification; this results in loss of definition; or

(3) Microradioscopy; the radiograph is either examined microscopically with a × 7–20 magnification, or by a magnifying eyepiece or loupe with a built-in millimeter scale using a standard X-ray Illuminator.

Radiographic

By increasing the distance of the object from the film a × 3–4 magnification can be obtained. The technique requires a microfocus tube and extra large film. It can be applied to thicker parts other than the hands or feet.

Assessment

The assessments can be by a semiquantitative grading or by quantitative measurements.

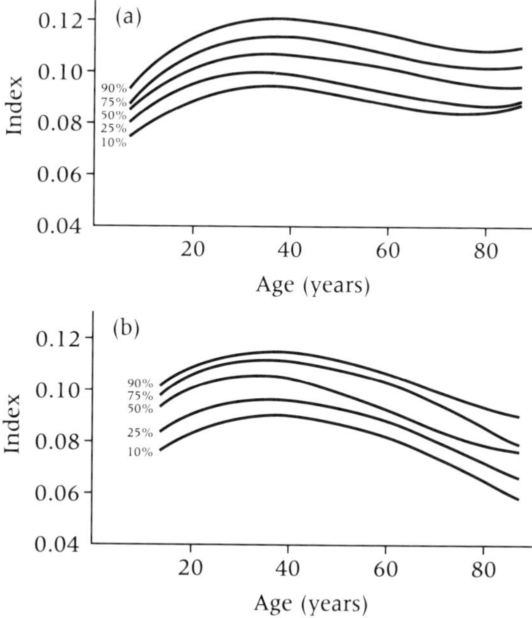

Figure 10 *Exton-Smith Index: distribution curves for age in normal males (top) and females (bottom)*

Semiquantitative grading

Semiquantitative grading is adequate for clinical practice.

Intracortical resorption This is usually assessed taking the second, third and fourth metacarpals.

- Grade 0 Solid cortex;
- Grade 1 Few intracortical striations;
- Grade 2 Radiolucent striations occupying more than half of the cortical area in the middle third of the shaft; and
- Grade 3 Striations occupying the whole cortex.

Periosteal resorption Assessment of the second and third phalanges of the second, third and fourth fingers:

- Grade 0 Normal smooth periosteal surface;
- Grade 1 Periosteal cortical defects in the proximal third of the shaft of the second phalanx;
- Grade 2 Periosteal cortical defects in mid- or distal sections of the second and third phalanges; and
- Grade 3 Periosteal resorption found in the first phalanges and elsewhere (e.g. clavicle).

Quantitative measurements

These are best applied to intracortical resorption. The intracortical absorption spaces (IRS) are counted over a zone 2 mm above and below the mid-point of the metacarpal or phalanx. If the spaces are branching the stem and branches are counted separately. Adjustment is made for cortical width giving the resorption factor as IRS/C. The upper limits for normal are 0.7 and 2.2 for the second and third metacarpals and for the phalanges, respectively. There is, however, considerable intraobserver error, the coefficient of variation being 20%.

Periosteal resorption is of particular value in the diagnosis and assessment of the progress of hyperparathyroidism (e.g. secondary to renal disease).

PHOTODENSITOMETRY

The large element of error that occurs in the subjective assessment of bone density on X-ray examination can be overcome by photodensitometry. The optical density of the X-ray image is compared with a reference wedge. Several bone sites have been used: the proximal phalanx, metacarpal, ulna, radius, femur, tibia and the os calcis.

A wedge with an atomic number close to bone is preferred[16,34–38]. The commonest is aluminium or an aluminium–zinc alloy, but ivory, bone and solutions of K_2HPO_4 and $CaSO_4$ have been used. The wedge may be of a ramp or step form.

Several methods have been utilized for estimating the bone density with a photodensitometer:

(1) *The Spot Method* The density at a fixed point in the bone (e.g. mid-point of a metacarpal)

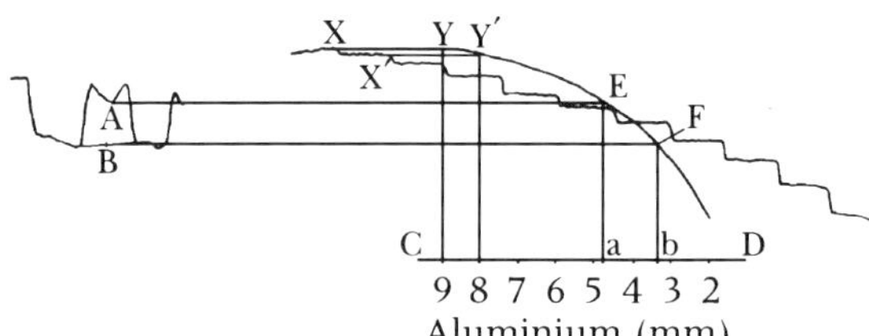

Figure 11 *Actual densitometer tracing of third metacarpal (left) and step wedge (right). To estimate the aluminium equivalent, first draw a horizontal line CD on any convenient part of the millimeter graph paper, CD being below the lowest step of the aluminium step wedge tracing. Mark off in centimeters the thickness of the step wedge along CD. Now graph the height of each step, e.g. XY X′Y′ and draw a horizontal line AE (A being the lowest point on the trough) from the metacarpal tracing to meet the curve of the step wedge at E. The base-line of the metacarpal tracing is taken from the mid-point B of the line joining the two lowest points of the metacarpal tracing. Draw the horizontal line BF to meet the curve of the step wedge at F. From E and F drop perpendiculars to meet CD at a and b. ab is then the equivalent thickness of aluminium. This procedure is essential as the response is not linear; reproduced with permission from reference 35*

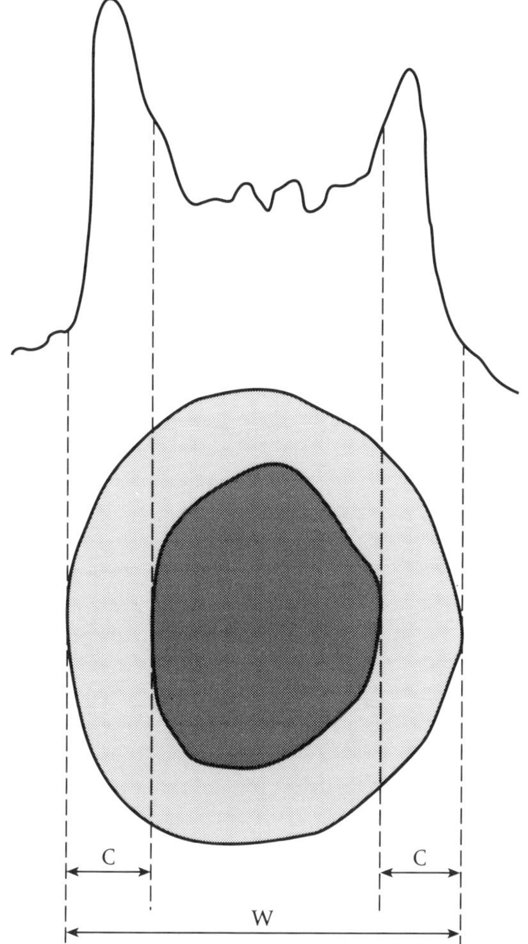

Figure 12 *Diagram showing a typical densitometer scan trace of the femur at the metaphysis: W = bone width, C = cortical width*[39]

as determined by caliper is measured with a microdensitometer and compared with the wedge;

(2) *Line Photodensitometry* (Figure 11) The bone is scanned along a line with a moving light spot; and

(3) *Area Photodensitometry* A line-by-line scan at fixed intervals is done over a given length of bone.

The X-ray dosage varies according to the bone site, whether a tank is used and with the dose preference of the center. A non-screen film or a screen film with no screen can be used. The latter has the advantage that it can be developed with an automatic processor[35].

There are three main sources of error:

(1) There is absorption of the X-ray beam by soft tissue and fat;

(2) A polychromatic low-energy X-ray beam is used and this may harden between observations; and

(3) Scatter of the X-ray beam may occur, being worse when the bone covering is thick.

The problem of absorption can be overcome by immersing the part being X-rayed in a tank of water of uniform depth, water having approximately the same absorption as soft tissues. A wetting agent obviates the problem of small air bubbles sticking to hairs.

Scatter can be reduced by limiting the field with a lead sheet and appropriate aperture above the tank. Water, although compensating for absorption, increases the scatter. Some prefer not to use it, and Pridie and co-workers[36,37] limits the volume to 500 ml. The effect of scatter can be minimized also by increasing the distance of the cassette from the bone being scanned.

When X-raying the hand, there may be a heel effect if the wedge is placed longitudinally alongside the hand or between the fingers, the bottom of the wedge thereby appearing darker than the upper part. This can be avoided by placing the wedge transversely opposite the mid-point of the bone being measured. Increasing the focus–film distance and limiting the field size also reduces the heel effect. Alternatively, a plastic convex spherical filter reduces the effect by producing uniform field[38]. It is important that the tube is never tilted.

Measurements of cortical thickness

An advantage of photodensitometry is that it can be used with a high degree of accuracy for measurements of cortical thickness[39,40]. The photodensitometric tracing can be used to measure the thickness of the bone and also the medullary

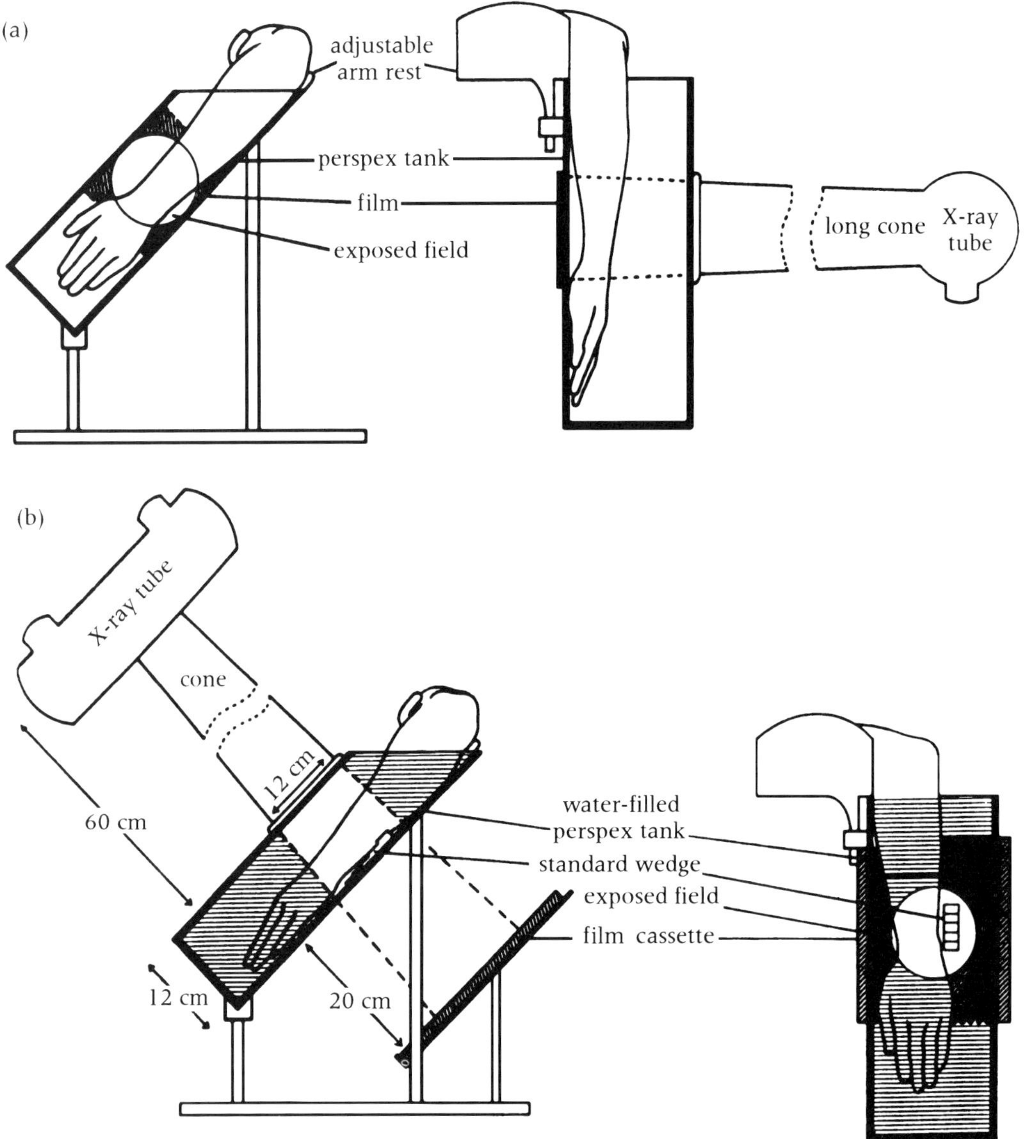

Figure 13 *(a) Lateral positioning: tank not filled with water, upper arm kept horizontal by arm rest; (b) Postero-anterior positioning: tank filled with water, X-ray tube and hand moved through 90°, standard wedge placed near ulna; reproduced with permission from reference 41*

width (Figure 12). The measurements are best made with a caliper because the light spot of the photodensitometer is too wide for a sharp end-point[36]. Morgan and co-workers[16], however, found little advantage in using this method compared with making visual measurements on the radiograph with a caliper.

Particular sites

Metacarpal A metacarpal is the commonest bone to be used[39] and, being cylindrical, does not require an orthogonal film for bone thickness (T)[36]. The usual index is a measurement of the density equivalent (D) of the wedge used divided by the cortical thickness (C) plus a correction for the medullary width (M). Pridie[36] showed the absorptive power of the medulla to be one-quarter that of the cortex, from which he derived a density index of D/[C + (M/4)]. Anderson and co-workers[35] used a different index of [D + (0.105 × C) + (0.018 × M)]/T.

Radius Meema and Meema[27] chose to use the proximal end of the radius in preference to the distal end, because they regarded measurements of cortical bone to be more reliable than cancellous bone in detecting osteoporosis. They related bone density to cortical thickness in preference to total width as this allowed for variation in bone thickness according to skeletal size. An orthogonal film was required to measure the cortical width. The diameter of the head of the radius was measured and measurements were made at sites two, two and a half and three times its diameter distal to the head. The density of the cortex at its mid-point was measured with the photodensitometer. Meema used a wedge containing K_2HPO_4, calibrated against hydroxyapatite equivalents as mg/cm^2 (N). He used an index of N/C which gave the bone salt equivalent in mg/cm^3. The normal value was 1200 ± 200 mg/cm^3.

Ulna Keane and colleagues[41] chose the distal ulna on the basis that demineralization is shown more readily in cancellous bone. A posterior and anterior film was taken with the arm immersed alongside an aluminium wedge in a tank of water and scanned at three distances from the lower end. An orthogonal film was taken in air to measure bone thickness (Figures 13a and b). Doyle[42] and Mayo[43] both used similar techniques.

Os calcis Mayo[43] used the os calcis with the foot immersed in water for measurements, but this use is open to criticism because the os calcis is subject to the stresses of weight bearing.

CONCLUSION

These methods have been largely superseded by modern techniques of dual photon absorptiometry and dual-energy X-ray absorptiometry but these detect osteopenia and do not differentiate between the causes. Measurements of cortical thickness are the only ones specific for osteoporosis, and in areas of the world with limited access to more sophisticated techniques these measurements may still be of value in population surveys[44]. They are less suitable for longitudinal studies, particularly involving response to treatment, because the degree of accuracy is not sufficient to detect small changes over short periods of time.

References

1. Andran GM. Bone destruction not demonstrable by radiography. Br J Radiol 1951; 24: 107–9.
2. Lachman E. Osteoporosis. The potentialities and limitations of its roentgenologic diagnosis [Editorial]. Am J Roentgenol 1955; 74: 712–15.
3. Urist MR, Zaccalini PS, MacDonald NS, Skoog WA. New approaches to the problem of osteoporosis. J Bone Jt Surg 1962; 44B: 464–84.
4. Barnett E, Nordin BEC. The radiological diagnosis of osteoporosis: a new approach. Clin Radiol 1960; 11: 166–74.
5. Raymakers JA, Kapelle JW, Berensteinjn ECH, Duursma SA. Assessment of osteoporotic spinal deformity. Skeletal Radiol 1990; 19: 91–7.
6. Caldwell RA. Observations on the incidence, aetiology and pathology of senile osteoporosis. J Clin Pathol 1962; 15: 421–31.
7. Virtama P, Gästrin G, Telkkä A. Biconcavity of the vertebrae as an estimate of their bone density. Clin Radiol 1962; 13: 128–31.
8. Singh M, Nagrath AR, Maini PS. Changes in trabecular pattern of the upper end of the femur as an index of osteoporosis. J Bone Jt Surg 1970; 52A: 457–67.
9. Singh M. Femoral trabecular pattern index for grading osteoporosis. In: Jaworski ZFG, ed. Proceedings of the 1st Workshop on Bone Morphometry. Ottawa: University of Ottawa Press, 1973: 86–8.

10. Singh M, Riggs BI, Beabout JW, Jowsey J. Femoral trabecular pattern index for evaluation of spinal osteoporosis. Ann Int Med 1972; 77: 63–7.
11. Dequeker J, Gautama K, Roh YS. Femoral trabecular patterns in asymptomatic spinal osteoporosis and femoral neck fracture. Clin Radiol 1974; 25: 243–6.
12. Dequeker J, Gautama K, Roh YS. Evaluation of the femoral trabecular pattern grading system, its value in spinal osteoporosis and femoral neck fracture. In: Jaworski ZFG, ed. Proceedings of the 1st Workshop on Bone Morphometry. Ottawa: University of Ottawa Press, 1973: 89–93.
13. Adams P, Davies GT, Sweetman PM. Observer error and measurements of the metacarpal. Br J Radiol 1969; 42: 192–7.
14. Horsman A, Simpson M. The measurement of sequential changes in cortical bone geometry. Br J Radiol 1975; 48: 470–5.
15. Naor E, Di Segni V, Robin G, Makin M, Meneze J. Intra-observer variability in the determination of the metacarpal cortical index. Br J Radiol 1972; 42: 213–17.
16. Morgan DB, Spiers FW, Pulvertaft CN, Fourman P. The amount of bone in the metacarpal and the phalanx according to age and sex. Clin Radiol 1967; 18: 101–8.
17. Garn SM, Poznanski AK, Nagy JM. Bone measurement in the differential diagnosis of osteopenia and osteoporosis. Radiology 1971; 100: 509–18.
18. Garn SM. An annotated bibliography on bone density. Am J Clin Nutr 1962; 10: 59–67.
19. Garn SM. The Earlier Gain and Later Loss of Cortical Bone. Springfield: Charles C. Thomas, 1970.
20. Exton-Smith AN, Millard PH, Payne PR, Wheeler EF. i Method of measuring quantity of bone. Lancet 1969; 2: 1153–7.
21. Exton-Smith AN, Millard PH, Payne PR, Wheeler EF. ii Pattern of development and loss of bone with age. Lancet 1970: 1; 360.
22. Dequeker J. Quantitative radiology: radiogrammetry of cortical bone. Br J Radiol 1976; 49: 912–20.
23. Dequeker J. Quantitative radiology of cortical bone at the second metacarpal. Influence of skeletal size – bone loss in different populations. In: Jaworski ZFG, ed. Proceedings of the 1st Workshop of Bone Morphometry. Ottawa: University of Ottawa Press, 1973: 44–7.
24. Dequeker J, Johnston CC. Non-invasive bone measurements: Methodological problems. Radiogrammetry, single and dual photon absorptiometry, neutron activation and CT densitometry. 16th European Symposium on Calcified Tissue Research, Belgium 1981. Oxford: IRC Press.
25. Dequeker J. Precision of the radiogrammetric evaluation of bone mass at the metacarpal bones. In: Jaworski ZFG, ed. Proceedings of the 1st Workshop on Bone Morphometry. Ottawa: University of Ottawa Press, 1973: 28–32.
26. Meema S, Meema HE. Improved recognition of bone loss by concurrent measurements in the 2nd metacarpal and radius. In: Jaworski ZFG, ed. Proceedings of the 1st Workshop on Bone Morphometry. Ottawa: University of Ottawa Press, 1973: 48–53.
27. Meema HE, Meema S. Measurable roentgenologic changes in some peripheral bones in senile osteoporosis. J Am Geriatric Soc 1963; 11: 1170–82.
28. Virtama P, Helelä T. Radiographic measurements of cortical bone variations in a normal population between 1 and 90 years of age. Acta Radiol Suppl 1969; 293: 1: 23–4.
29. Helelä T. Age dependent variation of the cortical thickness of the clavicle. Ann Clin Res 1969; 1: 140–3.
30. Garn SM, Poznanski AK, Larson K. Metacarpal lengths, cortical diameters and areas from the 10 State Nutrition Survey. In: Jaworski ZFG, ed. Proceedings of the 1st Workshop on Bone Morphometry. Ottawa; University of Ottawa Press, 1973: 367–80.
31. Meema HE. Cortical bone atrophy and osteoporosis as a manifestation of aging. Am J Roentgen 1961; 89: 1287–95.
32. Gryfe CI, Exton-Smith AN, Payne PR, Wheeler EF. Pattern of development of bone in childhood and adolescence. Lancet 1971; 1: 523–5.
33. Nordin BEC, MacGregor J, Smith D. The incidence of osteoporosis in normal women: its relation to age and the menopause. Quart J Med 1966; 35 No 137: 25–7.
34. Cohn SH. Non-invasive measurements of bone mass and their clinical application. Boca Raton, Florida: CRC Press, 1981; Chap.2: 5–50.
35. Anderson JB, Shimmins J, Smith DA. A new technique for the measurement of metacarpal density. Br J Radiol 1966; 39: 443–50.
36. Pridie RB. The diagnosis of senile osteoporosis using a new bone density index. Br J Radiol 1967; 40: 251–5.
37. Pridie RB, Higgins P McR, Yates JM. Bone changes following gastrectomy. Clin Radiol 1968; 19: 148–53.
38. Meema HE, Harris CK, Porrett RE. A method for determination of bone salt of cortical bone. Radiology 1964; 82: 986–97.
39. Atkinson PJ. Relevance of peripheral, axial or total skeletal mass measurement. In: Jaworski ZFG, ed. Proceedings of 1st Workshop on Bone Morphometry. Ottawa: University of Ottawa Press, 1973: 142–53.

40. Inoue J, Kusida K, Miyamoto S, Sumi Y, Orimo H, Yamashita G. Quantitative assessment of bone density on an X-ray picture. J Jpn Orthop Assoc 1983; 57: 1923–36.
41. Keane BE, Spiegler G, Davies R. Quantitative evaluation of bone mineral by a radiographic method. Br J Radiol 1959; 33: 162–7.
42. Doyle FH. Involutional osteoporosis. Clin Endocrinol Metab 1972; 1: 143–67.
43. Mayo KM. Quantitative measurement of bone mineral content in normal adult bone. Br J Radiol 1961; 34: 693–712.
44. Walker ARP, Walker BF, Richardson BD. Metacarpal bone dimensions in young and aged South African Bantu consuming a diet low in calcium. Postgrad Med J 1971; 47: 320–5.
45. Thompson PW. Assessment of the Skeleton. In Stevenson J. 'Osteoporosis' Update Postgraduate Center Series 1991; 19–22. Guildford: Reed Healthcare Communications
46. Meema HE, Meema S. Involutional (physiologic) bone loss in women and the feasibility of preventing structural failure. J Am Geriatr Soc 1974; 72: 443–57.

Quantitative measurements in osteoporosis

8

J. E. Adams

INTRODUCTION

As we get older, a certain amount of age-related bone loss, or osteopenia, is both inevitable and normal[1–8], and continues to the ninth decade[9]. The rate of bone loss is increased in women at the time of the menopause and this loss of bone can be prevented by the administration of hormone replacement therapy[10–17] (Figures 1 and 2). Osteoporosis occurs when there is a reduction in the amount of bone tissue with associated thinning or loss of trabeculae resulting in increased fragility and consequent increase in fracture risk[18,19] (Figure 3). The osteopenia may be generalized or focal (i.e. disuse, reflex sympathetic osteodystrophy). Generalized osteoporosis occurs either as a primary disorder, or secondary to endocrine and metabolic diseases known to affect the skeleton (e.g. corticosteroid excess, hyperparathyroidism, hyperthyroidism, hypogonadism), or be related to certain risk factors (e.g. excessive alcohol consumption, smoking, lack of exercise, amenorrhea[20–23]). Primary osteoporosis is idiopathic (juvenile, young adults) or involutional[24]. Involutional osteoporosis is divided into Type 1 (postmenopausal) and Type 2 (age-related). The bone loss, which occurs in both men and women with age, can result in Type 2 osteoporosis. The condition occurs in those 70 years of age or more and is characterized by a reduction in both cortical and trabecular bone density. Fractures occur in the femoral neck, spine, humerus, pelvis and proximal tibiae. The increased bone loss which occurs in women at the time of the menopause (Type 1 osteoporosis) affects principally trabecular

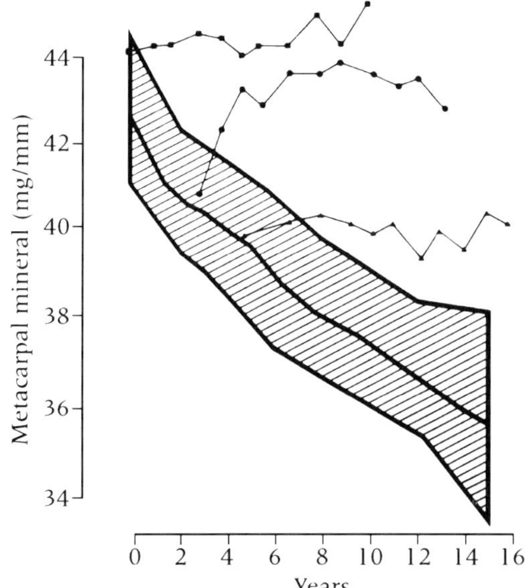

Figure 1 *Changes in bone mass by single photon absorptiometry in placebo-treated patients (hatched area: mean ± SD) and in three groups of estrogen-treated patients (from Lindsay, 1988 reference 10 – with permission)*

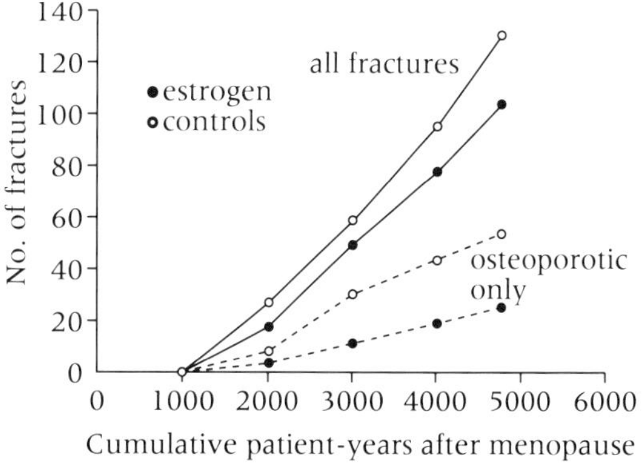

Figure 2 *A 50% reduction in osteoporotic fractures is observed in estrogen-treated women (from Ettinger et al., 1985 reference 12 – with permission)*

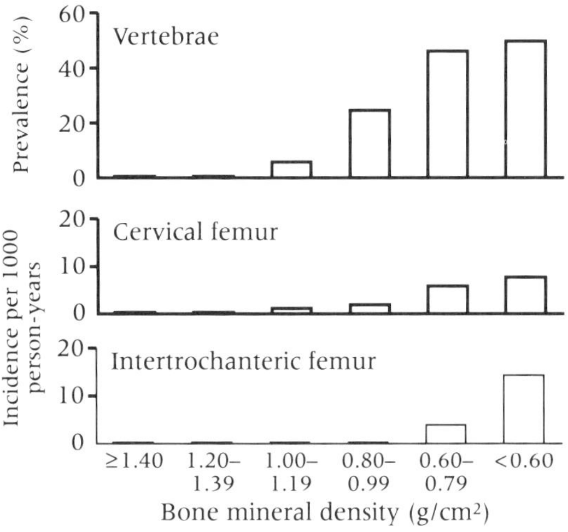

Figure 3 *Estimated prevalence of vertebral fractures by lumbar spine bone mineral density (BMD) and estimated incidence of cervical and intertrochanteric hip fractures by cervical and intertrochanteric BMD, respectively, among Rochester, Minnesota women 35 years of age (from Riggs and Melton, 1986 reference 19 – with permission). There is increase in fractures as BMD falls*

bone. As a consequence, fractures occur in areas of the skeleton rich in trabecular bone including the spine (vertebral body), distal radius and hip. It is this loss of bone which can be prevented by the administration of hormone replacement therapy. Such osteoporotic fractures, and principally those which occur in the hip, are responsible for considerable morbidity and even mortality, with enormous financial consequences for health care systems[25–27]. In the USA osteoporosis affects 20 million individuals and accounts for 1.5 million fractures in total per annum including 250 000 hip fractures. The estimated cost associated with fractures is 18 billion dollars, almost half of which (7 billion) is due to hip fractures alone. The incidence of hip fracture rises with age being greater in women than men. Caucasian women surviving to the age of 90 have a 30% lifetime risk of sustaining a hip fracture. There is appreciable mortality (20%) after hip fracture in the elderly and the costs of the acute care of such fractures in England and Wales has been estimated at 165 million pounds. Over the past three decades there has been a doubling of hip fractures in many Western populations, and this is only partly related to the increasing proportions of the population who are aged 65 years and over[28]. The explanation for this secular increase of hip fractures is unknown. However, these data emphasize the need for effective preventive strategies to limit this increasing burden of hip fractures.

Treatment of established osteoporosis is difficult and often unsatisfactory, although there have recently been encouraging results reported with the use of diphosphonates in established osteoporosis[29,30]. Treatment strategies have therefore favored prevention of osteoporosis by maximizing peak bone mass, minimizing age-related and postmenopausal bone loss (hormone replacement therapy), avoidance of risk factors, adequate dietary intake of calcium and adequate physical activity. There is a growing demand from patients, general medical practitioners and specialists (obstetricians, orthopedic surgeons, rheumatologists) for clinical services that provide for the detection, assessment and management of osteoporosis[31–33]. Whether a fracture is sustained depends upon a variety of factors including the propensity to fall and the way in which a patient falls[34–36]. However, bone mineral density (BMD) is the single most important determinant as to whether or not a fracture occurs[37–41]. Since breaking strength of bone is related to its mineral content, reduced bone mass is a useful predictor of increased fracture risk. The lower the peak bone density, the higher the risk of fracture in later life. Methods of measuring bone density are therefore relevant to the study of skeletal development, the detection of osteopenia and assessment of efficacy of treatment of osteoporosis.

BONE MINERAL DENSITOMETRY

Non-invasive methods for measuring bone mass *in vivo* are pertinent to the detection of osteopenia, identification of patients at risk of easy fracture and assessment of the efficacy of either prevention or treatment of osteoporosis[42–45]. Methods for measuring BMD should be accurate, precise, sensitive, inexpensive and involve a minimal exposure to ionizing radiation.

Accuracy expresses how close are the measured and actual bone mineral densities. It is usually expressed as the standard error of the estimate of linear regression between the measured and actual BMD, as a percentage of the mean BMD value. In the quantitative methods to be described, some inaccuracies are caused by variable fat content within the marrow of trabecular bone (single energy quantitative computed tomography) and by fat content of extraosseous soft tissues (photon absorptiometric techniques). Changes in body composition or marrow fat may therefore introduce errors in the measurement dependent upon the technique and measurement site used.

Precision assesses the reproducibility of the measuring technique and is usually expressed as a percentage coefficient of variation (% CV) and calculated from the standard deviation of the difference between pairs of repeat measurements as a percentage of the mean of all the measurements. A high precision (low % CV) is essential in longitudinal studies of bone mineral density. Precision can be estimated for repeat measurements over a period of minutes or hours (short-term precision) or over periods of weeks or months (long-term precision). Short-term precision reflects principally repositioning errors, whilst long-term precision using a calibration phantom reflects machine stability. The precision quoted by manufacturers of bone densitometry equipment is generally derived from repeated measurements of phantoms or in healthy young volunteers. Such good precision may not be achievable in patients, particularly those with osteoporosis in whom positioning may be difficult. Departments providing bone mineral density measurements should estimate the 'in-house' precision to be able to assess the significance of change in BMD with time in longitudinal studies.

Sensitivity is the capacity of the technique to separate an abnormal (fracture) from a normal (non-fracture) population, or to detect readily changes in BMD with time and therapy.

PAST METHODS

Early non-invasive methods of bone mass measurement included measurement of cortical thickness, the Singh Index and radiographic densitometry. Although these methods are simple to perform, cheap and widely available, they are relatively crude and imprecise. They have been dealt with in greater detail in Chapter 7, but the following comments are relevant.

X-ray densitometry

Qualitative assessment of the spinal bone mineral content from bone density on conventional radiographs is insensitive and inaccurate, since the subjective assessment is influenced by patient size, radiographic exposure factors and film processing techniques[46]. Some of the variations in bone density on radiographs caused by these variations can be compensated for by including on the film a calibration reference wedge of similar effective atomic number and specific gravity to that of bone. A photodensitometer is then used to measure optical density of the radiograph at a selected anatomical site and of the reference wedge, to determine mineral concentration. This technique has been applied to various anatomical sites including the metacarpal, phalanx, radius, ulna, femur and tibia. With this method, it is essential that there is standardization of the radiographic technique, exposure and processing. Despite such standardization, the method is of limited precision.

Radiographic morphometry

Radiographic morphometry is a simple technique in which the cortical diameter of the diaphyses of tubular bones is measured[47–56]. The method is usually applied to the mid-shaft of the bone, but other sites including the proximal humerus have also been used[57]. A large amount of data are available on age-related changes of total bone width, medullary width and cortical width for almost every tubular bone, but the most widely used was the second metacarpal. Such morphometric data from cross-sectional studies demonstrated endosteal resorption which occurred from middle age onwards and subperiosteal apposition throughout life[58,59]. This is a simple examination to perform, and is widely available with a low radiation dose and a large amount of reference data available. However, the technique does not reflect intracortical porosity nor trabecular bone resorption and is therefore insensitive to these changes. The method is also imprecise as endosteal resorption thins the bone cortex making accurate measurements difficult to obtain[60,61].

Singh Index

In the femoral neck there are two principle arches of trabeculae: the compressive group lie in the medial portion of the femoral neck and the tensile group in the lateral aspect. Trabeculae predominate and are thicker in areas of maximum stress. The number, thickness and arrangement of these trabeculae alter with aging due to resorption. On radiographs the change in trabecular pattern of the femoral neck can be graded to assess the loss of trabeculae as an index of osteopenia[62,63] (Figure 4). However, the subjectivity of the Singh grading scale makes it of limited reproducibility. Whether more sophisti-

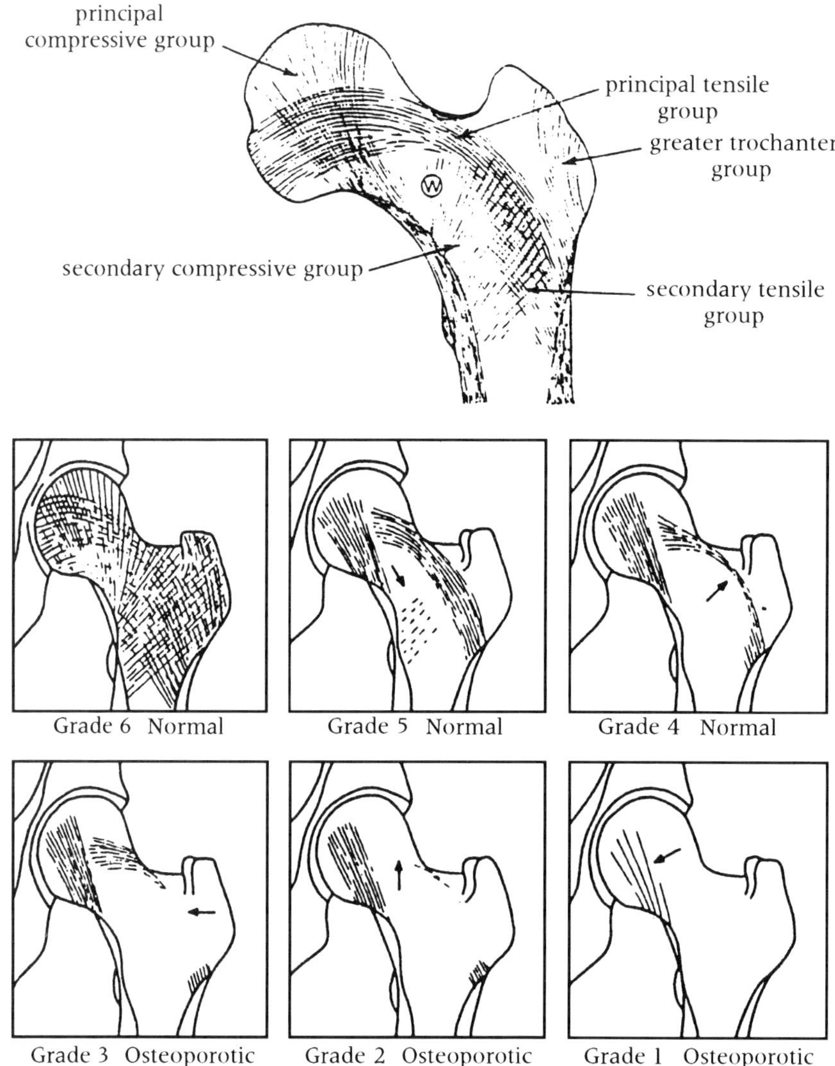

Figure 4 *The proximal femoral trabecular (Singh) Index based on changes in the trabecular pattern of the upper end of the femur: grades 3 and under indicate significant osteopenia (Singh et al., 1970 reference 62 – with permission)*

cated methods of image analysis can improve precision of the technique remains to be established.

Single photon absorptiometry

Photon absorptiometric techniques were introduced to overcome the problems described for the photodensitometric techniques when using polychromatic X-rays and radiographic film. The use of a single energy γ-ray source eliminates variation in photon output and the effects of beam hardening. Transmitted photons are measured by a scintillation detector scanning across the site of measurement and eliminates the problems of radiation scatter and the non-uniformity of film sensitivity and development.

This technique was first described by Cameron and Sorenson in 1963[64]. The mono-energetic γ photons are produced by a radionuclide source. The source most commonly used is ^{125}I which emits photons at an energy of 27.3 KeV. The radionuclide has a relatively short half-life of 60 days which requires a replacement source two or three times per annum at a cost of £800–£1000 for each renewed source. The 60 KeV radiation from ^{241}Am is preferred for application of the technique to areas of thicker tissue such as the thigh and has been used for the forearm. This radionuclide has a considerably longer half-life than ^{125}I.

Due to the low photon flux and energy from such radionuclide sources, the technique is generally only applicable to peripheral skeletal sites, usually the forearm[65–69]. However, the technique has also been applied to bone density measurement in the calcaneum, femur, humerus and finger. To correct for overlying soft tissue, the anatomical site in which the bone density is being measured has to be surrounded either by water, water bags or water equivalent mouldable material. The forearm is usually immersed in a water bath (Figure 5). The beam photon count obtained through the water bath alone is used as a baseline measurement. Scanning is then repeated with the non-dominant forearm positioned within the water bath. The difference in photon count below the baseline is assumed to be due to bone. Since skeletal muscle has an attenuating effect similar to that of water, the effects of varying amounts of muscle are eliminated by the water bath. An additional correction for adipose tissue has to be applied. Since fat has a less attenuating effect on the photon beam than water, photon counts will be higher than for the water baseline in regions scanned of high fat content. This effect is demonstrated in Figure 6a. The graph shows two large areas of reduced count which correspond to the radius and ulna. Between these bones and adjacent to their outer margins, the transmission of photons is elevated above the baseline. With the assumption that this effect of fat is present across the width of the forearm scanned a correction can be made to the baseline which is proportional to the amount of adipose tissue present[69]. The equipment measures the total area under the curve which is directly proportional to the amount of bone present. Results are provided as either bone mineral content (BMC) in g/cm of bone length or as bone mineral density (BMD) in g/cm^2. The margins of the bone are detected automatically from the graph permitting calculation of BMD of bone area by dividing BMC by bone width. This is an areal rather than a true volumetric density. This measurement partially compensates for the effect on bone density of patient size. Additional measurement errors introduced by using bone width for this calculation make BMD a rather less precise measure than BMC, but it is a better indicator of fracture risk.

Early equipment used an horizontal scan with the palm in a pronated position. The operator had to measure the distance from the olecranon to the ulna styloid and scanning was performed in the mid-point (the 50% site) of the radius which is composed wholly of cortical bone. Subsequently it was recognized that a vertical scan with the hand gripping a rod in the water bath (Figure 5) avoided rotation of the wrist with consequent improvement in precision of positioning. The radionuclide source is coupled to the detector by a C-arm and scans in a rectilinear fashion across the area of interest. Collimators fitted to both the source and the detector provide a narrow beam of γ radiation. Pulses from the scintillation detector are passed through an amplifier to a pulse height analyzer so as to

(a)

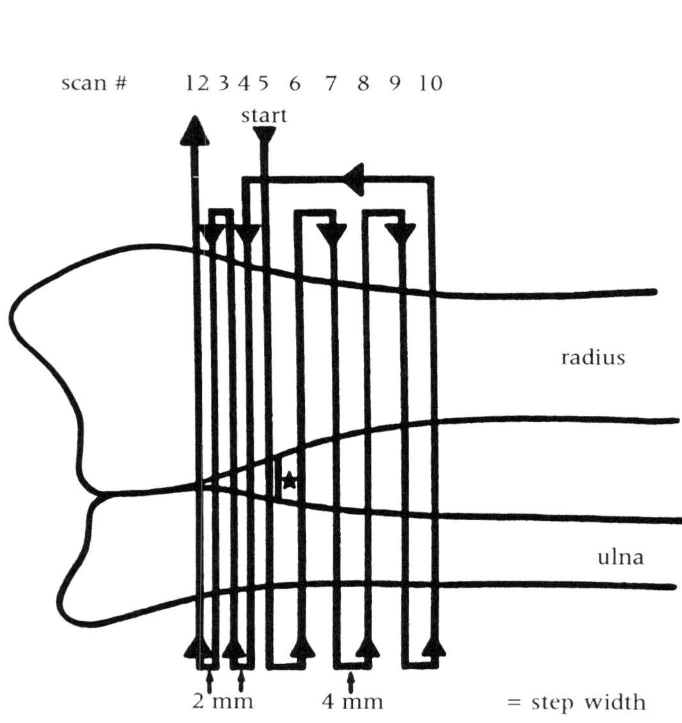

(b)

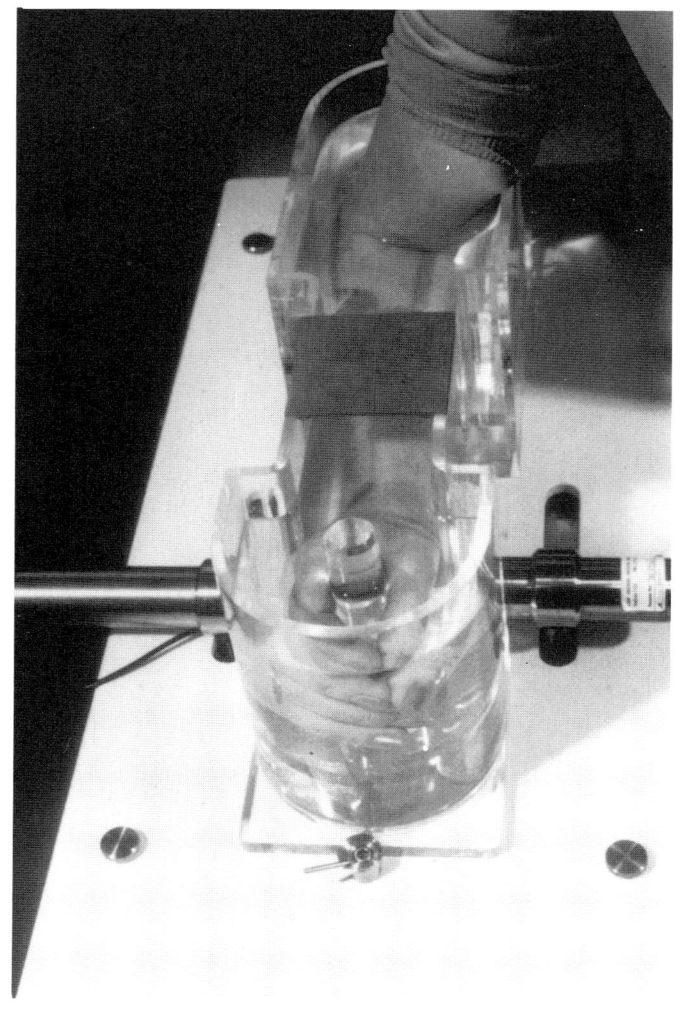

Figure 5 *(a) Single photon absorptiometry (Nuclear Data scanner). The non-dominant forearm is placed in a water bath with the hand gripping a rod to avoid rotation of the wrist. (b) The radionuclide source (^{125}I) scans in a rectilinear fashion in two sites (proximal and ultradistal) of the distal forearm, after determination of the site of the 8 mm gap between radius and ulna (*)*

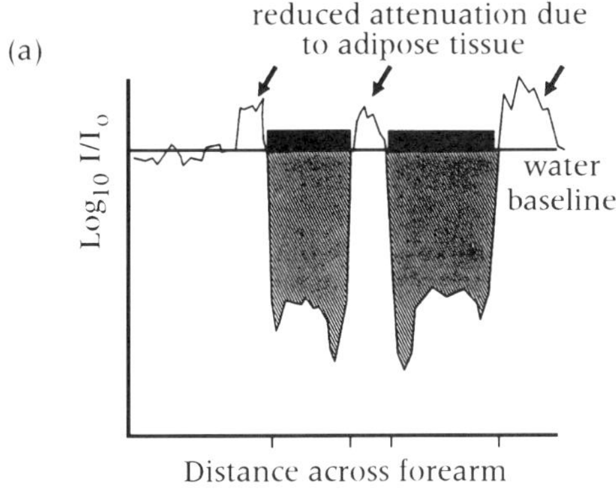

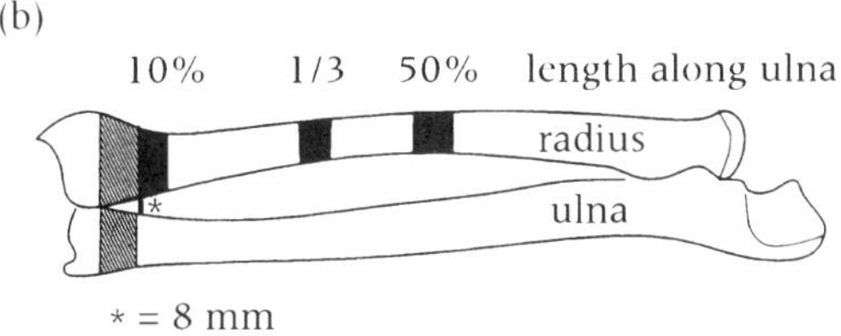

Figure 6 *(a) Graph of SPA log_{10} transmitted photon intensity against distance across the forearm. (b) Typical sites for single photon absorptiometry forearm densitometry. The sites have different percentages of trabecular and cortical bone; the mid-shaft is entirely cortical bone, the most distal site is predominantly (approximately 75–80%) trabecular bone (from Whitehouse, 1991 reference 69 – with permission). ■, Baseline adjustment for fat; ▒, attenuation due to bone*

minimize scatter radiation and select the appropriate energy for counting. Although the original scanners measured bone density in the midpoint of the forearm, the equipment developed subsequently used progressively more distal measurement sites with concomitant increasing relative proportions of trabecular bone. To scan consistently at the same anatomical site, current equipment uses an automated search procedure to locate a fixed gap (8 mm) between the distal radius and ulna. Several rectilinear scans (beam diameter 2 mm) using scanning speeds of 2 mm per second at 1 mm incremental steps are performed both proximal and distal to the fixed gap. The ratios of cortical to trabecular bone vary in these two sites, the more proximal being predominantly cortical bone and the ultradistal site containing a higher proportion of trabecular bone (Figure 6b). As the two sites of measurement are in close proximity, the source and detector of the scanner only need to travel a few centimeters, thus simplifying the design. Precision of 1% (% CV) can be achieved in BMC at the proximal site. Since the shape of the bones is less uniform in the more distal site used in the metaphysis, repositioning errors are more critical and the precision of both BMC and BMD in this ultradistal site is 2–3%. The accuracy of the technique is 4–5%. The cost of such equipment is approximately £20 000 and the radiation dose is negligible (effective dose equivalent < 0.6 mSv). Scanning time is 10–15 min.

Dual photon absorptiometry

A limitation of single photon absorptiometry is that it can only be applied to peripheral skeletal sites. The simultaneous measurement of the transmission of γ radiation of two different energies can compensate for the different thickness of soft tissue in measurement of bone mineral in clinically relevant sites such as the spine, hip and whole body[70–74]. The technique was introduced and developed during the late 1960s. The optimum combination of photon energies is dependent on soft tissue thickness and bone mineral density. For an average trunk thickness of 20 cm and a bone mineral content of 1 g/cm^2, the optimum lower energy is 40 KeV and for the higher energy < 100 KeV. ^{241}Am (60 KeV) with ^{137}Cs (662 KeV) were used initially because of their long half-life and relatively low cost. However, there were some disadvantages of this combination and a single radionuclide, ^{153}Gd provides energies close to the ideal. ^{153}Gd however has a rather short half-life (240 days) and the radionuclide source therefore needed to be replaced every 12–18 months at a cost of approximately £2000. The cost of the equipment was approximately £60 000. During rectilinear scanning, the detector system has a pulse height analyzer to separate the two energies, allowing photons of each energy to be counted separately. The difference in relative attenuations of these two photon energies allows the mass of bone mineral in the beam to be estimated. Any site of the body can be scanned, but the technique is generally applied to the lumbar spine, femoral neck and whole body. From the latter can be derived total body bone mineral, lean (muscle) and fat contents. The equipment scans in a rectilinear fashion and because of the low photon flux, images are of low spatial resolution and take a considerable scanning time to obtain (lumbar spine 30 min; whole body 40–60 min). Measurements are expressed as either bone mineral content in g/cm or as an areal measurement of mineral content per unit of projected area by using computerized edged detection with or without operator adjustment (BMD in g/cm^2). The precision of the technique is 2–4%. An assumption is made in dual photon absorptiometry scanning that soft tissue is of uniform composition but of unknown thickness. However, in practice this is not so and accuracy errors of up to 9% may occur due to non-uniform thickness of adipose tissue in the region scanned. Because of the low photon flux, the protracted scanning time and limited precision, this technique has now been superseded by dual energy X-ray absorptiometry.

DUAL ENERGY X-RAY ABSORPTIOMETRY

The physical principles of dual energy X-ray absorptiometry (DXA) are similar to those of dual photon absorptiometry, except that a low output X-ray tube replaces the gadolinium as a source of photons[75–77]. X-ray beams of two peak energies are produced by a variety of techniques by different manufacturers. The scanner manufactured by Lunar (Lunar Corporation, Madison, Wisconsin, USA) uses K-edge filtration with rare earth filters; equipment manufactured by Hologic (Hologic, Waltham, Massachusetts, USA) rapidly switches the tube potential from 70–140 kVp alternating at 60/s. The energies used are optimal for separating the mineralized and soft tissue components of the area analyzed. The problems of beam hardening and background radiation usually associated with polychromatic beams produced by X-ray tubes in quantitative applications are overcome by appropriate corrections and internal calibrations such as the hydroxyapatite bone reference disc which rotates through the beam synchronously with the generation of X-rays (Hologic, Waltham, Massachusetts, USA) (Figure 7a).

The technique is applied to scanning of the lumbar spine, femoral neck and whole body (Figures 8 and 9). With the increased photon flux from the X-ray tube as compared with a radionuclide source, image quality is improved, scanning time reduced (to 5 min or less) with consequent improvement in precision[78–81]. Precision of measurement in the spine is between 0.5 and 1%; in the femoral neck the precision is between 2 and 5% depending upon the anatomical site analyzed. Different manufacturers provide various regions of analysis within the proximal femur. These include the femoral neck, the usual site analyzed, with a precision of approximately 1.5–2%, the trochanter and Ward's triangle. The latter area may be sensitive to age-related changes in bone mass, but it is the least precise (CV = 5%). The accuracy of the technique is similar to that of dual photon absorptiometry (3–6%)[82,83]. Precision is not affected by changes in the antero-posterior (AP) diameter of patients over a wide range, except in children (when the diameter is below 10 cm, extra soft tissue equivalent material should be added) or when patients are very obese (AP diameter over 28 cm). The precision for whole body scanning is 1%.

Antero-posterior DXA presents the bone mineral data as linear or area measurements (BMC or BMD) in g/cm or g/cm^2. All the mineral within the path of the photon beam contributes to this measurement. Extraneous calcification such as within the wall of the aorta and degenerative and hyperostotic changes in the lumbar spine will cause inaccuracies and overestimation of bone mineral density[84,85] (Figure 8b). Degenerative disc disease is the most significant of these abnormalities to affect DXA measurement. This has led to the development of lateral DXA scanning of the lumbar spine[86–88] (Figure 8c). On some scanners the patient has to be repositioned lying on their side for scanning (Lunar) whereas on others a mobile C-arm is used to allow for lateral scanning with the patient remaining in the supine position.

(a)
X-ray detector system
display
computer
collimator
X-ray source
X–Y drive
(b)

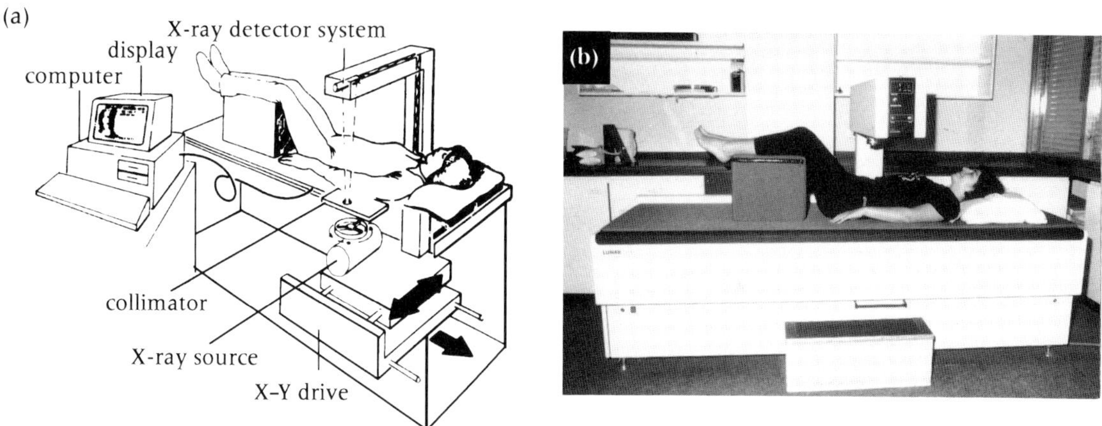

Figure 7 *(a) Schematic diagram showing principles of dual energy X-ray absorptiometry (DXA), with the X-ray source passing through the rotating calibration disc and the patient (Hologic Inc. – with permission). (b) Patient positioned on DXA scanner (Lunar DPX-L) for scanning of the lumbar spine*

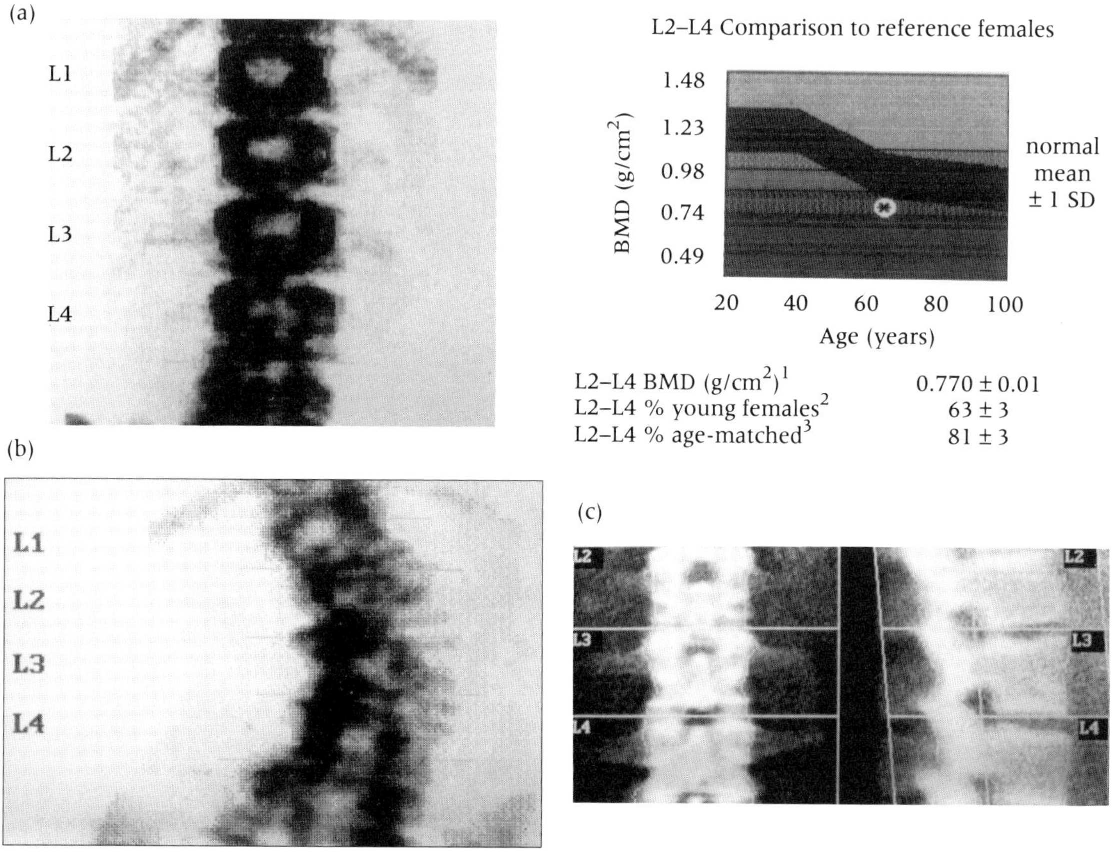

(a)
L1
L2
L3
L4
L2–L4 Comparison to reference females
BMD (g/cm²)
1.48
1.23
0.98
0.74
0.49
normal
mean
± 1 SD
20 40 60 80 100
Age (years)
L2–L4 BMD (g/cm²)¹ 0.770 ± 0.01
L2–L4 % young females² 63 ± 3
L2–L4 % age-matched³ 81 ± 3
(b)
L1
L2
L3
L4
(c)
L2
L3
L4

Figure 8 *(a) Antero-posterior scan of the lumbar spine with the mean bone mineral density (BMD) result calculated from the measurement of L2–L4 depicted on the normal reference range for females (± 1 SD) (Lunar Corporation – with permission). (b) Antero-posterior dual energy X-ray absorptiometry (DXA) scan of the lumbar spine with a marked scoliosis and associated hyperostotic changes with osteophytes at L2/3 and L3/4. The scoliosis makes scanning difficult and the osteophytes cause inaccuracies. (c) Antero-posterior (left) and lateral (right) DXA scan (Hologic Inc. – with permission)*

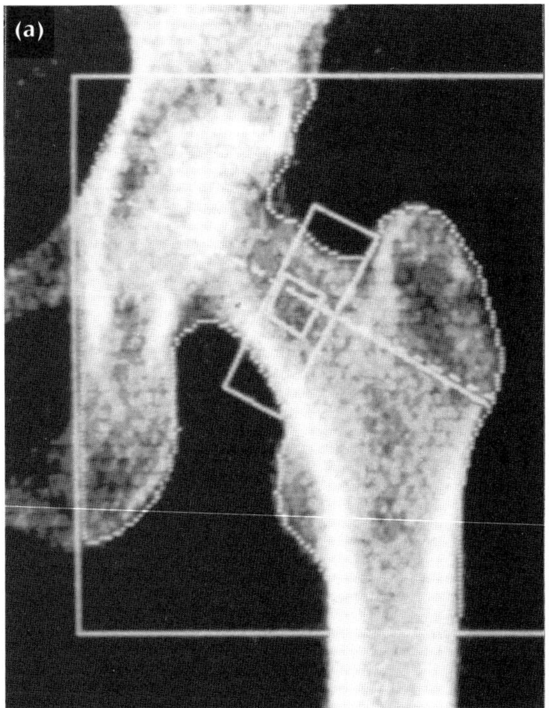

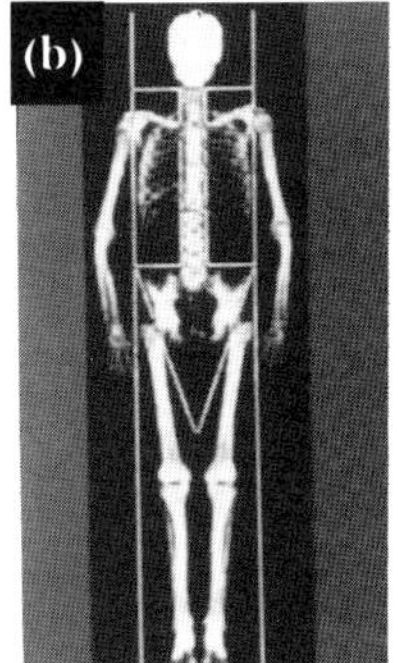

Bone results

Region	BMD g/cm^2
Head	2.024
Arms	0.959
Legs	1.302
Trunk	0.903
Ribs	0.742
Pelvis	1.051
Spine	1.019
Thoracic	0.967
Lumber	1.137
Total	1.151

Figure 9 *(a) Dual energy X-ray absorptiometry (DXA) scan of the hip showing automated boundary detection and regions of analysis which include the femoral neck (oblong region of interest (ROI)), trochanter and Ward's triangle (boxed ROI)) (Hologic Inc. – with permission. (b) Whole body DXA scan. From this the whole body and regional bone mineral density (BMD) can be measured, in addition to providing information on lean (muscle) and fat mass (Lunar Corporation – with permission)*

Higher X-ray tube outputs are required for such lateral scanning. Although this lateral technique is more sensitive than antero-posterior DXA in detecting age-related bone loss, often such a lateral measurement can be made in only one vertebral body (L3) because of overlying rib or iliac crest. The technique has poorer precision (2–5%) than conventional antero-posterior DXA and its role in clinical practice has still to be established. Marked scoliosis can also cause difficulties in scanning and analysis of DXA scan (Figure 8b).

In addition to lateral lumbar spine scanning there have been other rapid technological developments in DXA. These include orthopedic applications including the measurement of BMD around femoral hip prostheses[89] and in more localized anatomical sites such as the forearm (Figure 10a). DXA can now provide measurements previously made by single photon absorptiometry, but without the necessity of a water bath[90,91]. The technique can now be applied to small bone specimens and also to neonates with some software adaptations (Figures 10b and 10c). More recent scanners utilize fan beams instead of a pencil beam of photons and multiple detectors reducing scan times further to less than a minute. Methods to integrate lateral and AP scan data to derive a volume corrected integral bone mineral density are also available.

The most recent development is the use of DXA with improved image quality to produce lateral images of the vertebral bodies from T4 to L4 for vertebral morphometry[92] (Figure 11). If established as a valid technique, this would have the advantage over conventional radiographic vertebral morphometry of eliminating radiographic magnification and allowing automated analysis of vertebral dimensions to assess the prevalence and incidence of vertebral fractures at entry and during therapeutic trials in established osteoporosis.

The cost of DXA equipment is currently approximately £70 000, although scanners which permit vertebral morphometry may be closer to £90 000. Radiation dose (effective dose equivalent) is extremely low at 1 μSv per site examined in males; this value is slightly higher in females (up to 6 μSv) if the ovary is included in the field for scanning of the femoral neck.

BMC measurement obtained for the whole skeleton can be analyzed in localized regions of interest (arms, legs, pelvis, thorax) (Figure 9b). Information on body composition including lean body (muscle) and fat mass is obtained with good precision (1%) and correlation with other established indirect measures of body mass[93–96]. Errors in body composition measurements can be caused by edema since edematous fat will have the same X-ray attenuation characteristics as muscle.

Technique

For DXA scanning, the patient is positioned supine on the scanning table. When the lumbar spine is being examined the hips and knees are flexed over a support so as to eliminate the lumbar lordosis (Figure 7b). For scanning of the femoral neck the leg is slightly abducted and internally rotated by use of a positioning device so as to bring the femoral neck parallel to the top of the scan table and to avoid foreshortening of the femoral neck. Different leg positions can cause significant variations in DXA measurements[97]. Recent technical developments permit optimal scanning of the femoral neck by tube and detector angulation on a mobile C-arm.

Recently, one of the single photon absorptiometry scanners for measuring forearm bone densitometry has been adapted so that the radionuclide source has been replaced by an X-ray source (Figure 12a) (Osteometer, Hologic, Waltham, Massachusetts, USA). Such equipment is relatively compact and can be applied only to the forearm site (Figure 12b) and costs approximately £26 000.

In a detailed study, the panel for Diagnostic and Therapeutic Technology Assessment (DATTA) found DXA to be a safe, accurate and precise technology for assessing BMD[77]. Additionally, although the evidence was less direct, data also suggested that a single DXA measurement of BMD at the time of the menopause does predict future fracture risk[77,98].

QUANTITATIVE COMPUTED TOMOGRAPHY

The introduction of quantitative computed tomography (QCT) for imaging the brain in 1972 made it possible to demonstrate cross-sectional anatomy and to make precise measurements of the linear X-ray attenuation coefficients of small elements (voxels) of tissue *in vivo*, expressed as Hounsfield Units (HU). This permitted identification of substances with specific attenuation characteristics and the implication for quantitative measurement of BMD was soon appreciated[99–103]. Measurement of bone mass in the forearm on one of the original CT brain scanners showed QCT to be a precise method (reproducibility 0.2% *in vitro*; 2% *in vivo*)[99].

With the introduction of general purpose scanners in the mid-1970s, QCT could be applied to more clinically relevant sites in the axial skeleton (generally spine) and its use expanded from that time when the only alternative quantitative methods of bone densitometry available were single or dual photon absorptiometry. QCT is unique amongst all the methods of bone densitometry in that it allows separate estimation of trabecular and cortical bone as opposed to the integral (trabecular and cortical) bone density measurements provided by other photon absorptiometric techniques. In addition, QCT provides this measurement as a true mineral density per unit volume of bone, rather than the linear or areal measurements of photon absorptiometry[103–110].

The technique is generally applied to the lumbar spine. To perform the measurement the patient is positioned supine on the scanning table with the knees flexed over a triangular support so as to diminish the lumbar lordosis which is normally present. The arms are elevated out of the scanning field. A lateral scan projection radiograph is obtained and the cursor is placed to define the scanning plane through the mid-vertebral body, parallel to the end-plate (Figure 13). An antero-posterior projection radiograph may be obtained to check for the presence of scoliosis which may result in end-plates being included in the CT section. Sections are performed through four adjacent vertebrae, generally T12–L3 or alternatively L1–L4. Usually 10 mm sections are used, but if vertebral fractures are present, then thinner (5 mm) sections may be required to avoid more densely mineralized end-plate being included in the section scanned causing overestimation of BMD (Figure 14). A low-dose scanning technique (80 kV,

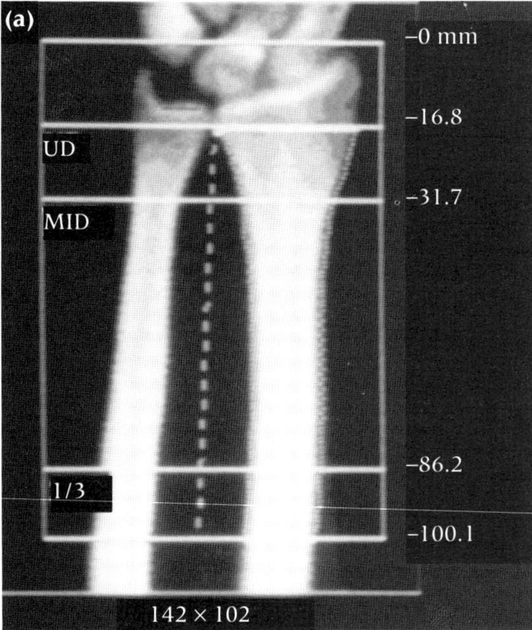

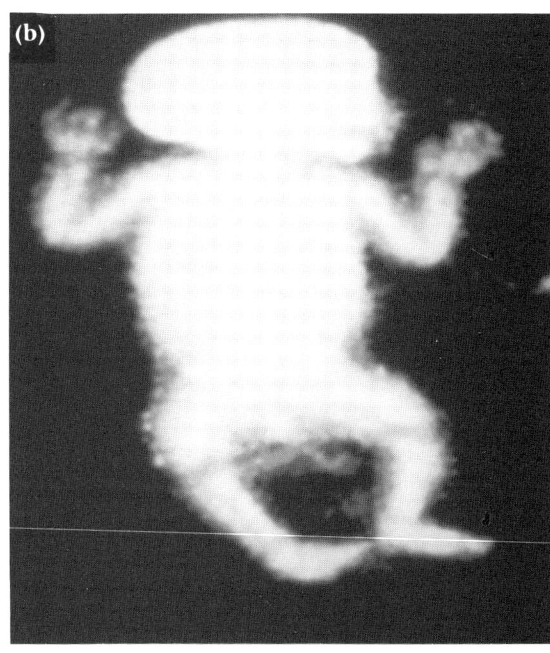

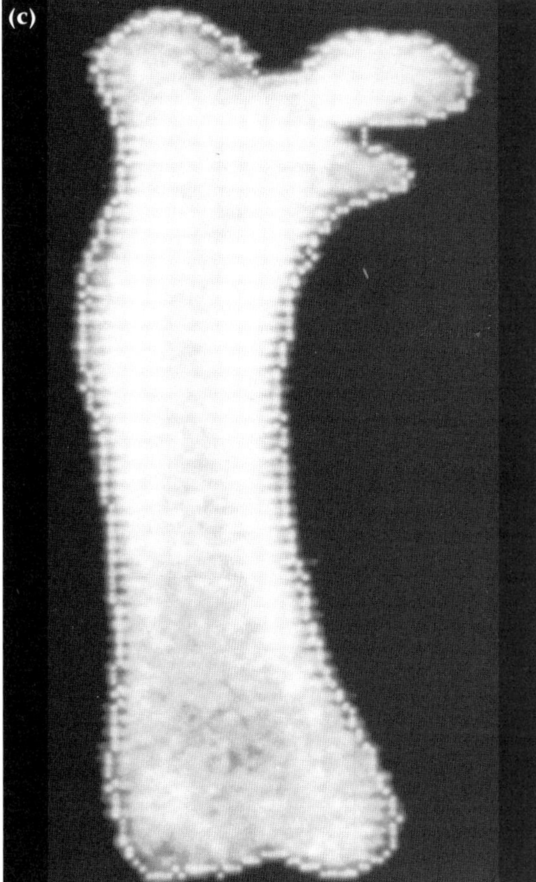

Figure 10 *(a) Dual energy X-ray absorptiometry (DXA) scan of the forearm providing bone density measurements at various sites. The proximal (1/3) provides a measure of cortical bone; the ultradistal (UD) site includes trabecular bone. (b) DXA scan in a neonate. (c) In vitro DXA scan of a bone specimen (all from Hologic Inc. – with permission)*

70 mA, 2S) can be used[111]. The section can be confirmed as being in the mid-plane of the vertebra by the presence of an area of reduced bone density posteriorly in the region of the entry of the basivertebral vein; a region of interest is selected for analysis (Figure 13). This is generally an oval region within the vertebral trabecular bone, which does not include either the cortical rim or the entry of the basivertebral vein. Because of the polychromicity of the X-ray beam of commercial CT scanners, beam hardening effects occur. To correct for this and for any scanner instability, QCT examinations have to be performed with a calibration reference phantom containing various concentrations of material with similar X-ray attenuation characteristics to bone[112]. From the regression of attenuation and concentration of calibration substance, the attenuation measured in the trabecular bone can be converted to bone mineral equivalents in mg/cm^3 (g/l). Originally,

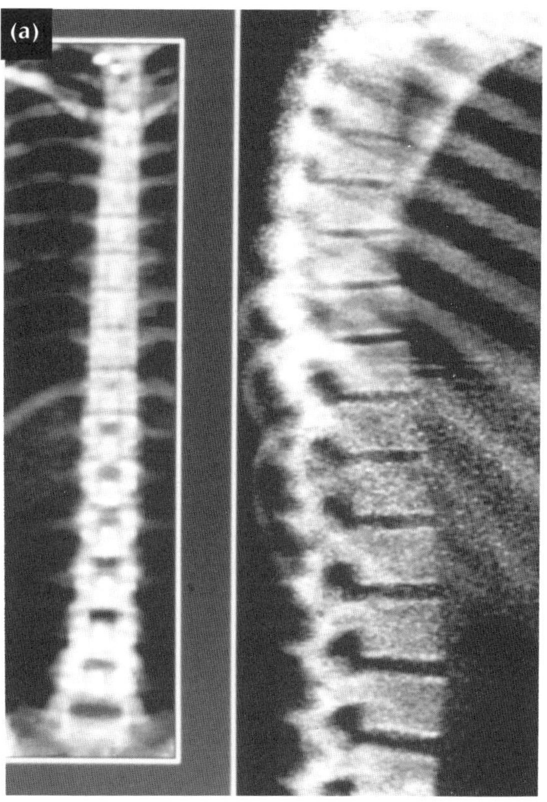

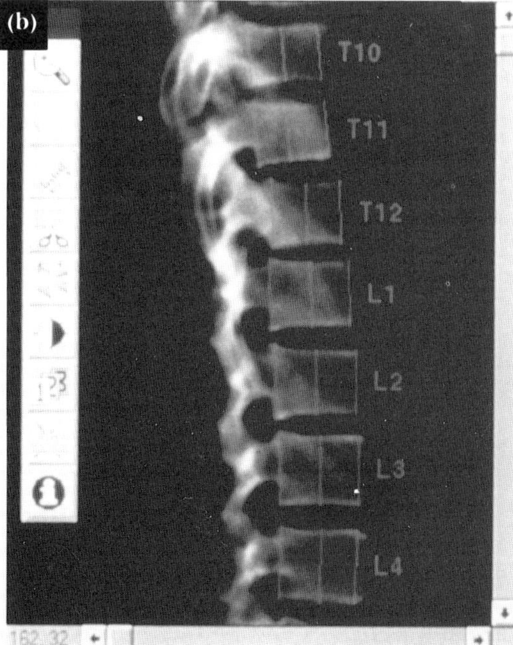

Morphometric results
Lateral spine

	Central Ht		A/P Rabo		Fracture
	% Normal	Z-score	% Normal	Z-score	Index
T5	98	−0.2	98	−0.3	Normal
T6	99	−0.1	102	+0.3	Normal
T7	101	+0.1	94	−0.3	Normal
T8	98	−0.2	102	+0.4	Normal
T9	94	−0.7	94	−0.9	Normal
T10	98	−0.3	99	−0.2	Normal
T11	95	−0.6	96	−0.6	Normal
T12	94	−0.8	98	−0.3	Normal
L1	95	−0.6	97	−0.5	Normal
L2	93	−1.0	84	−2.7	Normal
L3	93	−1.0	93	−1.2	Normal
L4	95	−0.7	98	−0.3	Normal

Figure 11 *(a) Antero-posterior (left) and lateral (right) dual energy X-ray absorptiometry (DXA) scan of the thoracic and lumbar spine for vertebral morphometry (from Hologic Inc. – with permission). (b) In vitro lateral thoraco-lumbar DXA scan showing morphometric measurements and results (Lunar Corporation – with permission)*

(a)

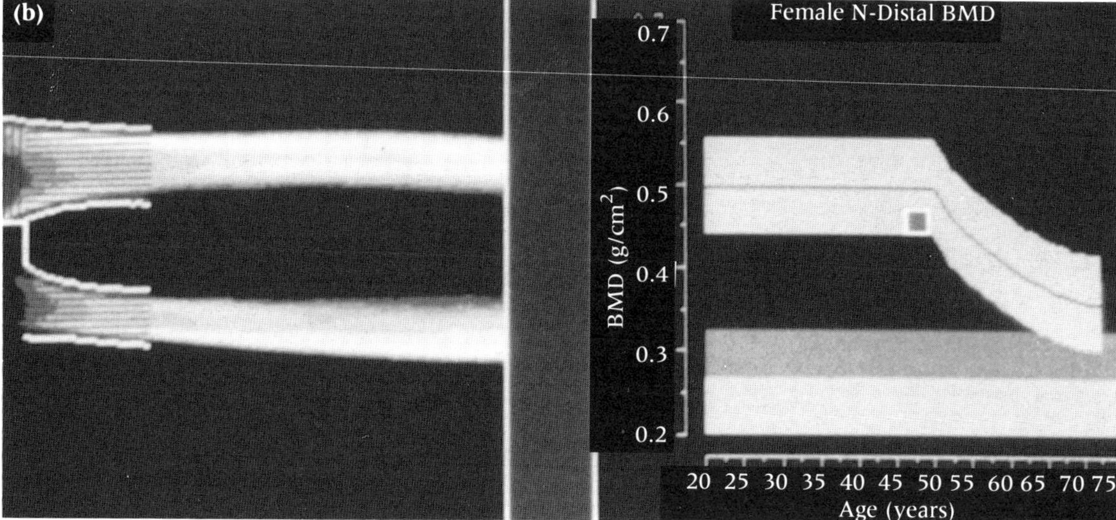

Figure 12 *(a) Patient having a scan performed by single energy X-ray absorptiometry. This provides a measure of bone mineral density (BMD) in a distal site (b) of the non-dominant forearm. The patient's result is displayed in relation to a normal reference range. (Osteometer from Hologic Inc. – with permission)*

fluid calibration phantoms with varying concentrations of dipotassium-hydrogen-phosphate (K_2HPO_4) were used. However, because of leakage or transpiration of fluid from the solutions into the perspex of the phantom, air bubbles developed in the solutions making scanning difficult or inaccurate. This led to the development of calibration phantoms in the solutions making scanning difficult or inaccurate. This led to the development of calibration phantoms using solid materials (hydroxyapatite), which are now generally preferred[113]. The results from different types of calibration phantoms are not interchangeable[114,115] unless a cross-calibration calculation can be made[113] (Figure 15). In longitudinal studies it is preferable that the same reference phantom be used.

Scanning takes approximately 10–15 min, and analysis 5–10 min. On some CT scanners (Siemens AG; Erlangen, Germany) software programs have been developed which allow automated selection of both the scan plane and the region of interest, resulting in improved precision and shorter scanning and analysis time[116]. More detailed areas of analysis can be made with QCT, to include separate estimates of BMD of the

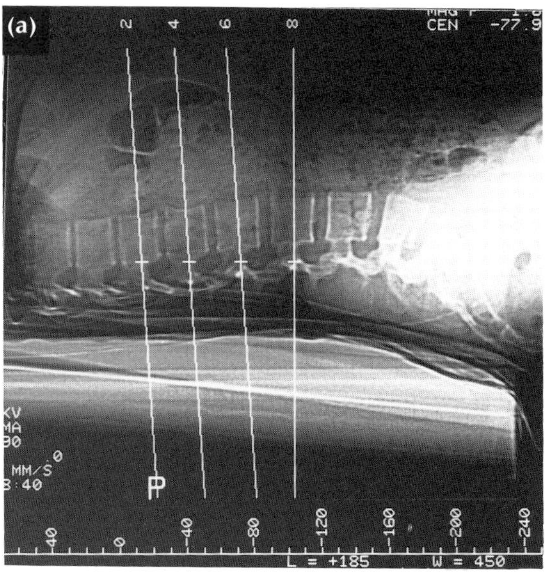

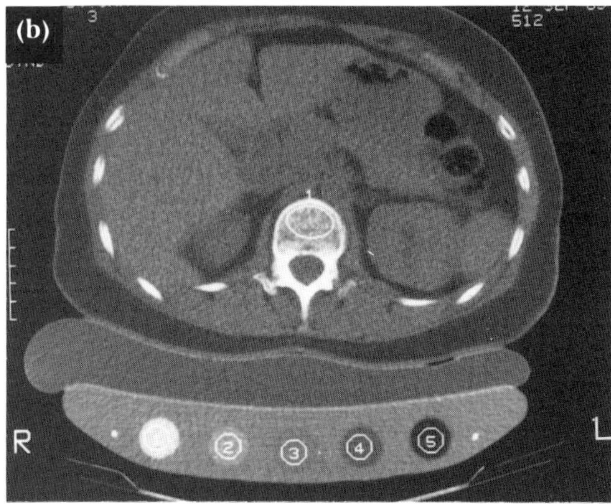

Figure 13 *(a) See lateral scan projection radiograph annotated with planes of section through the mid-vertebral planes of T12–L3. (b) Computed tomography section through mid-vertebral plane showing region of analysis of trabecular bone. Below the patient is the dipotassium-hydrogen-phosphate calibration phantom and between this and the patient is a water bag*

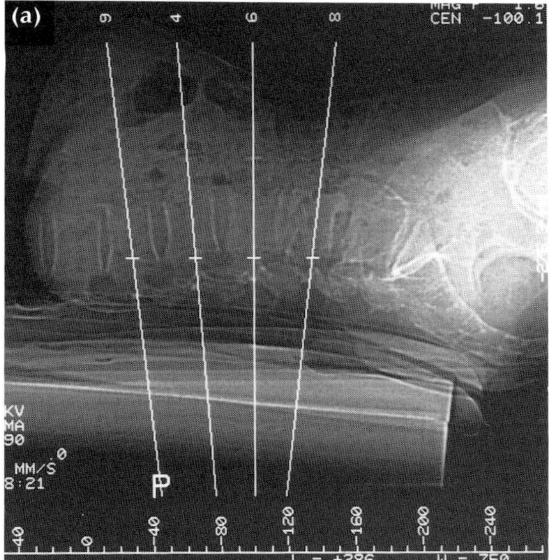

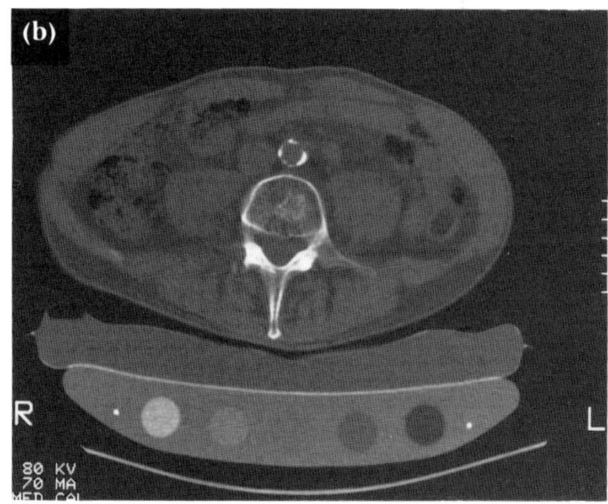

Figure 14 *(a) Computed tomography lateral scan projection radiograph showing upper end-plate fractures of L1 and L4. (b) The section through L4 has included part of the upper end-plate causing overestimation of bone mineral density. The value from this vertebral body would have to be excluded from analysis*

trabecular bone, the cortical rim of the vertebral body, and integral bone which includes the neural arch.

The precision of QCT *in vivo* is 1–3%, with an accuracy of 1–2% for K_2HPO_4 solutions and 5–15% for human vertebrae. The cause of the inaccuracy is the presence of marrow fat within trabecular bone which can cause single energy QCT to underestimate BMD[117]. This can be overcome and accuracy improved by applying a dual energy QCT technique[118–120], using either pre-[121,122] or postprocessing[123–127] methods. However, this bears the penalties of poorer precision and increased radiation dose and is not necessary in routine clinical practice. To achieve good precision with QCT, meticulous care is

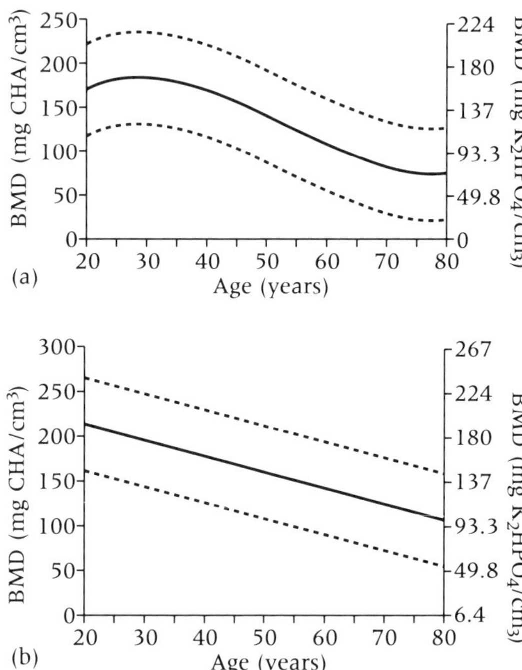

Figure 15 *Reference bone mineral density (BMD) data for (a) women and (b) men scanned on a GE 9800 at 80 kVp with a solid hydroxyapatite calibration standard (CHA axis) and with the liquid calibration standard (K_2HPO_4 axis) 95% confidence limits are also shown (from Faulkner et al., reference 113, Osteoporosis International 1993 – with permission)*

required to maintain constant scanning factors. This includes consistency of the scanner table height, exposure factors, gantry angle and field size, all of which should be recorded at each visit throughout longitudinal studies. To achieve this consistency, it is best to have a few, highly motivated and skilled radiographers performing the scans and analysis, rather than a large number of less experienced staff performing measurements infrequently. This dictum applies equally to all the quantitative methods of bone densitometry.

Although QCT has the highest radiation dose of any of the bone density techniques, this can be minimized by the use of a low-dose technique[111,128]. A lower kVp (70–80) than that routinely used in CT imaging (120–140 kVp) can be used with a lower mAs (e.g. 140 mAs). This can reduce patient radiation dose without significantly affecting measurement precision. The dose for QCT (90 μSv) is similar to that for a postero-anterior chest radiograph (60 μSv) which carries the lowest radiation dose of any conventional radiographic procedures[128]. Although a general purpose CT scanner may cost between £250 000 and £500 000, it is versatile in its clinical applications when not performing bone densitometry. For fairer comparison with other BMD techniques, one should compare the cost of the additional charges made by the companies for software to perform BMD which range between £10 000 and £16 000.

QCT has been generally and most widely applied to the measurement of vertebral trabecular bone. However, application to the appendicular skeleton has also been made in the forearm[129–131], tibia and femur[132]. Attempts to apply QCT to the femoral neck, a clinically important site from the point of view of osteoporotic fractures, have generally not been very successful or practical. Several special purpose, low-dose CT scanners have been built using a monoenergetic photon beam from a ^{124}I source. However, these are only applicable to the appendicular skeleton. A scanner has recently been developed in Germany (Stratec, Medizintechnik, Pforzheim, Germany) which has an X-ray source and provides QCT measurements (separate cortical and trabecular analysis) in the non-dominant forearm[131] (Figure 16). This equipment is relatively compact and costs approximately £35 000.

There is evidence that other factors additional to bone density contribute to bone strength. These include trabecular thickness and arrangement. With thin section, high resolution CT, such trabecular parameters can be assessed by image analysis techniques. Whether this has an additional role in predicting fracture risk remains to be established.

Despite the relatively high cost, and in some countries restricted availability, of CT scanners, QCT was widely applied to bone densitometry in the late 1980s when the only established alternative techniques were single and dual photon absorptiometry. With the developments and availability of DXA the number of centers using QCT will diminish. However, with its unique ability to measure separately trabecular bone

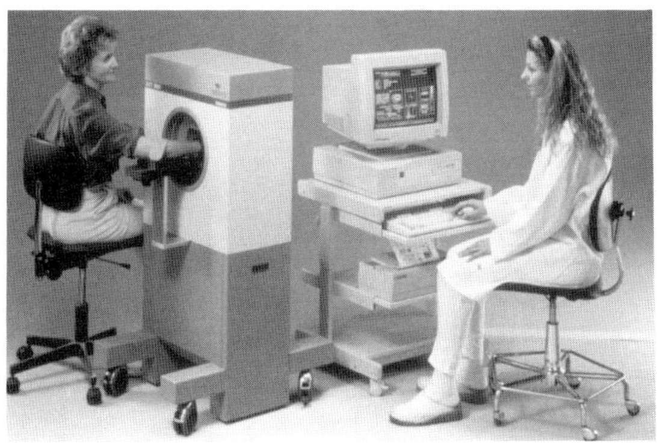

Figure 16 *Equipment for scanning a peripheral skeletal site (the non-dominant forearm) by quantitative computed tomography (pQCT) (from Stratec – with permission)*

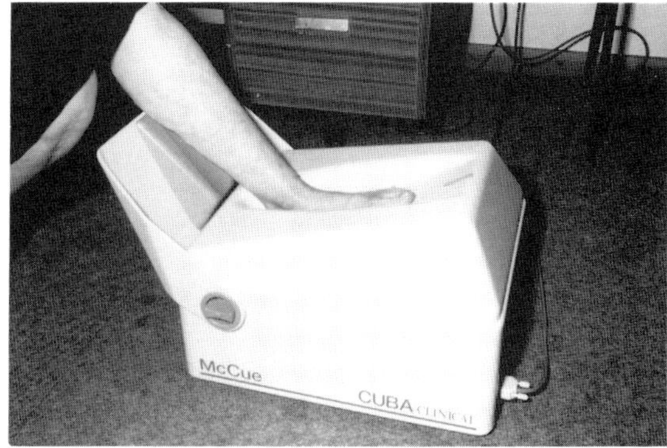

Figure 17 *Broadband ultrasound attenuation: foot in position for contact scanning for measurement of the os calcis (Cuba Clinical and McCue – with permission)*

which is metabolically some eight times more active than cortical bone, QCT may be more sensitive than other techniques which measure integral bone in studies assessing short-term changes in BMD[133,134].

POTENTIAL METHODS

Broadband ultrasound

Ultrasound was first applied to assess bone mass in 1984[135,136]. As ultrasound passes through a material, some energy is lost through mechanisms such as absorption and scattering. Since cancellous bone is highly attenuating, frequencies much lower than those used in diagnostic imaging ultrasound (1–10 MHz) have to be used, typically 0.2–0.6 MHz. Because of the high attenuation of ultrasound by trabecular bone, a transmission technique is used in which one ultrasound transducer acts as transmitter and a second as a receiver. The method is generally applied to the os calcis with these transducers positioned either side of the heel (Figure 17). Correction for soft tissue requires the heel to be placed in a water bath. The os calcis is chosen because of its high trabecular bone content, its ease of accessibility and its parallel sides across which the measurements are made. With the heel in position, ultrasound frequencies are transmitted either as a broad pulse with mixed frequencies with the received signal then being fed through a spectrum analyzer, or as a sequence of short transmissions each of a single frequency across the frequency range used (0.2–0.6 MHz) (Figure 18). Attenuation in decibels (dB) of ultrasound at a given frequency is defined as the ratio of signal amplitudes for the reference (water) and sample (bone). This relationship for trabecular bone is linear over the range of frequencies used. By linear regression analysis the slope of the relationship between attenuation and frequency is derived to give the broadband ultrasound index (dB/MHz). The speed of sound can also be measured both at the os calcis and in the patella (contact scanning). Not only does ultrasound not use ionizing radiation, the equipment is relatively portable and also reasonably low cost (approximately £20 000). Scanners presently available are manufactured by Walker Sonix (UBA 575), 'Achilles' (Lunar Wisconsin, USA) and the contact ultrasonic bone analyzer (Cuba-McCue)[137]. The first two require the foot to be placed in a water bath for measurement; the last does not and the contact technique was initially developed for the measurement of bone mass in the fetlock of thoroughbred racehorses where rapid data collection was essential. This contact scanning has also been used in neonates and infants for measurement of bone mass in the forearm. To improve precision of the conventional water bath technique, various foot restraints are used. A rectilinear scanning device to measure in a number of closely spaced sites through the os calcis have also been incorporated (Walker Sonix UBA

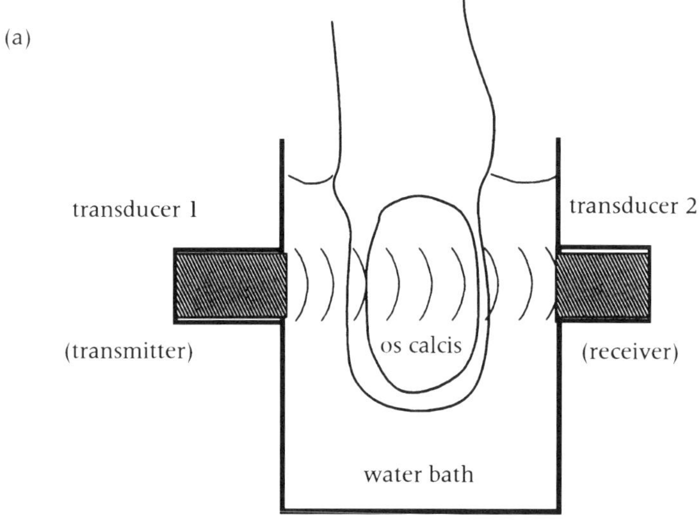

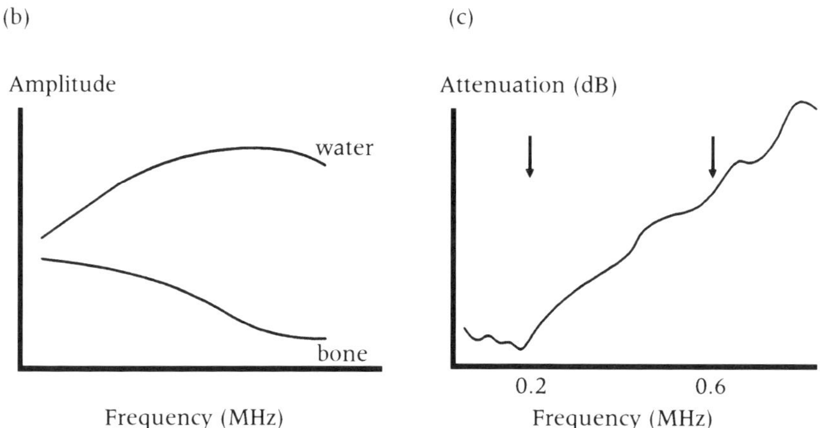

Figure 18 *(a) Diagram of equipment for os calcis broadband ultrasound attenuation (BUA) measurement. (b) Results of BUA measurement through water bath with and without the patient's heel in position. (c) Ultrasound attenuation plotted against frequency, the slope of which gives the BUA index (from Whitehouse, 1991 reference 69 – with permission)*

575). Broadband ultrasound scanning is simple and quick (> 5 min) to perform and has a short-term precision of 3–5%, and long-term precision of 5–10%[138].

Ultrasound has the potential for measuring several determinants of bone strength. There has been shown to be a close relationship between elasticity and speed of sound, but not broadband ultrasound. Several studies have documented a relatively close association between physical density and broadband ultrasound. The anisotropic arrangement of trabeculae is reflected by an orientational dependence found for both the speed of sound and the broadband ultrasound results. Fatigue damage of bone has been shown to correlate with elasticity and therefore should have a marked effect on the speed of sound although this still needs to be confirmed.

Studies *in vitro* have reported the association of broadband ultrasound and the speed of sound with bone strength and several studies indicate that ultrasound may yield information about bone strength and fracture risk independently of bone mass. However, this too requires experimental confirmation and further research is essential to determine the optimum method and site of measurement and the clinical applicability of the technique.

Broadband ultrasound has been found to correlate with other bone density measurements made in the same bone (with excised calcanei $r = 0.92$; with QCT of the spine $r = 0.80$, and with physical density $r = 0.85$)[139]. Some studies have been performed assessing the correlation between broadband ultrasound of the os calcis and DXA of the lumbar spine ($r = 0.83$) and femoral neck ($r = 0.87$)[140,141]. However, as with other correlations between methods of bone densitometry, these relationships are too weak to permit accurate prediction of BMD by another technique and in a different anatomical site from broadband ultrasound at the os calcis. *In vivo*, broadband ultrasound appears to separate patients with femoral neck fractures from control subjects[142–145]. The technique therefore shows potential, but further studies are required to verify its usefulness in the clinical assessment of osteoporosis and fracture risk.

Magnetic resonance imaging

Magnetic resonance imaging does not use ionizing radiation and has had immense impact in imaging in the brain, spine, soft tissues, heart and vessels. Although compact bone shows an absence of signal on magnetic resonance images, there have been recent developments in magnetic resonance techniques to study trabecular bone. The signal intensity from bone marrow is altered by the presence of trabecular bone matrix and such effects can be enhanced by using specific imaging sequences. The differences in magnetic properties between trabecular bone and bone marrow cause distortions of the magnetic lines of force which result in magnetic field heterogeneity. This heterogeneity alters the relaxation properties of tissue such as the transverse relaxation time ($T2^*$) in gradient echo images. Changes in $T2^*$ therefore relate to density and spatial geometry of the trabeculae. In preliminary studies, there has been shown to be an inverse relationship between trabecular density and $T2^*$[146]. Studies *in vitro* have demonstrated correlation between vertebral bone density (QCT) and the inverse of $T2^*$ relaxation ($1/T2^*$) ($r = 0.9$) with evidence that the parameter $T2^*$ is influenced not only by the density, but also the geometry, of trabeculae[147]. Magnetic resonance imaging has potential for providing information on both trabecular structure and architecture which has relevance in assessing bone strength and fracture prediction[148].

Recently developed magnetic resonance microscopy has research potential for the study of trabecular microarchitecture *in vitro*[149]. Images of trabecular bone specimens can be obtained with a resolution of between 33×33 μm to 66×66 μm. This demonstrates individual trabeculae, but requires a magnetic field strength of 9.4 Tesla, so can only be applied to bone specimens.

Quantitative magnetic resonance imaging and magnetic resonance microscopy hold potential for assessing bone density and structure and predicting fracture risk. However, at present the techniques remain in the research domain and further studies are required to assess their role in clinical practice. A limitation of magnetic resonance imaging at present is availability of scanner time to perform studies which are time-consuming and hence costly.

High resolution and micro-computed tomography

Additional information of the architecture of vertebral trabecular bone can be drawn from thin (1 mm) sections obtained during QCT with automatic regional evaluation of bone density[150]. These regional density measurements performed *in vitro* correlate with bone strength. However, the method involves a higher radiation dose than conventional QCT and requires sophisticated software programs for analysis. The technique can at present only be applied as a research, rather than a clinical, tool.

The spatial resolution of conventional CT images is 0.5–1.0 mm. Micro-CT equipment can provide a spatial resolution of 15 μm with tissue slices of 25 μm thickness[149,151]. This spatial resolution can identify Haversian canals and variations in mineralization. Although the technique provides potential for studying bone structure, it requires highly sophisticated equipment and involves high radiation doses and is at present limited to application to excised bone specimens only.

Finite element analysis

Finite element analysis is used in engineering to assess the strength of a new design from structural information. To define the mechanical behavior of a structure, knowledge of the geometry, the material properties and the load to which the structure is subjected are required. Finite element models have been derived from 3-dimensional QCT studies of the spine and hip[149,152]. Finite element analysis has been shown to correlate with the mechanical properties of bone specimens *in vitro*, and has been applied *in vivo* to estimate vertebral strength in order to distinguish between individuals with and without osteoporosis. Although the method shows promise, it presently utilizes considerable computer time for analysis and remains a research tool.

Compton scattering techniques

The inelastic scattering of X-rays by the electrons of an atom was initially described in 1923, and a Compton scatter densitometer for determination of electron densities of human tissues *in vivo* was introduced in 1959[153–155]. A variety of radionuclides have been used as the photon source but the techniques have relatively poor spatial resolution, require higher radiation doses than transmission (CT) imaging systems and have not become established as clinically useful tools[154–157]. Duke and Hanson[157] investigated the replacement of radionuclide sources with commercial X-ray tubes in Compton's scatter densitometry. As a result of the increased photon flux X-ray tubes might provide improved spatial resolution, precision and counting times. However, the polychromatic source provided by X-ray tubes results in problems of analysis.

Neutron activation analysis methods

This technique was first applied in 1964. By irradiating an individual with neutrons total body chlorine, sodium and calcium can be determined[158–162]. In the process of neutron activation, the nucleus absorbs a neutron which causes the nucleus to be in an excited state. The nucleus returns to its equilibrium state by emitting γ radiation and the photon intensities are proportional to the amounts of the elements present in the body[160]. Total body calcium determined in this way is expressed in grams of calcium normalized to body size. However, the equipment and resources required for such measurements are expensive, available in only a limited number of research centers and require significant expertise for operation.

RADIATION DOSE

The radiation doses involved in the photon absorptiometric techniques are extremely low. The effective dose equivalent for single photon absorptiometry < 0.6 μSv and for DXA is 1 μSv per site examined and up to 6 μSv per site in women, depending upon whether the ovary is included within the scanning field. The dose is relatively higher for QCT, but this can be minimized to between 60 and 90 μSv per examination if a low-dose scanning technique (80 kVp, 70 mA, 2 s scanning time) is used[111]. This compares favorably with conventional radiographic procedures, being similar to that for a postero-anterior chest radiograph (60 μSv) and considerably less than either background radiation (2400 μSv per annum), and other radiographic procedures commonly used in the investigation of osteoporosis (lateral lumbar spine radiographs between 700 and 2000 μSv)[128]. The extremely low doses involved in DXA make it a suitable tool for the investigation of skeletal development in neonates and children[163–165], and useful data are being acquired in this field. With the low radiation doses involved in DXA, the equipment does not have to be installed in designated radiation areas. However, it is essential that those clinically directing and operating the equipment comply with relevant radiation protection regulations.

CORRELATIONS BETWEEN ESTABLISHED BMD TECHNIQUES

The mineral content of the skeleton is stored in either cortical (compact) or trabecular (cancellous) bone. The skeleton is composed of cortical bone (80%), which predominates in the appendicular skeleton, and the remaining 20% is trabecular bone. Trabecular bone being porous has a large surface area per unit volume and is highly responsive to metabolic processes. As a consequence the turnover rate of trabecular bone is some eight times greater than that of the more stable and dense cortical bone. This factor makes trabecular bone a more sensitive measure for monitoring longitudinal changes in BMD with disease or therapy, and for the detection of early bone loss[105,133,134]. The rate of accretion of new bone during growth and development[165–167] and the rates of bone loss during aging and at the menopause in women vary in these different skeletal sites and with diseases[168–172]. The process of bone remodeling to replace old bone matrix with new may have an annual turnover of up to 25% in trabecular bone and 2–3% in cortical bone. Osteoporotic fractures tend to occur in sites in the skeleton composed predominantly of trabecular bone (vertebrae, femoral neck, distal radius), and the bone loss that occurs at the menopause affects predominantly trabecular bone. All such factors have to be considered when BMD is measured by the variety of techniques which are available. The methods measure either trabecular, cortical, or integral (cortical and trabecular) bone and may be applied to the axial or the appendicular skeleton (Table 1). Studies have shown that BMD measured by different techniques in the same individual are variously correlated ($r = 0.2–0.9$)[173–178] (Figure 19). Such variable correlations are to be expected if it is realized that the techniques are measuring different types of bone in variable skeletal sites. As a consequence of the dispersion around the regression line of correlations between BMD techniques results obtained by one method cannot be used to predict the result which would be obtained by using another method in the same, or at a different, anatomical site.

All the techniques established in clinical use (single photon absorptiometry, DXA and QCT) have precisions (0.5–4%) and accuracies (6–9%) which provide results which are clinically useful in assessing the effect of disease and therapy on the skeleton[43,149] (Table 1). However, all must be performed with meticulous care to ensure consistency of technique[45]. This applies perhaps most particularly to QCT, since BMD results will vary with inconsistency of scanning technique, and the use of different scanners and calibration phantoms. The BMD results from QCT using the hydroxyapatite phantoms are generally higher than those obtained from fluid K_2HPO_4 phantoms[113] (Figure 15). Similarly, measurements performed by dual photon absorptiometry and DXA, and between DXA scanners made by different manufacturers, are not interchangeable (Lunar DPX measuring approximately 12% higher than Hologic equipment)[175,176]. In longitudinal studies it is therefore essential that the technical aspects (scanner type, calibration system, software program) remain constant. Should changes in these technical parameters occur during established studies, then it may be possible to calculate a conversion factor to make results comparable[113] (Figure 15). Such variability of BMD values obtained by different techniques and in varying sites may result in some confusion and scepticism of their validity amongst clinicians requesting such measurements for use in clinical management. The necessity for standardization of BMD measurements[179] was the stimulus for the establishment of a multicenter study 'Quantitative Assessment of Osteoporosis' funded by the European Community (COMAC-BME-Comité d'Actions Concertée, project number MR4-0308-B). Anthropomorphic calcium hydroxyapatite phantoms were designed to simulate the lumbar spine and forearm[180]. These were

Table 1 *Comparison of currently used techniques for measuring bone mineral density*

Technique	*Cortical/ trabecular ratio*	*Precision* in vivo (%)	*Accuracy error* (%)	*Scanning time* (min)	*Effective dose equivalent* (μSv)
Single photon absorptiometry					
Distal third radius	95/5	1–2	4–6	10	< 1
Ultradistal radius	60/40	1–2	4–6	10	< 1
Os calcis	5/95	1–2	4–6	15	< 1
Dual photon absorptiometry					
Lumbar spine	50/50	2–4	5–10	30	5
Proximal femur	60/40	3–5	5–10	30	3
Total body	80/20	2–3	1–2	40	3
Dual energy X-ray absorptiometry (pencil beam)					
Lumbar spine					
antero-posterior	50/50	1	4–8	5–10	1
lateral	10/90	2–3	5–10	15–20	3
Proximal femur	60/40	1–2	4–8	5–10	1
Total body	80/20	1	1–2	20	3
Quantitative computed tomography					
Single energy spine	0/100*	2–4	5–15	20	50
Dual energy spine	0/100*	4–6	3–6	25	100

From Faulkner *et al.*, 1991, reference 149 – with permission.
*Depends on region of interest; the vertebral core is 100% trabecular bone

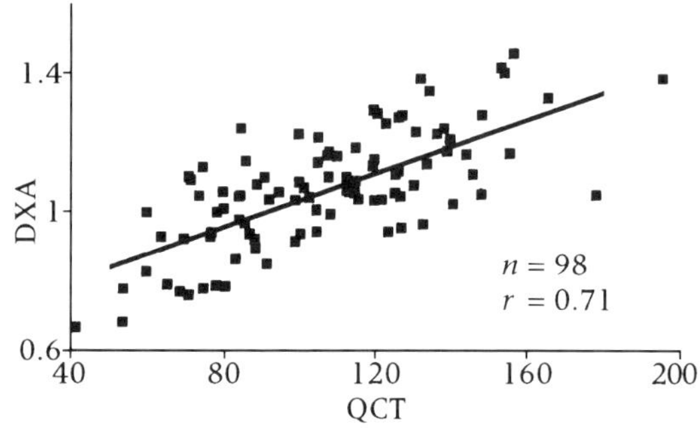

Figure 19 *Comparison of bone density measurements made in the same anatomical site (spine) but by different techniques quantitative computed tomography (QCT) (mg/cm^3) and dual energy X-ray absorptiometry (DXA) (g/cm^2) in the same individual showing correlation, but the results from one technique cannot be used to predict those which would be obtained by an alternative technique in the same anatomical site*

tributed to the participating centers within Europe for scanning by different techniques and scanners. The data are being analyzed to assess whether cross-calibration of scanners and techniques is feasible. Such cross-calibration and quality assurance are essential requirements for multicenter trials involved in the assessment of the efficacy of treatment in osteoporosis. Individual centers involved in such studies must measure their own long- and short-term precision *in vitro* and *in vivo* and have rigorous and regular programs to maintain quality assurance. Often, the precision quoted by manufacturers of BMD equipment has been measured either in phantoms or in young normal individuals. The precision which can be obtained in patients, particularly those with osteoporosis, will be less good because of the low bone mass and the difficulty in positioning the patient satisfactorily and the patient remaining still throughout the examination.

BMD REFERENCE RANGES

To be able to interpret whether the results of BMD in an individual, measured by any of the techniques, are normal requires appropriate BMD reference ranges to be available for comparison. Such reference ranges are either provided by the manufacturers of the scanning equipment or calibration phantom used, or can be drawn from published studies in both children[181–185] and adults[186–190] (Figure 20). Some variation has been observed between reference data drawn from an American Caucasian population and provided by equipment manufacturers and studies of different nationalities[191]. However, as the manufacturers' reference databases increase to include a greater number of subjects, such observed differences diminish and are probably negligible within the same racial group. It is essential that the reference range used for an individual is drawn from the appropriate racial group, since there are considerable differences in BMD between races[192,193].

BMD results can be expressed as a percentage, a percentile or preferably as a standard deviation score (Z-score) of age- and sex-matched reference range or of sex-matched peak bone mass (T-score)[194]. Comparison with such a reference range enables some arbitrary level of BMD to be selected for therapeutic intervention. For example a T-score of – 1 or less identifies women who would most benefit from hormone replacement therapy at the menopause. The result will also give an indication of the degree of osteopenia; a Z-score of – 2 or below indicating relative osteopenia, a T-score of – 2 or below indicating absolute osteopenia. This allows some prediction of fracture risk[195,196], there being a one to twofold increase in this risk for every one standard deviation the BMD falls below the lower range (– 2 SD) of sex-matched peak bone mass.

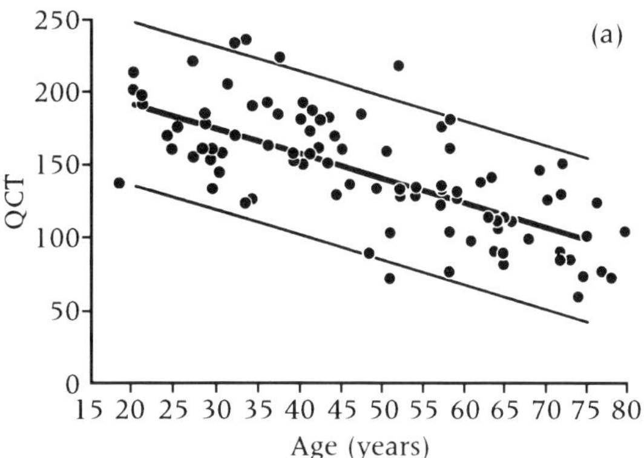

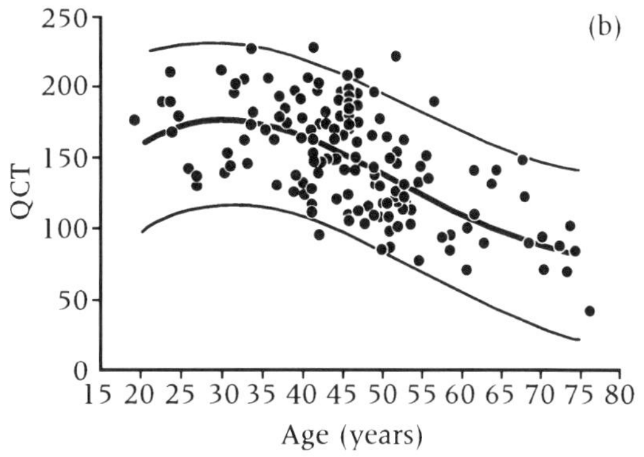

Figure 20 *(a) Reference male values for vertebral trabecular mineral content by quantitative computed tomography (QCT), using a linear regression with 95% confidence intervals. (b) Reference female values for vertebral trabecular mineral density by QCT, using a cubic regression with 95% confidence intervals; an accelerated bone loss is observed after the menopause (from Genant et al., 1988 reference 110 – with permission)*

APPLICATIONS OF BONE DENSITOMETRY

The methods of bone densitometry which are available in clinical practice (single photon absorptiometry, QCT and particularly DXA) are able to provide precise and reasonably accurate BMD results rapidly with low radiation dose and are all relatively easy to perform[45,149]. The cost and availability of the measurements vary, but the provision of DXA scanners has increased greatly over recent years. Whether this expansion in numbers of DXA densitometers will continue at the same rate is uncertain.

Bone mass measurements play an important role in research in studying the patterns of bone loss in both the normal population and in endocrine and metabolic diseases which affect the skeleton and in assessing the effect of therapies[197–203]. All techniques are able to demonstrate, in cross-sectional studies, the age-related change which occurs in both men[204,205] (Figure 20) and women and in all racial groups so far examined. The rate of bone loss shows a biphasic pattern with a slow phase accounting for rates of loss of 0.5–1% of peak bone mass each year in both men and women. An accelerated phase during which loss rates may be 5–6% of peak bone mass per annum occurs during the decade following the menopause in women (Figure 20). The rate of bone loss determines the interval between BMD measurements in an individual, adequate time being required to be certain that a change is real and not simply related to the precision error of the technique. In statistical terms the rate of change in BMD needs to be approximately 2.7 times the precision of the technique to be statistically significant. Except at times of high rates of bone loss, the interval between measurements needs to be at least 2 years.

There has been debate concerning the appropriate applications of bone densitometry. However, such measurements are established in certain clinical situations[206–209]. These are as follows:

(1) At the time of the menopause in women willing to take hormone replacement therapy BMD levels can be used to identify those who would most benefit from such treatment (those with BMD at a T-score of – 1 SD or below of peak bone mass);

(2) In those individuals in whom spinal or other radiographs suggest osteopenia, bone densitometry provides objective confirmation of reduced bone density;

(3) In asymptomatic primary hyperparathyroidism, reduced bone mass serves as a determinant for surgical treatment;

(4) In patients receiving corticosteroid therapy, bone densitometry can be used as a parameter to regulate the dose used, or to determine the need for additional therapy to prevent excessive bone loss; and

(5) An increasingly important application of bone densitometry is in identifying those individuals with osteopenia and increased fracture risk to permit early therapeutic intervention and to assess efficacy of such treatment.

Bone densitometry has now been widely applied to study age-related bone mass and the interventions which may prevent osteoporosis. These include dietary modifications to ensure adequate calcium intake[210] and the importance of adequate weight-bearing exercise and hormone replacement therapy at the menopause. In addition, the techniques have had important applications to assess the efficacy of compounds used in the treatment of established osteoporosis including calcitonin, bisphosphonates, fluoride and parathyroid hormone. BMD can be used to predict fracture risk. Any of the measurements can make general predictions of the risk of fracture[211–218]. However, fracture prediction is best made by BMD performed in that particular anatomical site[211,214,219–222]. QCT has therefore been found to be the most sensitive at predicting vertebral spine fractures, DXA of the hip the best predictor of hip fractures and a BMD measurement in the forearm the best predictor of wrist fractures. The combination of a single bone mineral measurement (by single photon absorptiometry) combined with biochemical measures of bone turnover (fasting urinary creatinine, calcium, hydroxyproline and serum alkaline phosphatase) can be used to predict actual bone loss[223]. Since bone strength depends on factors additional to bone mineral density (trabecular thickness and arrangement) measurement of these parameters may enhance the predictive BMD value for fractures of[149]. Information on bone structure can be obtained from BMD techniques which are influenced by trabecular arrangement (broadband ultrasound, quantitative magnetic resonance imaging), or by examining the regional distribution of trabeculae and BMD from radiographic images or QCT[224–228].

With the increasing number of bone density techniques now available, there has been considerable variation in the terms and abbreviations used for each technique. For example dual energy X-ray absorptiometry (DEXA) has been variously referred to as dual energy X-ray absorptiometry (DXA); dual energy radiography (DER); dual energy radiographic absorptiometry (DRA) and quantitative digital radiography (DQR). This leads to confusion, and some standardization of not only terminology, but also calibration and measurement units is desirable[229,230]. There is general agreement that the standard abbreviations should be:

(1) Single photon absorptiometry – SPA;

(2) Dual photon absorptiometry – DPA;

(3) Dual energy X-ray absorptiometry – DXA;

(4) Single energy X-ray absorptiometry – SXA;

(5) Quantitative computed tomography – QCT; and

(6) Peripheral quantitative computed tomography – pQCT.

For conformity it has been suggested that when ultrasound attenuation and magnetic resonance are applied to quantify BMD and structure then the acronym QUS for quantitative ultrasound and QMR for quantitative magnetic resonance imaging might be appropriate, but such terminology requires consensus for adoption.

BONE DENSITOMETRY IN POPULATION SCREENING

Considerable debate and controversy surround the application of BMD measurement to the general female population at the time of the menopause[231–236], and the cost effectiveness of such a program[237–240] has not been proved. Since the rationale for general population screening has not been established, the resulting polarized debates unfortunately detract from the important and established uses of bone densitometry in individual patients and appropriate clinical circumstances. This is unfortunate since the clinical screening of risk factors to predict the presence of osteopenia has been shown to be relatively insensitive[241].

WHICH TECHNIQUE TO USE?

With the variety of techniques now available, it may be confusing to those either requesting such measurements or purchasing bone densitometers, to know which method to select. In research studies assessing the effect of disease and therapy on the skeleton, the methods are complementary as they measure different types of bone (cortical, trabecular, integral) at various anatomical sites. In the assessment of small changes in BMD over short periods of time then a measurement of trabecular bone (QCT) may be more sensitive. Although any of the techniques can be used to assess general fracture risk, this prediction is more specific when the measurement is applied to that particular anatomical site such as the spine for vertebral fracture, and the femoral neck or forearm for fractures in these respective sites[241,242] (Figure 21). For screening of the population, the rationale for which bone densitometry has not yet been established, techniques that are relatively inexpensive and simple to perform (SPA, DXA of the forearm, pQCT, broadband ultrasound and even metacarpal index) may be adequate[243–245].

VERTEBRAL MORPHOMETRY

The aim of treatment of osteoporosis is to maintain or increase BMD and consequently reduce fracture rate. Assessing the effect of treatment on the rate of subsequent fracture of the femoral neck or forearm may require protracted periods of study (10–30 years) and large cohorts of patients. In therapeutic trials of shorter duration and a more limited number of subjects, the presence of vertebral fracture is an important criterion for entry to trials, and the assessment of vertebral deforming events (end-plate, wedge or crush fractures) has been used to assess treatment efficacy[28,29] (Figure 22). The assessments of these parameters can be made by both quantitative (morphometric) and semi-quantitative (visual) techniques[246–248]. These assessments are made from lateral spinal radiographs. In these there may be the problem of different magnifications when various X-ray focus-to-film distances are used and parallax, when the spine is not parallel to the radiograph. When such spinal assessments are being made, it is essential that the radiographic technique (film focus distance, patient positioning and X-ray tube centering) must be consistent to obtain reproducible results. Radiographs are generally obtained in the lateral projection of the thoracic (centered at T7–8 and including T4) and lumbar (centering L2–3 and including L5) spine. It is essential that the vertebral bodies can be accurately numbered. This may be aided by acquisition of antero-posterior projections which will also

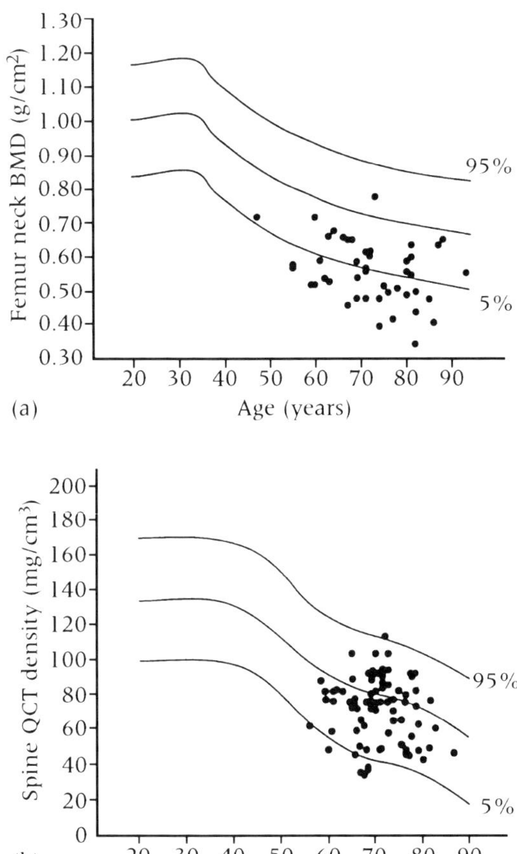

Figure 21 *(a) The femoral neck bone mineral density (BMD) by dual photon absorptiometry showing the values for those with hip fracture (n = 47) against the mean and 95% confidence limits of reference values (from reference 68, as adapted from Mazess et al., 1988, reference 211). (b) The vertebral trabecular bone density by quantitative computerized tomography (QCT) showing values in cases of hip fracture (n = 83) without concomitant spine fracture (from reference 68, as adapted from Firooznia et al., 1986 reference 214 – with permission). These figures illustrate that BMD measured in the femoral neck is a better predictor of hip fractures; data also exist to suggest that measurements of BMD in the spine, particularly QCT, better predicts vertebral fractures*

provide information concerning scoliosis and degenerative changes, but add to the cost and radiation dose. The prevalence of vertebral fractures is assessed from cross-sectional epidemiological studies or at entry to clinical trials. At present, there is no internationally accepted definition of the vertebral deformity which constitutes a vertebral fracture[249,250], and similar deformities may be the result of other diseases (degenerative, malignant) or congenital anomalies. Vertebral deformities can be defined visually or quantitatively by reduction in either anterior or mid-portion of a vertebra in relation to its posterior height (wedge, end-plate deformity), or by reduction of all the parameters (anterior, middle and posterior height) to either adjacent vertebra within the same individual, or when compared to data from a reference population (crush vertebrae) (Figure 22). Although there is no consensus at the present time as to what constitutes a vertebral fracture by these parameters a reduction of three standard deviations (3 SD) or more from such normal mean reference dimensions for individual vertebral bodies is emerging as a preferred criterion[250]. Deformities of less than this magnitude may result in a high incidence of false positive vertebral fractures. Alternatively the degree of wedging of a vertebra can be determined by comparison with other vertebrae within the same individual. There is debate on the degree of wedging (15%, 20% or 25%) that constitutes an osteoporotic fracture. Generally a 25% reduction or more in any of the height parameters is preferred since a 20% reduction may be normal. The prevalence of spinal osteoporosis in the community therefore varies according to the criteria used to define a vertebral fracture, and may be more common than previously appreciated, since only one-third of affected individuals are symptomatic and come to medical attention[251–253].

The incidence of vertebral fractures during a study is assessed by changes in the shape of vertebrae. For precision, it is essential that the radiographic technique is standardized. It is also preferable that the assessments are performed collectively at the end of the study rather than continuously during the study, again for consistency of results. Such assessment can be made visually or by manual morphometric measurements. The latter are time-consuming, and automated image analysis techniques are being developed and show promise[254]. Recent developments on DXA scanners enable lateral images of the vertebral bodies from T4 to L4 to be obtained (Figures 11a, 11b). From these im-

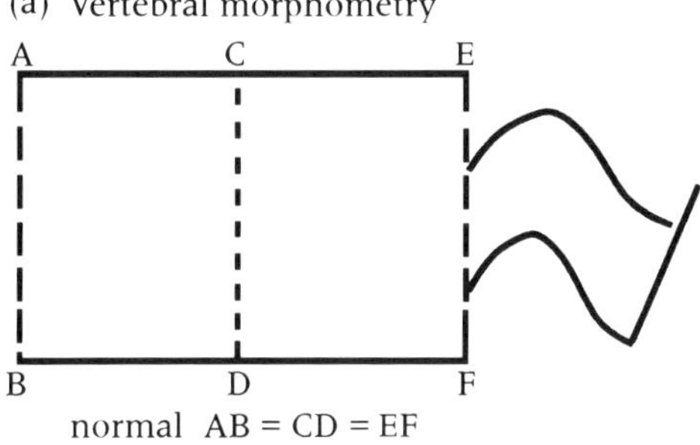

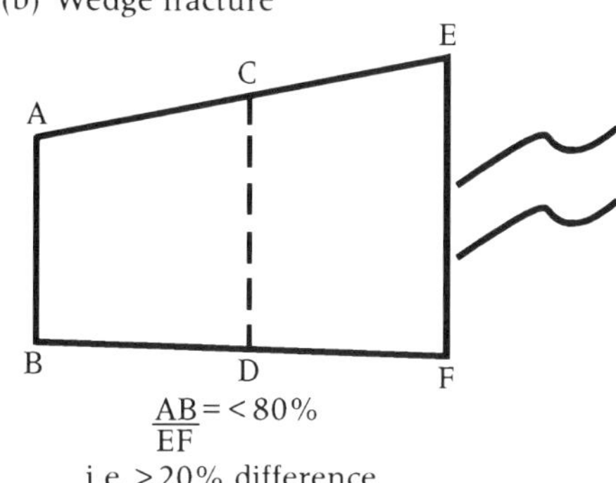

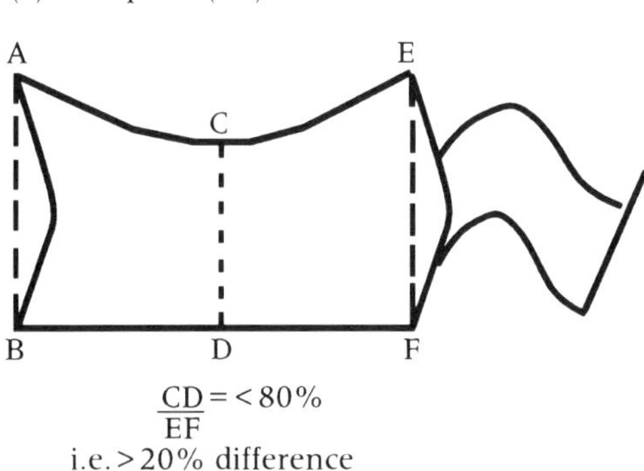

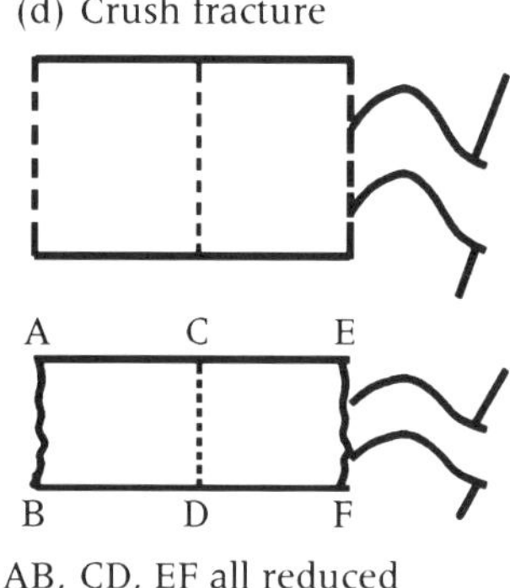

Figure 22 *(a) Vertebral morphometry. Line diagram to show the six points which are identified to assess the shape and size of the vertebral body on lateral radiograph. (b) Wedge fracture showing reduction in the anterior vertebral height (line AB) in comparison to posterior height (line EF). (c) End-plate fracture showing reduction in mid-vertebral height (line CD) when compared to anterior and posterior heights (line AB and EF, respectively). (d) Crush fracture, all the heights, anterior, mid- and posterior (lines AB, CD and EF, respectively) are reduced when compared to adjacent vertebrae*

ages, which avoid the magnification inherent in radiographs, automated identification of six points of the vertebral margin (both superior and inferior points of the anterior, middle and posterior vertebral margins) can be identified to provide quantification of vertebral morphometry with practical and theoretical advantages. The prevalence and incidence of vertebral fractures at commencement and during therapeutic trials of established osteoporosis could be determined at the same time as BMD was measured.

Magnetic resonance imaging also has potential for defining normal vertebral morphometry and identifying vertebral fractures without the use of ionizing radiation. However, the availability and cost may limit its development in this clinical area and its role in this field is still to be established.

FUTURE RESEARCH AND DEVELOPMENT

Technical developments with faster scanning, improved image quality and morphometric measurements will continue with DXA. To improve the discriminatory and predictive power of bone densitometry in assessing fracture risk, biomechanical and other parameters can be used. The thickness and arrangement of trabeculae are known to contribute to bone strength. Methods that can provide information on trabecular structure, including broadband ultrasound, high resolution CT and magnetic resonance imaging, require further studies to assess their application in the clinical arena. With the breadth of techniques, applications and developments in bone densitometry in health and disease, it becomes increasingly difficult for those with an interest to keep abreast of the field with relevant reports appearing in many and diverse journals. Journals in which all the articles are relevant to the subject of osteoporosis and bone densitometry or which provide precise or consensus summaries are therefore particularly welcome[255–257].

References

1. Newton-John HF, Morgan DB. Osteoporosis: disease or senescience. Lancet 1968; 1: 232–3.
2. Nordin BE. Clinical significance and pathogenesis of osteoporosis. Br Med J 1971; 1: 571–6.
3. Newton-John HF, Morgan DB. The loss of bone with age, osteoporosis and fractures. Clin Orthop 1970; 71: 229–52.
4. Mazess RB. On aging bone loss. Clin Orthop 1982; 165: 239–52.
5. Riggs BL, Melton LJ. Evidence for two distinct syndromes of involutional osteoporosis. Am J Med 1983; 75: 899–901.
6. Melton LJ, Riggs BL. Clinical spectrum. In: Riggs BL, Melton LJ, eds. Osteoporosis Aetiology, Diagnosis and Management, New York: Raven Press, 1988; 155–79.
7. Heath DA. Osteoporosis – its significance, prevention and treatment. Current Imaging 1991; 3: 221–5.
8. Dempster DW, Lindsay R. Pathogenesis of osteoporosis. Lancet 1993; 341: 797–801.
9. Steiger P, Cummings SR, Black DM, Spencer NE, Genant HK. Age related decrements in bone mineral density in women over 65. J Bone Min Res 1992; 7: 625–32.
10. Lindsay R. Sex steroids in the pathogenesis and prevention of osteoporosis. In: Riggs BL, Melton LJ eds. Osteoporosis, Aetiology, Diagnosis and Management. New York: Raven Press, 1988; 333–58.
11. Ruegsegger P, Dambacher MA, Ruegsegger E, Fischer JA, Anliker M. Bone loss in pre-menopausal and postmenopausal women. J Bone Joint Surg 1984; 66A: 1015–23.
12. Ettinger B, Genant HK, Cann CE. Long-term estrogen replacement therapy prevents bone loss and fractures. Ann Intern Med 1985; 102: 319–24.
13. Ettinger B, Genant HK, Cann CE. Postmenopausal bone loss is prevented by treatment with low-dosage estrogen with calcium. Ann Intern Med 1987; 106: 40–5.
14. Weiss NS, Ure CL, Ballard JH, Williams AR, Daling JR. Decreased risk of fractures of the hip and lower forearm with postmenopausal use of estrogen. N Engl J Med 1980; 303: 1195–8.
15. Hutchinson JA, Polansky SM, Feinstein AR. Postmenopausal oestrogens protect against fractures of hip and distal radius: a case–control study. Lancet 1979; 2: 705–9.
16. Riggs BL, Melton LJ. The prevention and treatment of osteoporosis. N Engl J Med 1992; 327: 620–7.
17. Lindsay R. Prevention and treatment of osteoporosis. Lancet 1993; 341: 801–5.
18. Cooper C, Barker DJP, Morris J, Briggs RSJ. Osteoporosis, falls, and age in fracture of the proximal femur. Br Med J 1987; 295: 13–15.
19. Riggs BL, Melton JJ III. Medical progress: involutional osteoporosis. N Engl J Med 1986; 314: 1676–86.
20. Cann CE, Martin MC, Genant HK, Jaffe RB. Decreased spinal mineral content in amenorrheic women. J Am Med Assoc 1984; 251: 626–9.
21. Wolman RL. Bone mineral density levels in elite female athletes. Ann Rheum Dis 1990; 49: 1013–16.
22. Gutin B, Kasper MJ. Can vigorous exercise play a role in osteoporosis prevention? A review. Osteoporosis Int 1992; 2: 55–69.
23. Ott SM. Should women get screening bone mass measurements (Editorial). Ann Intern Med 1986; 104: 874–6.
24. Cooper C, Eastell R. Bone gain and loss in perimenopausal women. Br Med J 1993; 306: 1357–8.
25. Grimley Evans J. The significance of osteoporosis. In: Smith R, ed. Osteoporosis. London: Royal College of Physicians of London, 1990; 1–8.
26. Gillespy T, Gillespy MP. Osteoporosis. Radiol Clin North Am 1991; 29: 77–84.
27. Cooper C. Who will develop osteoporosis? In: Smith R, ed. Osteoporosis. London: Royal College of Physicians of London, 1990; 163–71.
28. Wallace WA. The increasing incidence of fractures of the proximal femur: an orthopaedic epidemic. Lancet 1923; 1: 1413–14.

29. Watts, NB, Harris ST, Genant HK, Wasnich RD, Miller PD, Jackson RD, Licata AA, Ross P, Woodson GC, Yanover MJ, Mysiw WJ, Kohse L, Rad B, Steiger P, Richmond B, Chestnut CH III. Intermittent cyclical etidronate treatment of postmenopausal osteoporosis. N Engl J Med 1990; 323: 73–9.
30. Storm T, Thamsborg G, Steiniche T, Genant HK, Sorensen OH. Effect of intermittent cyclical etidronate therapy on bone mass and fracture rate in women with postmenopausal osteoporosis. N Engl J Med 1990; 322: 1265–71.
31. Stevenson JC, Whitehead MI. Postmenopausal osteoporosis. Br Med J 1982; 285: 585–8.
32. Wahner HW. Measurement of bone mass and bone density. Endocrin Metab Clin North Am 1989; 18: 995–1012.
33. Fogelman I, Rodin A, Blake G. Impact of bone mineral measurements on osteoporosis. Eur J Nucl Med 1990; 16: 39–52.
34. Prudham G, Evans JG. Factors associated with falls in the elderly; a community study. Age Ageing 1981; 10: 141–6.
35. Ray WA, Griffin MR, Schaffner W, Baugh K, Melton LJ. Psychotropic drug use and the risk of hip fracture. N Engl J Med 1987; 316: 363–9.
36. Kelsey JL, Hoffmann S. Risk factors for hip fracture. N Engl J Med 1987; 316: 404–6.
37. Wasnich RD, Ross PD, Heilbrun LK, Vogel JM. Prediction of postmenopausal fracture risk with use of bone mineral measurements. Am J Obstet Gynecol 1985; 153: 745–51.
38. Melton LJ, Chaom EYS, Lane J. Biochemical aspects of fractures in osteoporosis. In: Riggs BL, Melton LJ, eds. Osteoporosis Aetiology, Diagnosis and Management. New York: Raven Press, 1988; 111–31.
39. Melton LJ. Epidemiology of fractures. In: Riggs BL, Melton LJ, eds. Osteoporosis Aetiology, Diagnosis and Management. New York: Raven Press, 1988; 133–54.
40. Hui SL, Slemenda W, Johnston CC. Baseline measurement of bone mass predicts fracture in white women. Ann Intern Med 1989; 111: 355–61.
41. Ross PD, Davis JW, Vogel JM, Wasnich RD. A critical review of bone mass and the risk of fractures in osteoporosis. Calcif Tiss Int 1990; 46: 149–61.
42. Mazess RB. Measurement of skeletal status by noninvasive methods. Calcif Tiss Int 1979; 28: 89–92.
43. Wahner HW, Dunn WL, Riggs BL. Non-invasive bone mineral measurements. Semin Nucl Med 1983; 13: 282–9.
44. Lang P, Steiger P, Faulkner K, Gluer C, Genant HK. Osteoporosis: current techniques and recent developments in quantitative bone densitometry. Radiol Clin North Am 1991; 29: 49–76.
45. Adams JE. Osteoporosis and bone mineral densitometry. Curr Opin Radiol 1992; 4: 11–19.
46. Doyle FH, Gutteridge DH, Joplin GF, Fraser R. An assessment of radiological criteria used in the study of spinal osteoporosis. Br J Radiol 1967; 40: 241–50.
47. Barnett E, Nordin BEC. The radiological diagnosis of osteoporosis: a new approach. Clin Radiol 1960; 11: 166–74.
48. Morgan DB, Spiers FW, Pulvertaft CN, Fourman P. Amount of bone in the metacarpal and the phalanx according to age and sex. Clin Radiol 1967; 18: 101–8.
49. Meema HE, Meema S. Cortical bone mineral density versus cortical thickness in the diagnosis of osteoporosis. J Am Geriatr Assoc 1969; 17: 120–41.
50. Dequeker J. Bone loss in normal and pathological conditions. Leuven: Leuven University Press, 1972.
51. Morgan DB. The metacarpal bone: a comparison of the various indices for the assessment of the amount of bone and for the detection of loss of bone. Clin Radiol 1973; 24: 77–82.
52. Horsman A, Simpson M. The measurement of sequential changes in cortical bone geometry. Br J Radiol 1975; 48: 471–6.
53. Smith RW, Walker RR. Femoral expansion in aging women: implications for osteoporosis and fractures. Science 1964; 145: 156–7.
54. Evans RA, McDonnell GD, Schieb M. Metacarpal cortical area as an index of bone mass. Br J Radiol 1978; 51: 428–31.
55. Horsman A. Bone measurement by conventional radiographic techniques. In: Galasko CSB, Isherwood I, eds. Imaging Techniques in Orthopaedics. Berlin: Springer Verlag, 1988; 243–9.
56. Bloom RA, Pogrund H, Wilson E. Radiogrammetry of the metacarpal: a critical appraisal. Skeletal Radiol 1983; 10: 5–9.
57. Bloom RA, Laws JW. Humeral cortical thickness as an index of osteoporosis in women. Br J Radiol 1970; 43: 522–7.
58. Adams P, Davies GT, Sweetnam PM. Osteoporosis and the effects of aging on bone mass in elderly men and women. Q J Med 1970; 39: 601–15.
59. Dequeker J. Periosteal and endosteal surface remodelling in pathological conditions. Invest Radiol 1971; 6: 260–5.
60. Adams P, Davies GT, Sweetnam PM. Observer error and measurements of the metacarpal. Br J Radiol 1969; 42: 192–7.
61. Naor E, Di Segni V, Robin G, Makin M, Menczel J. Intra-observer variability in the determination of the metacarpal cortical index. Br J Radiol 1972; 45: 213–17.

62. Singh M, Nagrath AR, Maini PS. Changes in trabecular pattern of the upper end of the femur as an index of osteoporosis. J Bone Joint Surg 1970; 52A: 457–67.
63. Singh M, Riggs BL, Beabout JW, Jowsey J. Femoral trabecular-pattern index for evaluation of spinal osteoporosis. Ann Intern Med 1972; 77: 63–7.
64. Cameron JR, Sorenson J. Measurement of bone mineral *in vivo*: an improved method. Science 1963; 142: 230–2.
65. Cameron JR, Mazess RB, Sorenson JA. Precision and accuracy of bone mineral determination by direct photon absorptiometry. Invest Radiol 1968; 3: 141–50.
66. Tothill P. Photon absorptiometry. In: Galasko CBS, Isherwood I, eds. Imaging Techniques in Orthopaedics. Berlin: Springer Verlag, 1988; 251–7.
67. Christiansen C, Rodbro P, Jensen H. Bone mineral content in the forearm measured by photon absorptiometry: principles and reliability. Scand J Clin Lab Invest 1975; 35: 323–30.
68. Mazess RB, Wahner HM. Nuclear medicine and densitometry. In: Riggs BL, Melton LJ III, eds. Osteoporosis: Etiology, Diagnosis and Management. New York: Raven Press, 1988; 251–95.
69. Whitehouse RW. Methods for measuring bone mass. Current Imaging 1991; 3: 213–20.
70. Peppler WW, Mazess RB. Total body bone mineral and lean body mass by dual-photon absorptiometry. Calcif Tissue Int 1981; 33: 353–9.
71. Riggs BL, Wahner HW, Seeman E, Offord KP, Dunn WL, Mazess RB, Johnson KA, Melton LJ III. Changes in bone mineral density of the proximal femur and spine with aging. Differences between the postmenopausal and senile osteoporosis syndromes. J Clin Invest 1982; 70: 716–23.
72. Krolner B, Neilsen SP. Measurement of bone mineral content (BMC) of the lumbar spine, I. Theory and application of a new two-dimensional dual-photon attenuation method. Scand J Clin Lab Invest 1980; 40: 653–63.
73. Dunn WL, Wahner HW, Riggs BL. Measurement of bone mineral content in human vertebrae and hip by dual photon absorptiometry. Radiology 1980; 136: 485–7.
74. Wahner HW, Dunn WL, Mazess RB. Dual photon (Gd-153) absorptiometry of bone. Radiology 1985: 156: 203–6.
75. Cullum ID, Ell PJ, Ryder JP. X-ray dual-photon absorptiometry: a new method for the measurement of bone density. Br J Radiol 1989; 62: 587–92.
76. Kelly TL, Slovik DM, Schoenfeld DA, Neer RM. Quantitative digital radiography versus dual photon absorptiometry of the lumbar spine. J Clin Endocrinol Metab 1988; 67: 839–44.
77. Kellie SE. Measurement of bone density with dual-energy X-ray absorptiometry (DEXA). J Am Med Assoc 1992; 267: 286–94.
78. Sartoris DJ, Resnick D. Dual-energy radiographic absorptiometry for bone densitometry: current status and perspective. Am J Radiol 1989; 152: 241–6.
79. Nelson DA, Brown EB, Flynn MJ, Cody DD, Shaffer S. Comparison of dual photon and dual energy X-ray bone densitometers in a clinic setting. Skeletal Radiol 1991; 20: 591–5.
80. Mazess R, Chestnut CH III, McClung M, Genant H. Enhanced precision with dual-energy X-ray absorptiometry. Calcif Tiss Int 1992; 51: 14–17.
81. Lees B, Stevenson JC. An evaluation of dual-energy X-ray absorptiometry and comparison with dual-photon absorptiometry. Osteoporosis Int 1992; 2: 146–52.
82. Ho CP, Kim RW, Schaffler MB, Sartoris DJ. Accuracy of dual-energy radiographic absorptiometry of the lumbar spine: cadaver study. Radiology 1990; 176: 171–3.
83. Edmondston SJ, Singer KP, Price RI, Breidahl PD. Accuracy of dual energy X-ray absorptiometry for the determination of bone mineral content in the thoracic and lumbar spine: an *in-vitro* study. Br J Radiol 1993; 66: 309–13.
84. Laskey MA, Crisp AJ, Compston JE, Khaw KT. Short communication. Heterogenicity of spine bone density. Br J Radiol 1993; 66: 480–3.
85. Frohn J, Wilken T, Falk S, Stutte HJ, Kollath J, Hor G. Effect of aortic sclerosis on bone mineral measurements by dual-photon absorptiometry. J Nucl Med 1991; 32: 259–62.
86. Rupich R, Pacifici R, Griffin M, Vered I, Susman N, Avioli LV. Lateral dual energy radiography: a new method for measuring vertebral bone density: a preliminary study. J Clin Endocrinol Metabol 1990; 70: 1768–70.
87. Slosman DO, Rizzoli R, Donath A, Bonjour J-Ph. Vertebral bone mineral density measured laterally by dual-energy X-ray absorptiometry. Osteoporosis Int 1990; 1: 23–9.
88. Mazess BR, Gifford CA, Bisek JP, Barden HS, Hansen JA. DEXA measurement of spine density in the lateral projection. I Methodology. Calcif Tissue Int 1991; 49: 235–9.
89. McCarthy CK, Steinberg CG, Agren M, Leahy D, Wyman E, Baran DT. Quantifying bone loss from the proximal femur after total hip arthroplasty. J Bone Joint Surg 1991; 73B: 774–8.
90. Ryan PJ, Blake GM, Fogelman I. Measurement of forearm BMD in normal women by dual energy X-ray absorptiometry. Br J Radiol 1992; 65: 127–31.
91. Larcos G, Wahner HW. An evaluation of forearm bone mineral measurement with dual-energy X-ray absorptiometry. J Nucl Med 1991; 32: 2101–6.

92. Steiger P, Weiss H, Stein JA. Morphometric X-ray absorptiometry of the spine: a new method to assess vertebral osteoporosis. In: Christiansen C, Fourth International Symposium on Osteoporosis, Hong Kong, 1993; Abstract 715, 188.
93. Haarbo J, Gotfredsen A, Hassager C, Christiansen C. Validation of body composition by dual energy X-ray absorptiometry (DEXA). Clin Physiol 1991; 11: 331–41.
94. Herd RJM, Blake GM, Parker JC, Ryan PJ, Fogelman I. Total body studies in normal British women using dual energy X-ray absorptiometry. Br J Radiol 1993; 66: 303–8.
95. Fuller NJ, Laskey MA, Elia M. Assessment of the composition of major body regions by dual energy X-ray absorptiometry (DEXA) with special reference to limb muscle mass. Clin Physiol 1992; 12: 253–66.
96. Compston JE, Bhambharu M, Laskey MA, Murphy S, Khaw KT. Body composition and bone mass in postmenopausal women. Clin Endocrinol 1992; 37: 426–31.
97. Wilson CR, Fogelman I, Blake GM, Rodin A. The effect of positioning on dual energy X-ray densitometry of the proximal femur. Mineral 1991; 13: 69–76.
98. Ross PD, Wasnich RD, Heilbrun LK, Vogel JM. Definition of a spine fracture threshold based upon prospective fracture risk. Bone 1987; 8: 271–8.
99. Isherwood I, Rutherford RA, Pullan BR, Adams PH. Bone mineral estimation by computer assisted tomography. Lancet 1976; 2: 712–15.
100. Reich NE, Seidelmann FE, Tubbs RR, MacIntyre WJ, Meaney TF, Alfidi RJ, Pepe RG. Determination of bone mineral content using CT scanning. Am J Radiol 1976; 127: 593–4.
101. Pullan BR, Roberts TE. Bone mineral measurement using an EMI scanner and standard methods; a comparative study. Br J Radiol 1978; 51: 24–8.
102. Orphanoudakis SC, Jensen PS, Rauschkolb EN, Lang R, Rasmussen H. Bone mineral analysis using single energy computed tomography. Invest Radiol 1979; 14: 122–30.
103. Cann CE, Genant HK. Precise measurement of vertebral mineral content using computed tomography. J Comput Assist Tomogr 1980; 4: 493–500.
104. Lampmann LE, Duursma SA, Ruys JH. In: CT Densitometry in Osteoporosis. Boston: Martinus Nijhoff, 1984; 13–105.
105. Genant HK. Assessing osteoporosis: CT's quantitative advantage. Diagnostic Imaging 1985; 8: 52–7.
106. Gluer CC, Genant HK. Quantitative computed tomography of the hip. In: Genant HK, ed. Osteoporosis Update. San Francisco, California: Radiology Research and Education Foundation, 1987; 187–95.
107. Cann CE. Quantitative CT applications: comparisons of current scanners. Radiology 1987; 162: 257–61.
108. Cann CE. Quantitative CT for the determination of bone mineral density: a review. Radiology 1988; 166: 509–22.
109. Adams JE. Quantitative computed tomography (QCT). In: Galasko CBS, Isherwood I, eds. Imaging Techniques in Orthopaedics. Berlin, Heidelberg: Springer Verlag, 1988; 259–68.
110. Genant HK, Ettinger B, Harris ST, Block JE, Steiger P. Quantitative computed tomography in assessment of osteoporosis. In: Riggs BL, Melton LJ III, eds. Osteoporosis: Etiology, Diagnosis and Management. New York: Raven Press, 1988; 221–49.
111. Cann CE. Low-dose CT scanning for quantitative spinal mineral analysis. Radiology 1981; 140: 813–15.
112. Arnold BA. Automated software and phantom improvements for bone mineral analysis by quantitative computed tomography. In: Genant HK, ed. Osteoporosis Update. San Francisco, California: Radiology Research and Education Foundation, 1987; 197–207.
113. Faulkner KG, Glüer CC, Grampp S, Genant HK. Cross-calibration of liquid and solid QCT calibration standards: corrections to the UCSF normative data. Osteoporosis Int 1993; 3: 36–42.
114. Suzuki S, Yamamuro T, Okumura H, Yamamoto I. Quantitative computed tomography: comparative study using different scanners with two calibration phantoms. Br J Radiol 1991; 64: 1001–6.
115. Whitehouse RW, Adams JE. Single energy quantitative computed tomography: the effects of phantom calibration material and kVp on QCT bone densitometry. Br J Radiol 1992; 65: 931–4.
116. Kalendar WA, Klotz E, Suess C. Vertebral bone mineral analysis: an integrated approach with CT. Radiology 1987; 164: 419–23.
117. Adams JE, Chen SZ, Adams PH, Isherwood I. Measurement of trabecular bone mineral by dual energy computed tomography. J Comput Assist Tomogr 1982; 6: 601–7.
118. Gluer CC, Reiser UJ, Davis CA, Rutt BK, Genant HK. Vertebral mineral determination by quantitative computed tomography: accuracy of single and dual energy measurements. J Comput Assist Tomogr 1988; 12: 242–58.
119. Gluer CC, Genant HK. Impact of marrow fat on accuracy of quantitative CT. J Comput Assist Tomogr 1989; 13: 1023–35.
120. Reinbold WD, Adler CP, Kalender WA, Lente R. Accuracy of vertebral mineral determination by dual-energy quantitative computed tomography. Skeletal Radiol 1991; 20: 25–9.

121. Ritchings RT, Pullan BR. A technique for simultaneous dual energy scanning: a technical note. J Comput Assist Tomogr 1979; 3: 842–6.
122. Rutt B, Fenster A. Split-filter computed tomography: a simple technique for dual energy scanning. J Comput Assist Tomogr 1980; 4: 501–9.
123. Laval-Jeantet AM, Cann CE, Roger BM, Dallant P. A post-processing dual energy technique for vertebral CT densitometry. J Comput Assist Tomogr 1984; 9: 1164–7.
124. Nickoloff EL, Feldman F, Atherton MS. Bone mineral assessment: new dual energy approach. Radiology 1988; 168: 223–8.
125. Goodsitt MM, Kilcoyne RF, Gutcheck RA, Richardson ML, Rosenthal DI. Effect of collagen on bone mineral analysis with QCT. Radiology 1988; 167: 787–91.
126. Van Kuyk C. Evaluation of post processing dual energy quantitative computed tomography. Rotterdam: Erasmus University of Rotterdam, 1991.
127. Whitehouse RW. Compositional analysis of spinal trabecular bone by dual energy quantitative computed tomography (MD Thesis). University of Manchester, 1993.
128. Kalender WA. Effective dose values in bone mineral measurements by photon absorptiometry and computed tomography. Osteoporosis Int 1992; 2: 82–7.
129. Hosie CJ, Smith DAS. Precision of measurement of bone density with a special purpose computed tomography scanner. Br J Radiol 1986; 59: 345–50.
130. Ruegsegger P, Durand E, Dambacher MA. Localization of regional forearm bone loss from high resolution computed tomographic images. Osteoporosis Int 1991; 1: 76–80.
131. Schneider P. Development and testing of a tomography scanner for determination of trabecular density at the radius. Thesis, University of Wurzburg, 1984.
132. Sartoris DJ, Andre M, Resnick C, Resnick D. Trabecular bone density in the proximal femur. Work in progress. Quantitative CT assessment. Radiology 1986; 160: 707–12.
133. Reinbold WD, Genant HK, Reiser UJ, Harris ST, Ettinger B. Bone mineral content in early-postmenopausal and postmenopausal osteoporotic women: comparison of measurement methods. Radiology 1986; 160: 469–78.
134. Whitehouse RW, Adams JE, Bancroft K, Vaughan-Williams CA, Elstein M. The effects of Nafarelin and Danazol on vertebral trabecular bone mass in patients with endometriosis. Clin Endocrinol 1990; 33: 365–73.
135. Langton CM, Palmer SB, Porter RW. The measurement of broadband ultrasonic attenuation in cancellous bone. Engineer Med 1984; 13: 89–91.
136. Poll V, Cooper C, Cawley MID. Broadband ultrasonic attenuation in the os calcis and single photon absorptiometry in the distal forearm: a comparative study. Clin Phys Physiol Meas 1986; 7: 375–9.
137. Truscott JG, Simpson M, Stewart SP, Milner R, Westmacott CF, Oldroyd B, Evans JA, Horsman A, Langton CM, Smith MA. Bone ultrasonic attenuation in women: reproducibility, variation and comparison with photon absorptiometry. Clin Phys Physiol Meas 1992; 13: 29–36.
138. Salamone L, Zantos D, Makrauer D, Dawson-Hughes B. Short and longer term precision of broadband ultrasound attenuation measurements of os calcis. J Bone Min Res 1992; 7 (Suppl. 1): S178.
139. McKelvie ML, Fordham J, Clifford C, Palmer SB. *In vitro* comparison of quantitative computed tomography and broadband ultrasound attenuation of trabecular bone. Bone 1989; 10: 101–4.
140. Rossman P, Zaggebski J, Mesina C, Sorenson J, Mazess R. Comparison of speed of sound and ultrasound attenuation in the os calcis to bone density of the radius, femur and lumbar spine. Clin Phys Physiol Meas 1989; 10: 353–60.
141. McCloskey EV, Murray SA, Miller C, Charlesworth D, Tindale W, O'Doherty DP, Bickerstaff DR, Hamdy NAT, Kanis JA. Broadband ultrasound attenuation in the os calcis: relationship to bone mineral at other skeletal sites. Clin Sci 1990; 78: 227–33.
142. Baran DT, Kelly AM, Karellas A, Gionet M, Price M, Leahey D, Steuterman S, McSherry B, Roche J. Ultrasound attenuation of the os calcis in women with osteoporosis and hip fractures. Calcif Tissue Int 1988; 43: 138–42.
143. Heaney RP, Avioli LV, Chesnut CH, Lappe J, Recker RR, Brandenburger CH. Osteoporotic bone fragility. Detection by ultrasound transmission velocity. J Am Med Assoc 1989; 261: 2986–90.
144. Agren M, Karellas A, Leahey D, Marks S, Baran D. Ultrasound attenuation of the calcaneus: a sensitive and specific discriminator of osteopenia in post-menopausal women. Calcif Tissue Int 1991; 48: 240–4.
145. Baran DT, McCarthy CK, Leahey D, Lew R. Broadband ultrasound attenuation of the calcaneus predicts lumbar and femoral neck density in Caucasian women: a preliminary study. Osteoporosis Int 1991; 1: 110–13.
146. Wehrli FW, Ford JC, Attie M, Kressel HY, Kaplan FS. Trabecular structure: preliminary application of MR interferometry. Radiology 1991; 179: 615–21.
147. Ford JC, Wehrli FW. *In vivo* quantitative characterization of trabecular bone by NMR inter-

ferometry and localized proton spectroscopy. Magn Reson Med 1991; 17: 543–51.

148. Chen Y, Dougherty ER, Totterman SM, Hornak JP. Classification of trabecular structure in magnetic resonance imaging based on morphological granulometries. Magn Reson Med 1993; 29: 358–70.
149. Faulkner KG, Gluer CC, Majumdar S, Lang P, Engelke K, Genant HK. Noninvasive measurements of bone mass, structure and strength: current methods and experimental techniques. Am J Radiol 1991; 157: 1229–37.
150. Dickie-Cody D, Flynn MJ, Vickers DS. A technique for measuring regional bone density in human vertebral bodies. Med Phys 1989; 16: 766–72.
151. Elliot J, Dover S. X-ray microscopy using computerised axial tomography. J Microsc 1985; 138: 329–31.
152. Faulkner KG, Cann CE, Hasegawa BH. The effect of bone distribution on vertebral strength: assessment with patient specific non-linear finite element analysis. Radiology 1991; 179: 669–74.
153. Huddleston AL. Scattering methods in densitometry. In: Huddleston AL, ed. Quantitative Methods in Bone Densitometry. Boston: Kluwer Academic Publishers, 1988; 113–59.
154. Shukla SS, Leichter I, Karellas A, Craven JD, Greenfield MA. Trabecular bone mineral density measurement *in vivo*: use of the ratio of coherent to Compton-scattered photons in the calcaneus. Radiology 1986; 158: 695–7.
155. Webber CE, Kennett TJ. Bone density measurement by photon scattering: a system for clinical use. Phys Med Biol 1976; 21: 760–9.
156. Webster DJ, Lillicrap SC. Coherent-Compton scattering for the assessment of bone mineral content using heavily filtered X-ray beams. Phys Med Biol 1985; 30: 531–9.
157. Duke PR, Hanson JA. Compton scatter densitometry with polychromatic sources. Med Phy 1984; 11: 624–32.
158. Cohn SH, Dombrowski CS. Measurement of total body calcium sodium, nitrogen and phosphorus in man by *in vivo* neutron activation analysis. J Nucl Med 1971; 12: 499–505.
159. Harrison JE, MacNeill KG, Hitchman AJ, Britt BA. Bone mineral measurements of the central skeleton by *in vivo* neutron activation analysis for routine investigation of osteopaenia. Invest Radiol 1979; 14: 27–34.
160. Huddleston AL. Activation analysis methods. In: Huddleston AL, ed. Quantitative Methods in Bone Densitometry. Boston: Kluwer Academic Publishers, 1988; 161–78.
161. Palmer HE, Nelp WB, Murano R, Rich C. The feasibility of *in vivo* neutron activation analysis of total body calcium and other elements of body composition. Phys Med Biol 1968; 13: 269–79.
162. Cohn SH, Aloia JF, Vaswani AN, Yeun K, Yasumura S, Ellis KJ. Women at risk of developing osteoporosis: determination of total body neutron activation analysis and photon absorptiometry. Calcif Tissue Int 1986; 38: 9–15.
163. Salle BL, Braillon P, Glorieux FH. Lumbar bone mineral content measured by dual energy X-ray absorptiometry in newborns and infants. Acta Paediatr 1992; 81: 953–8.
164. Braillon PM, Salle BL, Brunet J. Dual energy X-ray absorptiometry measurement of bone mineral content in newborns: validation of the technique. Paediatr Res 1992; 32: 77–80.
165. Glastre C, Braillon P, David L, Cochat P, Meunier PJ, Delmas PD. Measurement of bone mineral content of the lumbar spine by dual energy X-ray absorptiometry in normal children: correlations with growth parameters. J Clin Endocrinol Metabol 1990; 70: 1330–3.
166. DeSchepper J, Derde MP, Van den Broeck M, Piepsz A, Jonckheer MH. Normative data for lumbar spine bone mineral content in children: influence of age, height, weight, and pubertal state. J Nucl Med 1991; 32: 216–20.
167. Ott SM. Bone density in adolescents. N Engl J Med 1991; 23: 1646–7.
168. Parfitt AM. Bone remodelling: relationship to the amount and structure of bone and the pathogenesis and prevention of fractures. In: Riggs BL, Melton LJ, eds. Osteoporosis, Etiology, Diagnosis and Management. New York: Raven Press, 1988; 45–93.
169. Riggs BL, Wahner HW, Dunn WL, Mazess RB, Offord KP, Melton LJ. Differential changes in bone mineral density of the appendicular and axial skeleton with ageing: relationship to spinal osteoporosis. J Clin Invest 1981; 67: 328–35.
170. Seeman E, Wahner HW, Offord KP. Differential effects of endocrine dysfunction on the axial and the appendicular skeleton. J Clin Invest 1982; 69: 1302–9.
171. Richardson ML, Genant HK, Cann CE. Assessment of metabolic bone diseases by quantitative computed tomography. Clin Orthop Rel Res 1985; 195: 224–38.
172. Ott SM, Kilcoyne RF, Chestnut CH. Longitudinal changes in bone mass after one year as measured by different techniques in patients with osteoporosis. Calcif Tissue Int 1986; 39: 133–8.
173. Sambrook PM, Bartlett C, Evans R, Katz D, Reeve J. Measurement of lumbar spine bone mineral: a comparison of dual photon absorptiometry and computed tomography. Br J Radiol 1985; 58: 621–4.
174. Adachi JD, Webber CE. The interchangeability of radioisotope and X-ray based measurements of bone mineral density. Br J Radiol 1991; 64: 217–20.

175. Blake GM, Tong CM, Fogelman I. Intersite comparison of the Hologic QDR-1000 dual energy X-ray bone densitometer. Br J Radiol 1991; 64: 440–6.
176. Laskey MA, Flaxman ME, Barber RW, Trafford S, Hayball MP, Lyttle KD, Crisp AJ, Compston JE. Comparative performance *in vitro* and *in vivo* of Lunar DPX and Hologic QDR-1000 dual energy X-ray absorptiometers. Br J Radiol 1991; 64: 1023–9.
177. Pouilles JM, Tremollieres F, Todorovsky N, Ribot C. Precision and sensitivity of dual-energy X-ray absorptiometry in spinal osteoporosis. J Bone Min Res 1991; 6: 997–1002.
178. Hannan MT, Felson DT, Anderson JJ. Bone mineral density in elderly men and women: results from the Framingham osteoporosis study. J Bone Min Res 1992; 7: 547–53.
179. Nord RH. Work in progress: a cross-correlation study on four DXA instruments designed to culminate in inter-manufacture standardization. Osteoporosis Int 1992; 2: 210–11.
180. Kalender WA. Standardization of bone mineral measurements of the lumbar spine using the European Spine Phantom. In: Ring EFJ, ed. Current Research in Osteoporosis and Bone Mineral Measurement, vol. 2. London: British Institute of Radiology, 1992; 24–5.
181. Gilsanz V, Gibbens DT, Roe TF, Carlson M, Senac MO, Boechat MI, Huang HK, Schulz EE, Libanati CR, Cann CC. Vertebral bone density in children: effect of puberty. Radiology 1988; 166: 847–50.
182. Bonjour JP, Theintz G, Buchs B, Slosman D, Rizzoli R. Critical years and stages of puberty for spinal and femoral bone mass accumulation during adolescence. J Clin Endocrinol Metab 1991; 73: 555–63.
183. Southard RN, Morris JD, Mahan JD, Hayes JR, Torch MA, Sommer A, Zipf WB. Bone mass in healthy children: measurement with quantitative DXA. Radiology 1991; 179: 735–8.
184. Katzman DK, Bachrach LK, Carter R, Marcus R. Clinical and anthropometric correlates of bone mineral acquisition in healthy adolescent girls. J Clin Endocrinol Metabol 1991; 73: 1332–9.
185. Theintz G, Bucks B, Rizzoli R, Slosman D, Clavien H, Sizonenko PC, Bonjour JP. Longitudinal monitoring of bone mass accumulation in healthy adolescents: evidence for a marked reduction after 16 years of age at the levels of lumbar spine and femoral neck in female subjects. J Clin Endocrinol Metab 1992; 75: 1060–5.
186. Thomsen K, Gotfredsen A, Christiansen C. Is postmenopausal bone loss an age-matched phenomenon? Calcif Tissue Int 1986; 39: 123–7.
187. Block JE, Smith R, Glueer CC, Steiger P, Ettinger B, Genant HK. Models of spinal trabecular bone loss as determined by quantitative computed tomography. J Bone Min Res 1989; 4: 249–57.
188. Hall ML, Heavens J, Cullum ID, Ell PJ. The range of bone density in normal British women. Br J Radiol 1990; 63: 266–9.
189. Karantanas AH, Kalef-Ezra JA, Glaros DC. Quantitative computed tomography for bone mineral measurement: technical aspects, dosimetry, normal data and clinical applications. Br J Radiol 1991; 64: 298–304.
190. Haddaway MJ, Davie MWJ, McCall IW. Bone mineral density in normal woman and reproducibility of measurements in spine and hip using dual energy X-ray absorptiometry. Br J Radiol 1992; 65: 213–17.
191. Kroger H, Heikkinen J, Laitinen K, Kotaniemi A. Dual-energy X-ray absorptiometry in normal women: a cross sectional study of 717 Finnish volunteers. Osteoporosis Int 1992; 2: 135–40.
192. Jano K, Wasnich RD, Vogel JM, Heilbrun LK. Bone mineral measurements among middle aged and elderly Japanese residents in Hawaii. Am J Epidemiol 1984; 119: 751–64.
193. Gilsanz V, Roe TF, Mora S, Costin G, Goodman WG. Changes in vertebral bone density in black girls and white girls during childhood and puberty. N Engl J Med 1991; 325: 1597–600.
194. Parfitt AM. Editorial. Interpretation of bone densitometry measurements: disadvantages of a percentage scale and a discussion of some alternatives. J Bone Min Res 1990; 5: 537–40.
195. Melton LJ, Chrischilles EA, Cooper C, Lane AW, Riggs BL. How many women have osteoporosis? J Bone Min Res 1992; 7: 1005–10.
196. Cummings SR, Black DM, Nevitt MC, Browner WS, Cauley JA, Genant HK, Mascioli SR, Scott JC, Seeley DG, Steiger P, Vogt TM and Study of Osteoporosis Fracture Group. Appendicular bone density and age predicts fracture in women. The Study of Osteoporotic Fractures Research Group. J Am Med Assoc 1990; 263: 665–8.
197. Kleerekoper M, Peterson EL, Nelson DA, Phillips E, Schork MA, Tilley BC, Parfitt AM. A randomized trial of sodium fluoride as a treatment for postmenopausal osteoporosis. Osteoporosis Int 1991; 1: 155–61.
198. Cundy T, Evans M, Roberts H, Wattie D, Ames R, Reid IR. Bone density in women receiving depot medroxyprogesterone acetate for contraception. Br Med J 1991; 303: 13–16.
199. Greenspan SL, Greenspan FS, Resnick NM, Block JE, Friedlander AL, Genant HK. Skeletal integrity in premenopausal and postmenopausal women receiving long-term L-thyroxine therapy. Am J Med 1991; 91: 5–14.
200. Franklyn JA, Betteridge J, Daykin J, Holder R, Oates GD, Parle JV, Lilley J, Heath DA, Sheppard

MC. Long-term thyroxine treatment and bone mineral density. Lancet 1992; 340: 9–13.
201. Compston JE, Laskey MA, Croucher PI, Coxon A, Kreitzman S. Effect of diet-induced weight loss on total body bone mass. Clin Sci 1992; 82: 429–32.
202. Love RR, Mazess RB, Barden HS, Epstein S, Newcomb PA, Jordan VC, Carbone PP, DeMets DL. Effects of tamoxifen on bone mineral density in postmenopausal women with breast cancer. N Engl J Med 1992; 326: 852–6.
203. Sambrook P, Birmingham J, Kelly P, Kempler S, Nguyen T, Pocock N, Eisman J. Prevention of corticosteroid osteoporosis: a comparison of calcium, calcitriol and calcitonin. N Engl J Med 1993; 328: 1747–52.
204. Gardsell P, Johnell O, Nilsson BE. The predictive value of forearm bone mineral content measurements in men. Bone 1990; 11: 229–32.
205. Finkelstein JS, Neer RM, Biller BMK, Crawford JD, Klibanski A. Osteopenia in men with a history of delayed puberty. N Engl J Med 1992; 326: 600–4.
206. Cummings SR. Bone mineral densitometry. Ann Intern Med 1987; 107: 932–6.
207. Genant HK, Block JE, Steiger P, Glueer CC, Ettinger B, Harris ST. Appropriate use of bone densitometry. Radiology 1989; 170: 817–22.
208. Johnston CC, Melton LJ, Lindsay R, Eddy DM. Clinical indications for bone mass measurements. A report from the Scientific Advisory Board of the National Osteoporosis Foundation. J Bone Min Res 1989; 4 (Suppl. 2): 1–28.
209. Johnston CC Jr, Slemenda CW, Melton LJ III. Clinical use of bone densitometry. N Engl J Med 1991; 324: 1105–9.
210. Dawson-Hughes B, Dallal GE, Krall EA, Sadowski L, Sahyoun N, Tannenbaum S. A controlled trial of calcium supplementation on bone density in postmenopausal women. N Engl J Med 1990; 323: 878–83.
211. Mazess RB, Barden H, Ettinger M, Schultz E. Bone density of the radius, spine and proximal femur in osteoporosis. J Bone Min Res 1988; 3: 13–18.
212. Gallagher C, Goldgar D, Mahony P, MacGill J. Measurement of spine density in normal and osteoporotic subjects using computed tomography: relationship with spine density to fracture threshold and fracture index. J Comp Assist Tomogr 1985; 9: 634–5.
213. Cann CE, Genant HK, Kolb FO, Ettinger BE. Quantitative computed tomography for prediction of vertebral fracture risk. Metab Bone Dis Res 1985; 6: 1–7.
214. Firooznia H, Rafii M, Galimbu C, Schwartz MS, Ort P. Trabecular mineral content of the spine in women with hip fracture: CT measurement. Radiology 1986; 159: 737–40.
215. Griffin MG, Rupich RC, Avioli LV, Pacifici R. A comparison of dual energy radiography measurements at the lumbar spine and proximal femur for the diagnosis of osteoporosis. J Clin Endocrinol Metabol 1991; 73: 1164–9.
216. Ross PD, Davis JW, Epstein RS, Wasnich RD. Pre-existing fractures and bone mass predict vertebral bone mass incidence in women. Ann Intern Med 1991; 114: 919–23.
217. Black DM, Cummings SR, Genant HK. Axial and appendicular bone density predict fractures in older women. J Bone Min Res 1992; 6: 633–8.
218. Kelsey JL, Browner WS, Seeley DG, Nevitt MC, Cummings SR. Risk factors for fractures of the distal forearm and proximal humerus. Am J Epidemiol 1992; 135: 477–89.
219. Cummings SR, Black DM, Nevitt MC, Browner WS, Cauley JA, Genant HK, Mascioli SR, Scott JC, Seeley DG, Steiger P, Vogt TM, and the Study of Osteoporotic Fracture Group. Appendicular bone density and age predict hip fracture in women. J Am Med Assoc 1990; 263: 665–8.
220. Aloia JF, Vaswani A, McGowan D, Ross P. Preferential osteopaenia in women with osteoporotic fractures. Bone Min 1992; 18: 51–63.
221. Johnell O, Cooper C, Melton LJ. How do we prevent hip fractures. Lancet 1993; 341: 89.
222. Cummings SR, Black DM, Nevitt MC, Browner W, Cauley J, Ensrund K, Genant HK, Palermo L, Scott J, Vogt TM for the Study of Osteoporotic Fracture Research Group. Bone density at various sides for prediction of hip fractures. Lancet 1993; 341: 72–5.
223. Christiansen C, Riis BJ, Rodbro P. Prediction of rapid bone loss in postmenopausal osteoporosis. Lancet 1987; 1: 1105–7.
224. McBroom RJ, Hayes WC, Edwards WT, Goldberg RR, White AA. Prediction of vertebral body compressive fracture using quantitative computed tomography. J Bone Joint Surg 1985; 67A: 1206–14.
225. Hayes WC, Piazza SJ, Zysset PK. Biomechanics of fracture risk prediction of the hip and spine by quantitative computed tomography. Radiol Clin North Am 1991; 29: 1–18.
226. Cann CE. Skeletal structure-function revisited. Radiology 1991; 179: 607–8.
227. Biggemann M, Hilweg D, Seidel S, Horst M, Brinckmann P. Risk of vertebral insufficiency fractures in relation to compressive strength predicted by quantitative computed tomography. Eur J Radiol 1991; 13: 6–10.
228. Chevalier F, Laval-Jeantet AM, Laval-Jeantet M, Bergot C. CT image analysis of the vertebral trabecular network *in vivo*. Calcif Tissue Int 1992; 51: 8–13.
229. Wilson CR, Collier D, Carrera GF, Jacobson DR. Acronym for dual-energy X-ray absorptiometry. Radiology 1990; 176: 875.

230. Genant HK, Gluer CC, Faulkner KG, Majumdar S, Harris ST, Engelke K, van Kuijk C. Acronyms in bone densitometry (Letter). Radiology 1992; 184 (3).
231. Woolf AD, Dixon A St J. The menopause and hormone replacement therapy in practical problems in medicine. In: Woolf AD, Dixon A St J, eds. Osteoporosis: A Clinical Guide. London: Martin Dunitz, 1988; 168–80.
232. Melton LJ, Eddy DM, Johnston CC. Screening for osteoporosis. Ann Intern Med 1990; 112: 516–28.
233. Rubin SM, Cummings SR. Results of bone density affect women's decisions about taking measures to prevent fractures. Ann Intern Med 1992; 116: 990–5.
234. Law MR, Wald NJ, Meade TW. Strategies for prevention of osteoporosis and hip fracture. Br Med J 1991; 303: 453–9.
235. Reed DM, Purdie DW. Bone density measurement. Lancet 1992; 339: 370.
236. Screening for osteoporosis to prevent fracture. In: Effective Health Care No. I January 1991. Inquiries to Nick Freemantle, Effective Health Care, School of Public Health University of Leeds, 32 Hyde Terrace, Leeds, LS2 9LN, UK.
237. Ross PD, Wasnich RD, McLean CJ, Hagino R, Vogel JM. A model for estimating the potential costs and savings of osteoporosis prevention strategies. Bone 1988; 9: 337–47.
238. Tosteson ANA, Rosenthal DI, Melton LJ, Weinstein MC. Cost effectiveness of screening perimenopausal white women for osteoporosis: bone densitometry and hormone replacement therapy. Ann Intern Med 1990; 113: 594–603.
239. Cummings SR, Rubin SM, Black D. The future of hip fractures in the United States: numbers, costs, and potential effects of postmenopausal estrogen. Clin Orthop 1990; 252: 163–6.
240. Chrischilles EA, Butler CP, Davis DS, Wallace RB. A model of lifetime osteoporosis impact. Arch Intern Med 1991; 151: 2026–32.
241. Cooper C, Shah S, Hand DJ, Adams JE, Compston J, Davie M, Woolf A. Screening for vertebral osteoporosis using individual risk factors. Osteoporosis Int 1991; 2: 48–53.
242. Aloia JF, McCowan D, Erens E, Miele G. Hip fracture patients have generalized osteopaenia with a preferential deficit in the femur. Osteoporosis Int 1992; 2: 88–93.
243. Need AG, Nordin BEC. Which bone to measure? Osteoporosis Int 1990; 1: 3–6.
244. Meema HE. Improved vertebral fracture threshold in postmenopausal osteoporosis by radiogrammetric measurements: its usefulness in selection for preventive therapy. J Bone Min Res 1991; 6: 9–14.
245. Wishart JM, Horowitz M, Bochner M, Need AG, Nordin BEC. Relationships between metacarpal morphometry, forearm and vertebral bone density and fractures in postmenopausal women. Br J Radiol 1993; 66: 435–40.
246. Virtama P, Gastrin G, Telkka A. Biconcavity of the vertebrae as an estimate of their bone density. Clin Radiol 1962; 13: 128–31.
247. Kleerekoper M, Parfitt AM, Ellis BI. Measurement of vertebral fracture rates in osteoporosis. In: Christiansen C, Arnaud CD, Nordin BEC, Parfitt AM, Peck WA, Riggs BL, eds. Osteoporosis Glostrup, Denmark: Department of Clinical Chemistry, Glostrup Hospital, 1984; 255–62.
248. Kanis JA, Minne WH, Meunier PJ, Ziegler R, Allende RE. Quality of life and vertebral osteoporosis. Osteoporosis Int 1990; 2: 161–3.
249. Smith-Bindman R, Cummings SR, Steiger P, Genant HK. A comparison of morphometric definitions of vertebral fracture. J Bone Min Res 1991; 6: 25–34.
250. Kanis JA, McCloskey EV. Epidemiology of vertebral osteoporosis. Bone 1992; 13: S1–S10.
251. Cooper C, Melton LJ. Vertebral fractures. How large is the silent epidemic? Br Med J 1992; 304: 793–4.
252. Nevitt MC, Cummings SR, Browner WS, Seeley DG, Cauley JA, Vogt TM, Black DM. The accuracy of self-report of fractures in elderly women: evidence from a prospective study. Am J Epidemiol 1992; 135: 490–9.
253. Silverman SL. The clinical consequences of vertebral compression fractures. Bone 1992; 13: 27–31.
254. Kalidis L, Felsenberg D, Kalender W, Eidloth H, Wieland E. Morphometric analysis of digitized radiographs: description of automatic evaluation. In: Ring EFJ, ed. Current Research in Osteoporosis and Bone Mineral Measurement, vol. 2. London: British Institute of Radiology, 1992; 14–16.
255. Reviews–various authors. Am J Med 1991; 91 (Suppl. 5B): 2S–68S.
256. Osteoporosis International Journal of The European Foundation for Osteoporosis, Editors Lindsay R, Meunier PJ, published by Springer International, Springer Verlag London Ltd, 8 Alexander Road, London SW19 7JZ, UK.
257. Osteoporosis Review Journal of the National Osteoporosis Society. Editor Woolf AD, Editorial Office Media Medica, The Chambers, Chapel Street, Chichester, West Sussex PO19 1DL, UK.

Conclusions

9

F. I. Tovey and T. C. B. Stamp

As will be seen from the previous chapters, the variety of methods available for bone measurements in metabolic bone disease is large and the choice depends on the purpose for which the measurement is to be used.

At the present time dual energy X-ray absorptiometry is the investigation most widely used for bone densitometry, particularly for screening in horizontal studies of a population or in longitudinal studies such as the monitoring of treatment. It is, however, only a measurement of bone mineral density, and does not differentiate between the various pathophysiological processes affecting bone density.

Many longitudinal studies in progress at present, however, were commenced before the advent of dual energy X-ray absorptiometry and in these series further measurements will have to be made using the original method of bone density measurement such as single or dual photon absorptiometry.

In certain circumstances, such as those presently existing in some developing countries, sophisticated methods are not available and there may still be a place for radiogrammetric methods. There is some evidence that the Singh Index[1] of the upper end of the femur may still be one of the most useful radiogrammetric parameters in the identification of people at risk of hip fractures.

BIOCHEMICAL CHANGES

The use of biochemical markers of bone turnover is increasing. Normally, bone resorption and bone formation are coupled and balanced, and the various markers for each have been described in Chapter 4. Bone-specific alkaline phosphatase is readily available as an index of bone mineralization, but serum osteocalcin gives better correlation with bone formation. Procollagen type 1 C-terminal propeptide is the ideal marker of bone formation but less easily available. Measurements of urinary hydroxyproline are indicators of bone resorption, but estimations of urinary deoxypyridinoline when available are more specific.

Biochemical markers are useful in monitoring the response to treatment and also the prediction of bone loss[2].

In the screening of a population for osteomalacia, such as a postgastrectomy population, plasma or serum bone-specific alkaline phosphatase levels are useful.

MANAGEMENT OF SUSPECTED OSTEOPOROSIS OR OSTEOMALACIA

The algorithim shown in Figure 1 (prepared by Professor Richard Eastell) is a guide to diagnosis and treatment based on dual energy X-ray absorptiometry measurements of bone mineral density. The spinal measurements are mostly used in the monitoring of efficacy of treatment regimens. Care must be taken to exclude artificially high readings as a result of osteophytes or osteoarthritic changes[3].

According to the recommendations of the Scientific Advisory Board of the National Osteoporosis Foundation, the lower end of the reference range with dual energy X-ray absorptiometry is 75% of the expected average for age and sex. A patient with bone density below this range is regarded as having a bone loss or deficit requiring investigation and treatment.

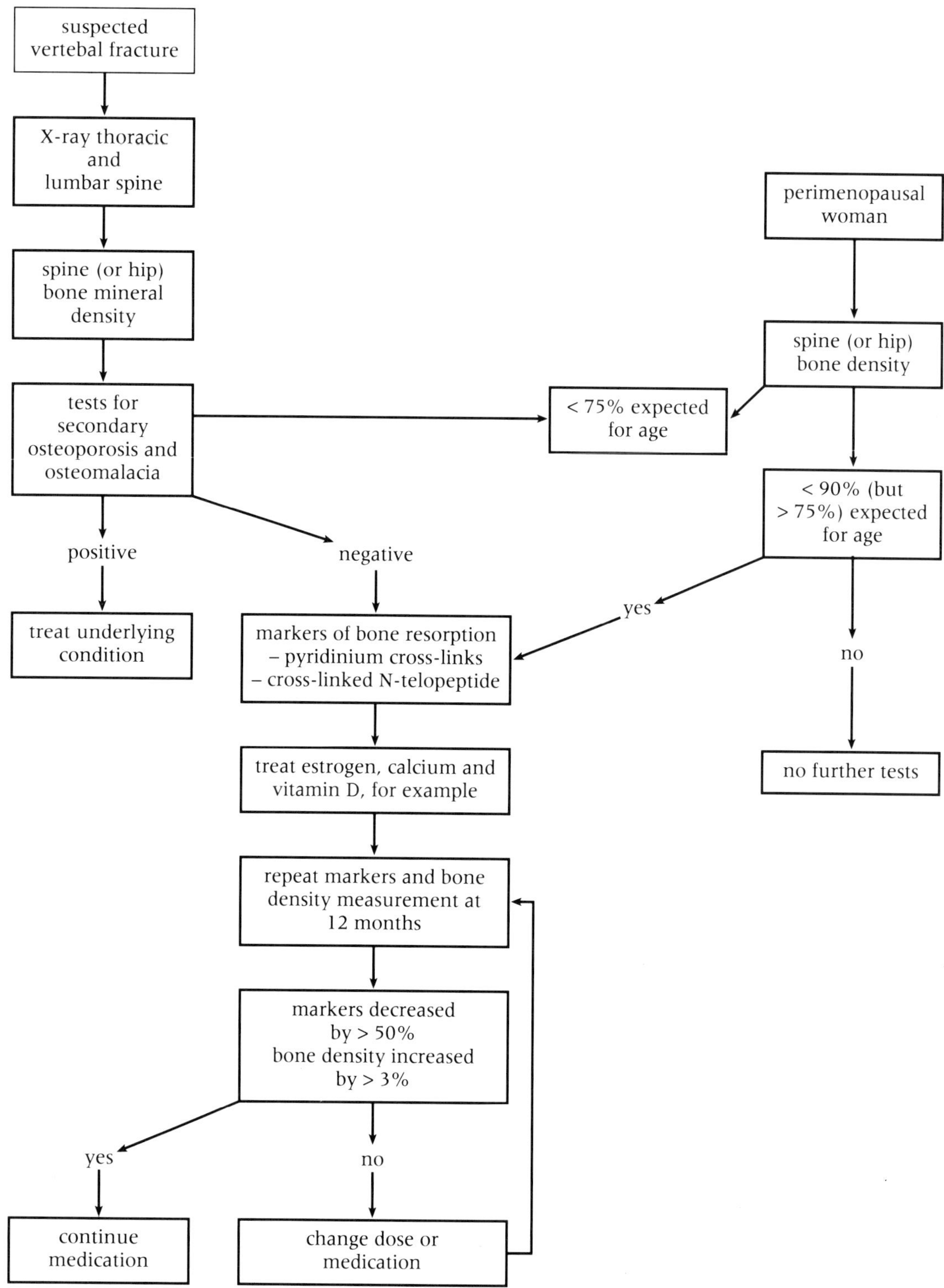

Figure 1 *Algorithm which is used as a guide to diagnosis and treatment of suspected osteoporosis or osteomalacia, based on dual energy X-ray absorptiometry measurements of bone mineral density*

The higher value of 90% of the average shown on the algorithim is regarded as an indication for preventive measures, particularly if markers for bone resorption are also positive.

Markers of bone resorption are preferred at present because they show a greater change with treatment than markers of bone formation.

PREDICTION OF BONE LOSS

Bone density measurements are of particular value in the early prediction of progressive bone loss, especially in identifying those at risk of postmenopausal osteoporosis[4]. It is uncertain as to whether measurements of the lumbar spine, hip or appendicular skeleton should be selected as the optimal sites. The selection depends partly on whether the investigator is primarily concerned with the prevention of fractures of the lumbar spine or of appendicular sites such as the hip or radius[5–8]. Changes in bone density may vary according to the site chosen. The problem is complicated by the availability of different standard ranges which vary according to sex, race and the Body Mass Index.

Law and colleagues question the predictive value of estimation of bone density in women as a means of prediction of hip fracture[1], saying that the standard deviation in the elderly between normal values for age and those with fractures is only 0.5 standard deviations or less. Cummings and colleagues however, state that for every standard deviation decrease in bone mineral density of the proximal femur there is a 2–3 fold increase in the risk of fractures[8].

If patients are to be selected for preventive treatment such as hormone replacement therapy it is important to be able to identify those at greater risk of developing severe osteoporosis and fractures. This may be made possible by the selection of those who are 'fast losers' by a combination of low estimations of bone density or of peak bone mass, plus a biochemical indication of increased bone loss[9].

Hansen and associates[10] reported the accurate prediction of postmenopausal bone loss from a combination of low peak bone mass, as measured by single photon absorptiometry of the distal forearm, plus an index rate of bone loss using three parameters. These were a measurement of fat mass calculated from weight and height, serum total alkaline phosphatase levels, and the ratio of fasting urinary calcium concentration to fasting creatinine concentrations.

More accurate biochemical estimations of the rate of bone loss nowadays can be given by bony alkaline phosphatase estimations, serum osteocalcin, procollagen type 1 C-terminal propeptide or urinary deoxypyridinoline levels[11].

HISTOMORPHOMETRY

Bone histomorphometry will give direct measurements of bone resorption and formation. It is an invasive procedure, however, and restricted to a small area of bone. It is of particular value in supporting a diagnosis when other parameters are equivocal. This may apply particularly to the diagnosis of early subclinical osteomalacia. It is useful also in certain conditions in providing an assessment of the extent of a disorder or of a defect in function of a particular cell type, enabling a decision as to whether any intervention is required. In addition, histomorphometry may be used to monitor the response to treatment, as in the management of the osteodystrophy associated with renal failure.

RELEVANT INVESTIGATIONS IN THE DIFFERENTIAL DIAGNOSIS OF METABOLIC BONE DISEASE

Table 1 lists the relevant investigations that are of significance in the diagnosis and management of metabolic bone diseases. The most frequent clinical conditions requiring diagnosis are osteoporosis, osteomalacia and Paget's disease. The important investigations and characteristics related to these are indicated by the tinted area.

Table 1 *Relevant investigations that are of significance in the diagnosis and management of metabolic bone disease. The shading indicates the important characteristics relating to osteoporosis, osteomalacia and Paget's disease*

Investigation	*Osteoporosis*	*Osteomalacia*			*Renal glomerular osteo-dystrophy*	*Hyperpara-thyroidism*	*Hypopara-thyroidism*	*Hyper-thyroidism*	*Hypophos-phatasia*	*Paget's disease*	*Metastatic bone disease*
		Privational	*Hypophos-phatemic*	*Acidotic*							
Bone densitometry											
Dexa scan	↓	↓	↓↑ if X linked	↓	↓	↓	↑	↓	↓	↑ or ↓	↑ or ↓
X-ray											
Specific changes	+	+ (Looser's zones)				+			±	+	+
Radio isotope scan	+ over recent fractures	+ (over Looser's zones)								+	+
biochemistry											
Ca	□	⬓ or □	□ occ ⬓	↓ or ⬓	↓ or ⬓	↑	↓	□ or ↑	□ or ↑	□	□ or ↑
PO_4	□	⬓ or ↓*	↓	↓ or ⬓	⬒ or ↑	↓ or ⬓	↑ or ⬒	□ or ↓	□	□	
Bony alkaline phosphatase	□	↑ occ ⬒	↑ or □**	↑ occ ⬒	↑	□ or ↑	□	↑	↓	↑ +++	↑ or ↓ if osteolytic
Osteocalcin	↑→↓	↑				↑	↓	↑		↑	□ or ↓ if Ca[††]
PICP	□					⬒				↑	
TRAP	↑					↑				↑	
Creatinine/urea				□ or ⬒	↑	□ or ↑			□ or ↑		
Vitamin D 25 OHD		↓ or [†]⬓	□	□	□ or ⬓	□ or ⬓	□		□		
1:25$(OH)_2D$		□ or [††]⬓	" or □	□[‡]	⬓ or ↓	□ or ↑	⬓ or ↓		□[‡]		□ or ↓ if Ca[††]
PTH		↑	□[‡‡]	□ or ↑	↑	↑	↓	↓	□[‡]		

Table 1 *continued*

Investigation	*Osteoporosis*	*Osteomalacia*			*Renal glomerular osteo-dystrophy*	*Hyperpara-thyroidism*	*Hypopara-thyroidism*	*Hyper-thyroidism*	*Hypophos-phatasia*	*Paget's disease*	*Metastatic bone disease*
		Privational	*Hypophos-phatemic*	*Acidotic*							
Urine biochemistry											
Deoxypyridinoline	↑					↑		↑		↑	
Hydroxyproline	↓	↑ or □	↑ or □	↑ or □		↑				↑	↑ if osteolytic
Ca	□ or ↓	↓ very low	□	⬒ or ↑	↓	□ or ↑	↓ or ↑°	□ or ↑	□ or ↑	□	□ or ↑
Histomorphometry											
Osteoblast number	↓	□ or ⬒	↓ or □	□	↓, □ or ↑	↑	↓	↓	↓	↑	□ or ↑
Osteoblast activity	↓ or □	□ or ⬒	□	↓	↓, □ or ↑	□ or ↑	↓	↓	↓	↑	□ or ↑
Osteoclast number	□ or ↑	⬒ or ↑	⬓ or ↓	↑	↑, □ or ↓	↑	↓	□ or ⬓	□	↑	↑
Osteoclast activity	□	□ or ⬒	↓	↑	↑, □ or ↓	↑	↓	□ or ↑	□	↑	↑
Osteoid	□ or ↓	↑	↑	↑	↓, □ or ↑	↑	↓	↓	↓	↑	↑
Bone mass	↓	□ or ↑	↑	□ or ↑	↓ or □	□ or ⬓	↓	↓	↓	↑	↓

*, Paradoxically increased if calcium is very low (in children) and rises rapidly in early healing stage; **, depends on disease activity, i.e. adults usually normal; †, depending on seasonal variation; ††, levels rise too briskly with recent vitamin D intake to provide diagnostic value; ‡, insufficient data for certainty; ‡‡, increases with large phosphate supplements, rarely spontaneously; °, may be raised if there is a renal tutular leak of Calcium PICP, procollagen type 1 C-terminal propeptide; TRAP, tartrate-resistant acid/phosphatase; PTH, parathyroid hormone; ↑, increase; ↓, decrease; □, normal range; ⬒, high normal; ⬓, low normal

References

1. Law MR, Wald MJ, Meade TW. Strategies for prevention of osteoporosis and hip fractures. Br Med J 1991; 303: 453–9.
2. Peel NFA, Eastell R. Measurement of Bone Mass and Turnover. Baillière's Clinical Rheumatology 1993; vol. 7, No. 3: 479–98.
3. Maseed T, Langley S, Wiltshire P, Doyle DV, Spector TD. Effect of spinal osteophytosis on bone mineral density measurements in vertebral osteoporosis. Br Med J 1993; 307: 172–3.
4. Johnston CC, Melton LJ, Lindsay R, Eddy DM. Clinical indications for bone mass measurement. J Bone Min Res 1989; 4(Suppl. 2): 1–28.
5. Riggs BL, Wahner HW, Seeman E, Offord KP, Dunn WL, Mazess RB, Johnson KA, Melton LJ. Changes in bone mineral density of the proximal femur and spine with ageing: differences between the postmenopausal and osteoporosis syndromes. J Clin Invest 1982; 70: 716–23.
6. Mazess RB, Wahner HW. Nuclear medicine and densitometry. In: Riggs BL, Melton LJ, eds. Osteoporosis, Diagnosis and Management. New York: Raven Press, 1988; 251–9.
7. Eastell R, Wahner HW, O'Fallen WM, Amadio PC, Melton LJ, Riggs BL. Unequal disease in bone density of lumbar spine in Colles' and vertebral fracture syndrome. J Clin Invest 1989; 83: 168–74.
8. Cummings SR, Black DM, Nevitt MC, Browner W, Cauley J, Ensrud K, Genant HK, Palermo L, Scott J, Vogt TM. Bone density at various sites for prediction of hip fractures. Lancet 1993; 341: 72–5.
9. Christiansen B, Riis B, Rodbro P. Prediction of rapid bone loss in postmenopausal women. Lancet 1987; ii: 1105–8.
10. Hansen MA, Overgard K, Christiansen C. Role of peak bone mass and bone loss in postmenopausal osteoporosis: 12 year study. Br Med J 1991; 303: 961–4.
11. Johnston J, Foo AY, Rosalki SB. Peak bone mass and bone loss in postmenopausal osteoporosis (Letter). Br Med J 1991; 303: 1549.

Index